Physical Activity and Cardiovascular Disease Prevention

Peter Kokkinos, PhD, FACSM, FAHA

Professor, Department of Cardiology
Veterans Affairs Medical Center
Georgetown University School of Medicine
George Washington University School of
Medicine and Health Sciences
Washington, DC

JONES AND BARTLETT PUBLISHERS

Sudbury, Massachusetts

BOSTON   TORONTO   LONDON   SINGAPORE

World Headquarters

Jones and Bartlett Publishers
40 Tall Pine Drive
Sudbury, MA 01776
978-443-5000
info@jbpub.com
www.jbpub.com

Jones and Bartlett Publishers
Canada
6339 Ormindale Way
Mississauga, Ontario L5V 1J2
Canada

Jones and Bartlett Publishers
International
Barb House, Barb Mews
London W6 7PA
United Kingdom

Jones and Bartlett's books and products are available through most bookstores and online booksellers. To contact Jones and Bartlett Publishers directly, call 800-832-0034, fax 978-443-8000, or visit our website, www.jbpub.com.

Substantial discounts on bulk quantities of Jones and Bartlett's publications are available to corporations, professional associations, and other qualified organizations. For details and specific discount information, contact the special sales department at Jones and Bartlett via the above contact information or send an email to specialsales@jbpub.com.

The author, editor, and publisher have made every effort to provide accurate information. However, they are not responsible for errors, omissions, or for any outcomes related to the use of the contents of this book and take no responsibility for the use of the products and procedures described. Treatments and side effects described in this book may not be applicable to all people; likewise, some people may require a dose or experience a side effect that is not described herein. Drugs and medical devices are discussed that may have limited availability controlled by the Food and Drug Administration (FDA) for use only in a research study or clinical trial. Research, clinical practice, and government regulations often change the accepted standard in this field. When consideration is being given to use of any drug in the clinical setting, the health care provider or reader is responsible for determining FDA status of the drug, reading the package insert, and reviewing prescribing information for the most up-to-date recommendations on dose, precautions, and contraindications, and determining the appropriate usage for the product. This is especially important in the case of drugs that are new or seldom used.

Production Credits

Acquisitions Editor: Shoshanna Goldberg
Senior Associate Editor: Amy L. Bloom
Senior Production Editor: Susan Schultz
Production Assistant: Tina Chen
Associate Marketing Manager: Jody Sullivan
Composition: Appingo
V.P., Manufacturing and Inventory Control:
  Therese Connell
Cover Design: Kristin E. Parker
Photo Research and Permissions Manager:
  Kimberly Potvin

Cover Image: © Marc Palmer/Dreamstime.com
Image Credits: 1-1 © Netfalls/ShutterStock, Inc;
  1-2 © topal/ShutterStock, Inc; 1-3 © Sean Nel/
  ShutterStock, Inc; 2-6 © Maciej Olesky/
  Dreamstime.com. Unless otherwise indicated, all
  photographs and illustrations are under copyright
  of Jones and Bartlett Publishers, LLC.
Printing and Binding: Malloy, Inc.
Cover Printing: Malloy, Inc.

Library of Congress Cataloging-in-Publication Data
Kokkinos, Peter.
  Physical activity and cardiovascular disease prevention / Peter Kokkinos.
    p. ; cm.
  Includes bibliographical references and index.
  ISBN 978-0-7637-5612-3
1. Heart—Diseases—Exercise therapy. 2. Heart—Diseases—Prevention. I. Title.
[DNLM: 1. Cardiovascular Diseases—prevention & control. 2. Exercise—physiology. WG 120 K79p 2010]
RC684.E9K65 2010
616.1'205—dc22

6048   20090195436048

Printed in the United States of America
13 12 11 10 09   10 9 8 7 6 5 4 3 2 1

Brief Contents

Contents

Preface

I t is now well established that regular physical activity or exercise protects against the premature development of cardiovascular disease and mortality. The primary reason for this protection is the innate capacity of the body to adapt to an imposed demand. More specifically, physical activity (work) increases the energy requirements for the body. The increased energy requirements place a greater demand on the cardiovascular system to deliver substantially more oxygen and nutrients to the working muscles. To accomplish this task, the cardiovascular system makes specific and immediate adjustments, such as increasing the heart rate and the force of contractions by the heart.

In addition to the immediate changes, physical work or exercise serves as the stimulus for chronic adaptations in both the cardiovascular and muscular systems. These changes are task-specific and designed to make both systems more efficient in their respective tasks. More specifically, the cardiovascular system becomes more efficient in delivering oxygen and nutrients to the working muscles, while the working muscles become more efficient in utilizing the oxygen and nutrients delivered. Consequently, the capacity of the individual to perform physical work increases significantly. These chronic adaptations render all systems involved in the task (and the entire organism) more resilient to injury or disease. They constitute the basis for all exercise-related health benefits. It is this premise upon which this book is based.

The energy required for all work is provided by the foods we eat. More specifically, fats and carbohydrates comprise the raw material for the energy needs of all cells. These raw materials are metabolized by specific systems found within cells into high energy compounds that the cells can use to meet their energy needs.

Exercise, diet, and the development of diseases are inextricably related. That is, exercise influences metabolism favorably and, in turn, metabolism influences diseases, such as diabetes, hypertension and heart disease. Therefore, for those who wish to pursue research or teach in this exciting and evolving field of exercise and health, it is imperative that they acquire a basic understanding of the physiologic changes that occur during physical work or exercise in the cardiovascular, muscular, and metabolic systems. This is also true for individuals involved in advising individuals on exercise and exercise-related health issues.

Accordingly, this book discusses the physiologic and metabolic processes that occur during physical work, the acute and chronic adaptations that come about as a result of that work and how these changes are related to chronic diseases. Ultimately, the aim of this book is to bridge the gap between epidemiology of disease and exercise physiology. The book is structured into three parts.

In Part I, the basic concepts of physical activity and nutrition are reviewed. In Part II, the structure and function of the muscular and cardiovascular system are discussed. Then, basic concepts of metabolism, energy utilization, and fuel preferences of the muscles during physical activity are covered. Finally, the discussion focuses on the acute changes and chronic adaptations of the muscular system and the exercise-related adaptations of the muscular and cardiovascular system.

In Part III, the basic concepts of epidemiology and the latest statistics on cardiovascular disease epidemiology are presented. The pathophysiology of atherosclerosis, plaque formation, ischemia and myocardial infarction, heart failure, and stroke are also covered. This is fol-lowed by discussion of the role of physical activity in the prevention of cardiovascular disease, including heart disease, stroke, and peripheral vascular disease. Finally, the effects of physical activity on blood lipids, hypertension, diabetes and obesity are discussed. The last chapter of the book deals with risks associated with physical activity.

■ THE AUDIENCE

The book is written for individuals in graduate and undergraduate programs in epidemiology, health promotion, kinesiology, exercise science, exercise rehabilitation and other health-care-related disciplines. The book can also serve as a reference for those involved in exercise/physical activity-related research, or exercise rehabilitation and healthcare science programs.

Acknowledgments

I would like to acknowledge the foresight, patience, and support of Amy Bloom, Senior Associate Editor at Jones and Bartlett Publishers.

I also wish to express special gratitude to Dr. Ben Hurley, professor, mentor, and friend; and to Drs. Vasilios Mougios, Paul McAuley, and Jonathan Myers for their friendship and for their gracious, insightful guidance. A special appreciation is extended to Lauren Korshak, MS, for her organizational skills and her critique of the book from a student's perspective; and to Monica Aiken, MA, for her assistance in the lab and the meticulous recording of data that resulted in numerous research projects, publications, and ultimately the expansion of knowledge. Finally, this book is the outcome of an arduous but rewarding journey, one that began on a winter morning over four decades ago, as a bus left a small village in Northern Greece. The course of this journey was determined by the kindness and foresight of a few and was guided by the love and sacrifices of my parents and my family.

■ DEDICATION

To Evangeline: wife, mother, and friend, your unconditional love, support, and gentle guidance over the years have left an indelible mark in my soul; and to our two sons, who have enriched our lives beyond all expectations.

Basic Concepts of Physical Activity and Nutrition

This book is based on the premise that physical activity leads to certain physiologic changes in the body. These changes lead to improved cardiovascular health, which positively affects the well-being of the human body.

Why does this occur? The simplest answer is that physical activity causes specific physiologic changes to occur that, in turn, lead to a more disease-resistant system. That is, physical activity is the stimulus that elicits a response by the organism, the result of which is a stronger, healthier system. To understand the different changes, one must learn the nature of the stimulus (physical activity) and the responses elicited by the stimulus.

Three major players are involved in the relationship between physical activity and cardiovascular health: the muscular system, the cardiovascular system, and the circulatory system. Part I defines physical activity and fitness; describes how physical activity is assessed and quantified; and explains the association between physical activity and health, and the physiologic principles governing physical activity and related health. This section also discusses the necessity of proper food and sufficient water to sustain life and build the energy requirements that have an integral role in energy formation and utilization. Because certain fats and carbohydrates are major factors in diseases such as diabetes mellitus and heart disease, the basic metabolic processes of carbohydrates and fats are described.

CHAPTER

History of Physical Activity and Health

Physical strength, endurance, and the overall ability to perform work have been an integral to human survival since the dawn of man on Earth. Even more, these factors have shaped the history of humankind.

For Paleolithic era (50,000–10,000 BC) humans, physical activity and fitness were not a matter of choice but of survival. On a daily basis, humans depended on their physical strength and endurance to find water and shelter; track and kill prey; harvest seeds, herbs, grains, and fruit; carry foods back to the family and clan; and at times fight fiercely to keep it. Women were not exempt from having to be physically hardy. Only the strongest survived the rigors of childbirth, child rearing, and daily crafting the clothing, household tools and eating implements, and the sheer labor to process and cook food for the entire family.

Food sources were fairly plentiful during Neolithic era (4,000–2,000 BC). As the hunter-gatherer societies transformed into the agricultural age, and sophisticated tribal societies, villages, and even cities began to form, the physical demands remained high for survival, cultural, and religious functions. These included dancing to pray for and/or celebrate a bountiful hunt as well as tribal and intertribal competitive games that involved mostly physical tasks.[1] Trade and visiting families over as much as 20 mile distances were quite popular. But being able to plant and harvest, cope with managing domesticated animals in addition to building more permanent shelters and maintaining farms remained a dangerous business. An early death or maiming of the primary worker often meant impoverishment and/or death for the entire family. Endurance and physical strength continued to be primary factors to be able to survive the skirmishes and warfare that swept across tribal societies.

■ PHYSICAL ACTIVITY IN ANCIENT SOCIETIES

As larger ancient civilizations began to develop, the influence of physical activity is evident in the culture, health, expansion, and even the rise and fall of their nations.

In the early Eastern and Near Eastern civilizations, physical activity and the quest for the development of fitness through structured programs mostly stemmed from the desire for conquest and expansion of territory. Military leaders of the Persian Empire recognized the link between the physical strength and endurance of the soldier on the battlefield with successful acquisition of land and resources. These leaders implemented rigid training programs designed to enhance the strength, endurance, and overall performance of their fighting men.[2,3]

Some historians believe that the first non-militaristic approach to physical conditioning was developed in China around the sixth century BC, following the downfall and collapse of the Persian Empire. This exercise system known as Tai Chi consists of graceful movements developed in accord with the principles of the Chinese philosophy of Taoism, a philosophy that advocates longevity through simple living.

In India, Hindu priests also developed a passive system of exercise aimed to promote stretching and flexibility as well as mental awareness, known as Yoga.[2] Stone tablets depicting these postures have been dated by archeologists to 3000 BC.[4] Although Yoga was intended more for religious and spiritual pursuits, certain health aspects were attached to it. Practitioners believed that the discipline required to achieve physical suppleness was essential in the pursuit of spiritual and emotional stability.

Many African nations developed systems of martial arts to enhance their social and religious culture that combined agility and flexibility with endurance.[5] To this day, running prowess in such tribes as the Kenyan Masai and Samburu is linked with social status and manhood.[6]

Across the Americas, from the earliest hunter-gatherer societies (~10,000–8,000 BC) found along the coastal and Andean regions of Peru (archeological evidence is sparse in the jungles east of the Andes), to the precursor nations of what is now the Iroquois (Northeast United States, Eastern Canada) and Inuit (Alaska-Canadian Northwest), all ran to hunt, combat invaders, and trade. A variety of versions of the modern game lacrosse were played, sometimes even by entire villages. Running was also a physical method to connect with their metaphysical world.[6]

Some researchers speculate that the harsh and physically demanding environments of the Late Paleolithic era favored the selection, regulation, and evolution of genes to support survival in such conditions. Consequently, the development of large, strong muscles and a robust cardiovascular system increased the likelihood of survival while the lack of such attributes can be regarded as a maladaptation and meant the elimination of the organism. The researchers hypothesize that in the mainly sedentary environment of modern times, our current genome is maladapted, resulting in abnormal gene expression, which in turn manifests itself as heart disease, diabetes, and other chronic diseases.[7] This is an area for future research.

■ PHYSICAL ACTIVITY DURING THE HELLENIC CIVILIZATION

Ancient Greeks also recognized the importance of physical conditioning and fitness for military purposes. Athletics and athletic competition in

the Greek culture is evident since 1200 BC. In Homer's *The Iliad*, physical attributes of muscular strength speed and endurance are exalted not only in the battlefield but also in competitions among the warriors. Homer describes contests held in honor of fallen heroes. Warriors competed in running, javelin throwing, and sword fighting contests. The motivation to be the best and the exaltation of physical qualities is evident in Homer's descriptions of the warriors as well as the surviving art in ceramics and statuary of the period.

The embodiment of the superb physical conditioning of the Greeks is the battle-hardened Spartan warriors, whose physical endurance and discipline were unrivaled. Perhaps the best testament to the physical conditioning of the Greeks is the grueling battle at Thermopolis, where for 3 days a handful of Spartans and other Greeks fought against wave after wave of attacks by thousands of Persians. Despite the final defeat of the Greeks on the third day of the battle, the Persian losses were so numerous that the troops were demoralized, which contributed to their eventual defeat.

To achieve a strong and stress-enduring body, the Greeks developed structured exercise programs that were systematically practiced by the youth in the *pallestra*, a precursor of the modern gym. Running, jumping, and wrestling were some of the activities that comprised such programs.[8,9] Because the participants performed without clothing (naked), these activities were referred to as *gymnastics* (from the Greek word for naked, *gymnos*) and the facilities were called *gymnasiums*, words that remain in use today.

Although this idealistic fitness program existed mostly within Athens, Sparta, and other city states also had similar facilities for their youths to pursue athletic endeavors. The popularity of fitness within these city states eventually gave birth to the idea of the Olympic

Games, established in 776 BC and held every four years in honor of the god Zeus, who dwelled in the mount Olympus with the other gods. The Games were held in ancient Olympia, located southwest of Athens (**Figure 1.1**). The stadium was the largest of its kind and could seat at least 20,000 people. During the Olympic Games, youths from all Greek city states competed in activities such as wresting, decathlon, triathlon, discus and javelin throwing, sports events that exist in modern Olympics (**Figure 1.2**). Winners received no other prize but a crown made from olive branches.

The Olympic Games served a greater purpose than a mere competition among athletes and city states. They were about peace, honor, respect, and the quest for perfection through struggle. As such, all conflicts among the Greek city states ceased during the Games. The olive branch crown awarded to the winners is evidence that they competed not for monetary gains but for the idealistic pursuit of perfection. The concept of competition for no monetary gains was inconceivable to *barbarians* (Greek word for non-cultured [i.e., non-Greeks]).

This is perhaps best depicted in a passage from the ancient historian Herodotus' writings about the Persian Wars. The Persians inquired from some locals what the Greeks were doing. They were told that the Greeks were holding the Olympic Games, competing in athletic sports and the chariot races. When the Persians inquired what prize was given to the man who wins, the locals replied "an olive wreath." The concept of competing not for money but for a

Figure 1.1 Ancient Olympia.

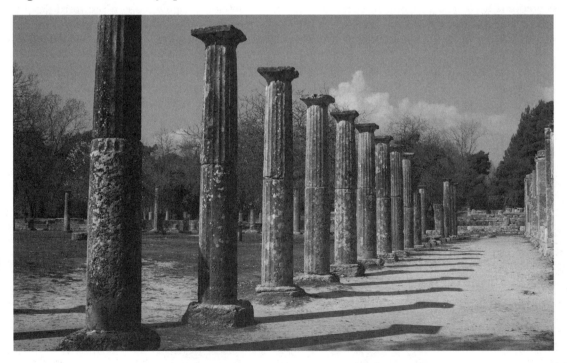

Figure 1.2 Ancient Olympic sports.

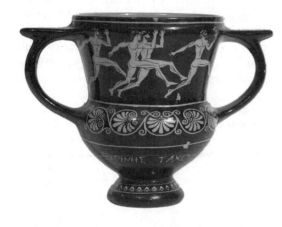

wreath of olive was incomprehensible. Realizing the significance of this in the battlefield, one of the Persian nobles exclaimed "Good heavens, what manner of men are these against whom you have brought us to fight—men who contend with one another, not for money, but for honor." His statement was later ridiculed by the Persian King Xerxes and he was dismissed as a coward.[10]

To promote fair competition and protect against the seductive powers of winning at any cost, athletes who cheated were dishonored. Their statues, paid for by those cheaters, were erected along the avenue leading to the gate of the stadium as an ethical reminder to those who were about to enter.

The Olympic Games were banned in 394 AD by the Roman Emperor Theodosius. The modern Olympic Games resumed in 1896, about 1,500 years later, in their birthplace: Athens, Greece. The modern-day marathon took place on the 11th day of the games. The race followed the same route that the messenger Phidippides ran about 2,500 years prior (from Marathon to Athens) to announce to the Athenians the victory against the invading Persians. The 1896 race was won by a Greek runner, Spiridon Louis.

As impressive as the physical conditioning of athletes or warriors may be, what distinguishes the Greeks most—especially the Athenians—are the concepts of physical activity that were developed in the gymnasium. Such ideals were a clear departure of the ordinary requirements of the battlefield. They defined all aspects of Greek life, including culture, beauty, and health. Their appreciation for the beauty of the body and the importance of health and fitness throughout society is unparalleled in history. No other civilization has held fitness in such high regard as did those during the Hellenic period. For this period in history, the development of a strong and enduring body was viewed not only as part of a military doctrine, but more importantly, as an integral aspect of the pursuit of perfection in both mind and body.

The pursuit of excellence that characterized the Greek spirit was applied to the body. Development of physical attributes such as muscular strength, endurance, and speed is epitomized in their creation of the extraordinary mythical hero, Heracles (Hercules) (**Figure 1.3**) Hercules (the equivalent to our modern day comic book Superman) was considered the "ultimate man," a person whom all should strive to emulate. He was stronger than the strongest lion, faster than the fastest deer, and brave beyond measure. More importantly, he combined his superhuman physical attributes with a clever mind and benevolent actions. As a young man, he made a decision to put his physical prowess and mental gifts to work for the good of the people. It is in Hercules that we first see the concept of mind and body working in harmony and for the good of humanity that is rooted in the Hellenic culture. The concept of this mind–body connection is discussed later in this chapter.

Figure 1.3   Statue of Hercules.

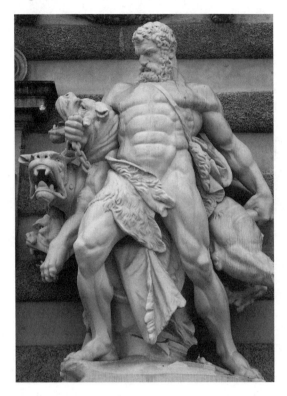

■ PHYSICAL ACTIVITY AND HEALTH CONNECTION

In addition to athletics, the overall health benefits of physical activity and fitness was recognized by founding medical practitioners who include Herodotus, Hippocrates, and Galen.[11,12] The most systematic recordings of observations, concepts, and statements describing health benefits attributed to physical activity are from these Greek physicians and philosophers. Their concepts have greatly influenced Western civilization and provide the basis for our modern views about the association between physical activity and health.

More importantly, it is their precise statements and details that emphasize not only the connection between fitness and health but also the implementation of fitness to a large population, something most civilizations struggle with today. For example, the Greek physician Hippocrates stated:

> "Speaking generally, all parts of the body which have a function, if used in moderation and exercised in labors to which each is accustomed, become thereby healthy and well developed and age slowly; but if unused and left idle, they become liable to disease, defective in growth, and age quickly."

It is truly astonishing that Hippocrates was able to conceive the relationship between physical activity, health, vigor, and aging at a time when epidemiologic research and statistical methods did not exist. Perhaps even more amazing is that he emphasized the importance of moderation in the pursuit of health through increased physical activity, something that was documented only recently after decades of research. Although these concepts are widespread today, it took us awhile to advance beyond the false perception of fitness depicted by the cliché "no pain, no gain" that echoed in high school, college, and other athletic training facilities across the United States during the 1950s through the 1980s.

Hippocrates is more direct in another profound statement:

> "Walking is a man's best medicine."

In the next two quotes, he emphasized the importance of combining diet and physical activity as the most effective and safest way to health.

> "Eating alone will not keep a man well; he must also take exercise."

"If we could give every individual the right amount of nourishment and exercise, not too little and not too much, we would have found the safest way to health."

In addition to combining diet and physical activity, Hippocrates' latter statement touches upon another important concept. He emphasizes the "right amount . . . , not too little and not too much," which clearly indicates his keen awareness that only the proper amount will yield health benefits. Too much is likely to cause harm and not enough will be ineffective.

Only recently and after years of research, health scientists have recognized that walking is the safest and most effective form of exercise that can be implemented in large populations to foster health.

■ THE MIND–BODY CONNECTION

In addition to the development of the body, the Athenians were the first people to recognize fitness as a way to promote physical and mental health. Perhaps more amazing is their recognition of the mind–body connection. The Greeks believed that physical well-being was necessary for mental well-being and that a strong, healthy body harbors a healthy, sound mind. Furthermore, they believed that both mind and body are equally important and therefore should be equally developed to complement each other. This enduring concept of a harmonious existence between mind and body and the importance of cultivating both equally is eloquently echoed by the philosopher Plato.

"Physical activity is not merely necessary to the health and development of the body, but to balance and correct intellectual pursuits as well. The mere athlete is brutal and philistine, the mere intellectual unstable and spiritless. The right education must tune the strings of the body and mind to perfect spiritual harmony."

Interestingly, it took centuries for Western civilizations such as ours to recognize the importance of this concept. Even now, we often concentrate in the development of one aspect at the expense of the other. For years, athletes were frequently referred to as "dumb jocks." With the help of modern science and the foresight of some bright scientists, we are beginning to appreciate the mind–body connection and recognize that physical activity promotes clarity of thought.

Studies show that physically active children perform much better in school when compared to their more sedentary classmates. Other findings from recent studies also support that higher levels of activity are associated with better cognitive performance for both women and men.[13,14] The risk of Alzheimer disease was a 1.8-fold higher in men who walked 2 miles or less per day (low-fit) versus those who walked more than 2 miles per day.[14]

■ PHYSICAL ACTIVITY AFTER HELLENISM

Following the decline of Greece and the rise of the Roman Empire, the Athenian concept of fitness as an integral part of a healthy individual and a healthy vibrant society perished. Physical conditioning for the Romans was strictly for military purposes while the fitness level of the general Roman population declined. Roman soldiers participated in activities such as running, marching, jumping, and discus and javelin throwing strictly to maintain their readiness for battle.[15] Materialistic acquisition and excess became higher priorities than physical condition. The Romans became enamored with wealth and entertainment. Overindulging in food and wine and watching gladiators slaughter each other in arenas throughout their country became more important for the individual than the development of a strong, athletic body. Some historians believe that this decadence eventually led to the downfall of the Roman civilization.[16]

After the fall of the Roman Empire, the lifestyle of the Northern European conquerors was similar to other hunter-gatherer people.[16] Thus, once again physical activity and fitness became a prerequisite for survival.

During the European Renaissance period between the 14th and 17th centuries, a renewed interest in the human body emerged. Once again, the ancient Greek ideals glorifying the human body and the importance of fitness for health gained widespread acceptance by educators, philosophers, and even religious leaders.[17,18] Many advocated the idea that good health led to intelligence and the value of fitness began to spread throughout Europe.

By the 18th century, individuals in countries such as Germany, Denmark, Sweden, and Great Britain recognized once again the importance of physical fitness gymnastics as a form of the fitness movement. The health benefits of physical activity were once again recognized by Per Henrik Ling in Sweden and Archibald MacLaren in England. Both men advocated exercise as a way to promote better health. Ling recognized that exercise programs should be tailored, based on individual differences. He also advocated that physical educators must possess knowledge of the effects of exercise on the human body. Several modern concepts of fitness can be traced back to educators of that time.[19]

In England, the observations of Archibald MacLaren's writings as a medical student provide the basis for present-day exercise recommendations. He conceptualized several principles that govern exercise and the body's adaptations to exercise. For example, he noted that adequate fitness cannot be attained by the occasional recreational exercise provided by games and sports, and so promoted the importance of a structured exercise program that offered consistency and progression. Like Ling, MacLaren also recognized the need for individual variation in fitness training programs. He developed an exercise training system that was used extensively throughout the army and public schools in England. He is credited for the transformation of the soft and slow British Army soldier to a swift, strong, and enduring warrior. His gymnasium at Oxford is credited for the promotion of extraordinary degree of health and vigor of the young men. MacLaren also realized that both growing boys and girls required regular physical exercise for the developing strong and healthy adults.[20]

■ PHYSICAL ACTIVITY IN THE UNITED STATES

Early fitness concepts in the United States were influenced to some extent by European tenets. Although regular physical activity for health purposes, was advocated by some,[21] German and Swedish gymnastic programs never attained the same levels of popularity as in Europe and physical activity was not promoted within the U.S. educational system until the latter part of the 19th century.[20,22] Despite the relative lack of interest in fitness existing during this period, several people did advocate for increased physical activity and fitness.

Benjamin Franklin and President Thomas Jefferson both viewed physical activity as importance for good health and encouraged physical activity for all Americans. In the 1800s, Dr. J.C. Warren, then a medical professor at Harvard, developed and recommended exercises such as gymnastics and calisthenics for men and women.[2] Catherine Beecher, a strong advocate for women's education, believed that women were responsible for the education and moral development of the next generation; she devoted most of her life to this cause. Beecher advocated physical activity for women as an avenue to better health, and warned against poor health and contemporary societal beliefs and practices that limited women's participation in physical activities. Her concepts were ahead of their time, especially when considering that women's athletics, physical activity, and involvement of women in sports has only been emphasized in the last few decades in North America. Beecher devised a system of calisthenics for women performed to music.[22]

Following the Civil War, a popular exercise, "The New Gymnastics," was introduced by the temperance lecturer, Dioclesian Lewis.[23] Edward Hitchcock, William Anderson, and Dudley Sargent also played significant roles in the development of fitness concepts during this time. Hitchcock introduced the concept of using anthropometric measurements to assess fitness progress. He also recognized the association between fitness and health. Sargent added scientific research to fitness instruction and developed organized instructor teaching methodologies. Anderson focused on physical education instruction.[2,22,23]

Interestingly, during this period, a number of physical educators with vision believed that physical education programs must not emphasize sports and games, but concentrate in exercise that would improve overall health-related fitness. However, the popularity of sports was increasing and consequently, the majority of physical education programs focused on particular sports and games. This mentality and the debate between health-related fitness and skill-related fitness physical education programs continues to exist.[22]

Following World War I, fitness took a back seat to overeating, drinking alcohol, partying, and other forms of entertainment.[24] The Second World War found American youth physically soft and unfit for combat. Nearly half of all draftees were either rejected or given noncombat positions.[23] These disturbing statistics helped focus the attention of the nation to the importance of fitness.

An important departure from the random approach to physical activity and fitness came during the 1940s. Dr. Thomas K. Cureton at the University of Illinois introduced the application of research to fitness. Cureton recognized the importance of the type and duration of exercise, and strived to answer questions about the basic requirements to achieve health. He also developed fitness tests for muscular strength, flexibility, and cardiorespiratory endurance. His research resulted in multiple recommendations for improving cardiorespiratory fitness, including the identification of exercise intensity guidelines necessary to increase fitness levels. His suggestions became the fundamental basis for future exercise programs. This is an enormous contribution because it propelled physical activity, human performance, and health from anecdotal evidence to a discipline governed by scientific principles.[7,9]

During this time, two reports prompted action towards a national emphasis on physical education and fitness. First, statistics gathered on draftees during World War II revealed a gloomy picture on the physical fitness of young men. Of the nine million registrants, almost three million were not qualified to serve for physical and mental reasons.[25] Shortly afterwards, the 1954 study findings of muscular fitness of schoolchildren were equally disturbing. The Kraus-Weber test consisted of six simple movements of key muscle groups was administered to U.S. children. Nearly 58% of the children failed the test compared to only 8.7% of

European children.[26] These alarming findings caught the attention of President Eisenhower. In June 1956, he called for a special White House Conference; its aim was to find ways to promote fitness in the United States. The result was the formation of the President's Council of Youth Fitness and the President's Citizens Advisory Committee on the Fitness of American Youth.

The 1950s marked the beginning of a broader scientific scrutiny of the association between physical activity and health. In 1953, a landmark study was published in *Lancet*.[27] In this British study, Dr. Morris and co-workers observed that bus conductors who climbed up and down the stairs of double-decker busses died from heart disease at half the rate of bus drivers whose activity was relatively sedentary, as they sat for most of the day behind the wheel. In addition, if conductors developed heart disease, it was less severe and appeared later in life than the bus drivers. The same investigators also reported similar findings in a comparison of mail-handlers who walked to deliver the mail to other government clerks with desk jobs. Morris and Crawford later provided additional evidence for the benefits of physical activity in their large necropsy study of British workers who died of heart disease.[28] Their findings sparked worldwide interest. A number of subsequent scientific investigations performed in different countries reached the same conclusion: The death rate for physically active individuals was about half that of those who were sedentary.

In 1954, the American College of Sports Medicine (ACSM) was formed, which perhaps is the most important and pivotal event in the U.S. history of physical activity and health. Throughout the decades since its inception, the ACSM has established position stands on various exercise-related issues based on scientific research. The college has been one of the premier organizations in the promotion of health and fitness to American society and worldwide. ACSM among other organizations such as the American Medical Association; the American Association for Physical Education, Recreation, and Dance; and the President's Council on Youth Fitness and later the President's Council on Physical Fitness would provide merit and legitimacy to the coming fitness movement.[22]

During the 1960s, President John F. Kennedy was a major proponent of fitness and its health-related benefits. He spoke openly about the need for American citizens to improve their fitness levels and published an article in *Sports Illustrated* entitled, "The Soft American." He wrote, "We are under-exercised as a nation; we look instead of play; we ride instead of walk."[29]. Kennedy prompted the federal government to become even more involved in national fitness promotion and started many local youth programs. In a statement reminiscent of ancient Greek philosophical concepts, Kennedy said, "Physical fitness is the basis for all other forms of excellence."[30]

In 1968, the book entitled *Aerobics* was published. Its author, Kenneth Cooper, a retired Air Force physician, introduced fitness concepts to the public that until that time were known only by professionals. His book extended the concept of fitness beyond the high school and college gyms. Almost overnight, exercise and fitness became the "in thing." He coined the term *aerobics* for such activities as running, biking, swimming, and walking, and proclaimed that such activities are the best exercises to promote fitness. In addition, Cooper's book sent a powerful message to the American public that to prevent the development of chronic diseases, one must exercise regularly and maintain high fitness levels throughout life.[31] Cooper advocated a philosophy that shifted away from disease treatment to one of disease prevention. "It is easier to maintain good health through proper exercise, diet, and emotional balance than it is to regain it once it is lost."[31]

Dr. Cooper became internationally known, and is perhaps the most influential individual for the popularization of exercise and fitness in modern times.

In addition to the promotion and popularization of exercise and physical activity, the Cooper Institute of Aerobic Research, under the direction of Dr. Steve Blair, has provided and continues to provide a wealth of epidemiologic evidence to support the association and benefits of regular exercise and health.

As a wealth of scientific evidence accumulated over the years, it became increasingly more convincing that physical activity is the cheapest and perhaps the single most powerful deterrent for a number of chronic disease that plague the human race. For example, physical activity reduces the risk for developing high blood pressure, diabetes mellitus, obesity, arthritis, osteoporosis, and stroke; it strengthens the immune system; prevents the formation of blood clots, and much more. In addition to disease prevention, exercise has therapeutic properties. It lowers blood pressure in those with high blood pressure, improves blood sugar levels in diabetics, and blood lipids (fats) in those with abnormalities in that area. It also reduces the risk for a second heart attack and death in heart patients.

The contributions of Dr. Ralph S. Paffenbarger, Jr., an internationally renowned epidemiologist and professor at both Stanford University School of Medicine and Harvard University School of Public Health, and Dr. John O. Holloszy, professor of medicine at Washington University in St. Louis cannot go unmentioned. Paffenbarger's classic studies provided strong evidence on the physical activity and its association with cardiovascular risk and longevity, and shaped future research in this areas. This work, along with work by Drs. Art Leon, William Haskell, and Jerry Morris provided the evidence necessary for physical inactivity to be officially recognized by the

American Heart Association as a major risk factor.

Finally, the work by Drs. John O. Holloszys, Charles Tipton, and Phil Gollnick shaped the biochemical approach to exercise physiology research. Holloszy's gerontology research contributed in our understanding the exercise-induced biochemical adaptations, exercise metabolism, and the impact of exercise training on glucose metabolism and the quality of life of the elderly. Many distinguished researchers and scholars including Drs. James Hagberg, Bernard Hurley, Andrew Goldberg, and Douglas Seals, trained in Holloszy's laboratory and continued their distinguished careers in a number of universities and hospitals across the United States. Their work greatly expanded our understanding of exercise-related health benefits. For his contributions to health, Holloszy was awarded the 2000 Olympic Prize.

In 1996, the *Surgeon General's Report on Physical Activity and Health*,[32] the Centers for Disease Control and Prevention, the American College of Sports Medicine, and a number of other health agencies declared physical inactivity as a health hazard for all people. It is now recognized by authorities that increasing physical activity is a public health objective that is of equal importance as sound nutrition, the use of seat belts, and the adverse health effects of tobacco use. The main message that the government and these health organizations want to communicate is that:

> "People can substantially improve their health and quality of life by including moderate amounts of physical activity in their daily lives."[32]

The report continues by stating the amount of physical activity recommended:

> "Every U.S adult should accumulate 30 minutes of moderate intensity physical activity on most, preferably all, days of the week."[32]

The report also emphasized the fact that more vigorous activity or greater amounts of activity (to a certain extent) can yield additional health benefits.

Finally, in the summer of 2007, the American Heart Association and the American College of Sports Medicine issued two reports on exercise recommendations for the public.[33,34] The central message of these reports is that all adults should participate in daily physical activity.

■ FINAL NOTE

Some dared to say that the decline of the great empires of the world coincide with the decline of their people's physical fitness.[35] If these pundits are correct, we are in a perilous path.

As history indicates, physical fitness and the appreciation of it have been sporadic throughout nations and cultures. It took the modern world 1,500 years to reinstitute the Olympic Games, while most are still struggling to embrace the concepts of fitness, health, and beauty—even in modern Athens the birthplace of such concepts. In this regard, the efforts of the Hellenic Heart Foundation, under the direction of Professor Toutouzas, present an exception. For years the foundation has operated a program to promote physical activity and an overall healthy lifestyle throughout modern Greece through the schools and publications geared for physicians and the general public.

The evidence connecting a physically active lifestyle to health benefits is overwhelming and certainly indisputable. Despite this fact, it is difficult to find any progress in our fitness status as a nation since the *Surgeon General's Report* in 1996. On the contrary, all indications are that we are becoming fatter and less fit by the day. In fact, the epidemic proportions of obesity that are sweeping across the United States and the galloping increase in the prevalence of Type 2 diabetes, even in children as young as 10 years, are directly and indirectly related to the physical inactivity epidemic that prevails.

According to the National Health and Nutrition Examination Survey (NHANES) age-adjusted prevalence of overweight and obesity was 64.5% in 1999–2000 and increased to 66.3% in 2003–2004. The prevalence of obesity alone increased during this period from 30.5% to 32.2% and for extreme obesity from 4.7% to 4.8%.[36]

Many businesses allow or at least tolerate multiple "smoke breaks" throughout the day. This is certainly the right approach, as it protects non-smokers from smoke exposure. Although some employers allow time for their employees to exercise, many do not. Perhaps it is in order to give equal time to those who wish to walk as those who wish to smoke. Such policy will not only be fair but most likely a wise business decision over time.

Even more alarming is that children are becoming overweight and obese at a progressively younger age. This trend in childhood obesity raises concerns that their sedentary and overeating habits will continue into adulthood, which will contribute to the number of cases of chronic diseases that are already stressing our public healthcare system.

The increase in the popularity of electronic games and gadgets that promote a sedentary existence, coupled with an increasing reliance on transportation methods that require minimal physical exertion are other lifestyle factors affecting young people today. This, along with minimum and often inadequate requirements for physical education training in primary and secondary education schools, are likely to perpetuate the epidemic of obesity.

Attempts to reverse these trends have begun on the national level. Parents, educators, and even children themselves have helped to shift attention to programs in schools that promote physical fitness for the many instead of focusing only on athletics for the few. Concerned parent-teacher organizations have successfully removed sugared soft drink machines and instituted more nutritious lunch options at school cafeterias. Some school systems have increased the training requirements for physical education teachers and coaches, and encouraged the entire student body to participate in classes and after-school physical activities. Professional athletes continue to volunteer in their communities to encourage young people to find success in a variety of athletic activities.

Although these changes represent a welcome and long overdue approach, they fall short of a long-lasting solution. It is vital that parents and educators become involved in promoting physical activity and healthy lifestyles for children. For a long-term solution, it is imperative that our attitudes toward fitness, sports, and diet change. For too long, we have devoted a great deal of resources in our schools to promote competitive sports for the few and only a fraction is spent to promote physical activities and cultivate lifelong fitness attitudes for the many. For too long, we have debated whether physical education programs should emphasize sports or health-related fitness. This should never have been debated. The two should and must coexist, for each complements the other. Our pursuit of sports and athletics should not be solely for entertainment but for the increased health benefits, quality of life, and prosperity of the individual as well as the health of our nation. Think of what we could accomplish nationwide if a small fraction of the profits from professional sports were allocated to promote fitness on the state and national level.

■ SUMMARY

- Physical fitness before the Hellenic civilization was an integral part of survival as primitive hunter-gatherers sought food and migrated with their food sources.
- As civilizations developed, the quest and development of fitness through structured programs were primarily for military purposes, and ultimately for the expansion of land and resources for an empire.
- The first people to recognize fitness as a way to promote physical and mental health were the Athenians during the Hellenic era; later, the other Greek city states of ancient Greece embraced these ideals.
- Hellenic era Greeks believed that physical well-being was necessary for mental well-being and that a strong, healthy body harbors a healthy, sound mind. These concepts have endured over the centuries.
- The development of Olympic Games to honor their god Zeus served a more compelling ideal than a mere competition among athletes and between city states. The Olympics stood for honor, peace, respect, and the quest for perfection through struggle.
- In addition to athletics, the ancient Greeks recognized the health benefits of physical activity and fitness. Hippocrates and Galen described the relationship between physical activity and health and concepts that govern that relationship. These concepts had a great influence on Western civilization and provide the basis for our modern views about this association.
- Despite their admiration for the Greek civilization and attempts to emulate it, the Romans failed to conceptualize the value

of fitness for the general public, using it strictly for military purposes.

- Eventually, the lavish lifestyle and decadence of the Romans led to a decline of interest in fitness and physical decay ensued. Some historians believe that this decay led to the downfall of the Roman civilization.
- A renewed interest in the human body emerged during the European Renaissance. Ancient Greek ideals glorifying the human body gained widespread acceptance by educators, philosophers, and even religious leaders throughout Europe.
- In the United States, concepts about fitness to some extent were influenced by Europeans. However, structured physical education, particularly for women, remained missing from the public education system until the latter part of the 19th century.
- With the advent of World War II, the nation realized the poor physical condition of its youth and efforts were made to reverse this trend. Attention on fitness was paid by the highest level of government. This led to the development of a number of organizations that promoted scientific research and the implementation of sound principles regarding physical activity, fitness, and health.
- In the 1960s, President John F. Kennedy was a major proponent of fitness and its health-related benefits to the American people. Kennedy prompted the federal government to become more involved in national fitness promotion and started many youth programs.
- Perhaps the most influential individual to popularize exercise and fitness in the United States as well as the world was Dr. Kenneth Cooper. He is generally credited with encouraging more individuals to exercise than any other individual in

history and is widely recognized as "the father of the modern fitness movement."

- The wealth of information gathered in the last four decades on physical fitness and health compelled the government once again to take action against the epidemic of physical inactivity. In 1996, the *Surgeon General's Report on Physical Activity and Health*, the Centers for Disease Control and Prevention, the American Heart Association, and a number of other health agencies declared physical inactivity as a health hazard for all people.
- The government and a number of businesses allow or at least tolerate multiple "breaks" throughout the day for smoking. However, few allocate time for exercise. Perhaps it is in order to give equal time to those who wish to walk as well as to those who wish to smoke.
- Attempts to reverse the trend towards a sedentary lifestyle have begun on a national level. Although this is a long overdue approach, it falls short of a long-lasting solution. Physical education programs should emphasize sports and health-related fitness. The two should and must co-exist, for each complements the other.

■ REFERENCES

1. Eaton SB, Shostak M, Konner M. *The Paleolithic Prescription: A Program of Diet and Exercise and a Design for Living*. New York: Harper and Row; 1988.
2. Wuest DA, Bucher CA. *Foundations of Physical Education and Sport*. St. Louis, MO: Mosby; 1995.
3. Green P. *Classical Bearings: Interpreting Ancient History and Culture*. London: Thames and Hudson; 1989.
4. Bance S. *History of Yoga—A Complete Overview of the Yoga History*. Available at

http://www.abc-of-yoga.com/beginnersguide/yogahistory.asp. Accessed March 2, 2009.

5. Desch Obi TJ. *Fighting for Honor. The History of African Martial Arts in the Atlantic World*. Columbia, SC: The University of South Carolina Press Inc; 2008.

6. Historical background and evolution of physical activity recommendations (Chapt 2). In *Physical Activity and Health. A Report of the Surgeon General*; 1999. Available at http://www.cdc.gov/NCCDPHP/sgr/intro2.htm. Accessed March 2, 2009.

7. Booth FW, Chakravarthy MV, Spangenburg EE. Exercise and gene expression: physiological regulation of the human genome through physical activity. *J Physiol* 2002;543(2):399–411.

8. Forbes CA. *Greek Physical Education*. New York: The Century Company; 1929.

9. Dalleck LC, Kravitz L. History of fitness. *IDEA Health and Fitness Source* 2002;20(2): 26–33.

10. Herodotus, *The Persian Wars*, VIII, 26.

11. Grant M. *A Short History of Classical Civilization*. London, UK: Weidenfeld and Nicolson; 1991.

12. Grant M. *The Birth of Western Civilization: Greece and Rome*. New York: McGraw-Hill; 1964.

13. Weuve J, Kang JH, Manson JE, et al. Physical activity, including walking, and cognitive function in older women. *JAMA* 2004;292 (12):1454–1461.

14. Abbott RD, White LR, Ross GW, et al. Walking and dementia in physically capable elderly men. *JAMA* 2004;292(12):1447–1453.

15. Harris HA. *Sport in Greece and Rome*. Ithaca, NY: Cornell University Press; 1972.

16. Randers-Pehrson JD. *Barbarians and Romans: The Birth Struggle of Europe, AD 400–700*. Norman, OK: University of Oklahoma Press; 1993.

17. Hay D. *The Age of the Renaissance*. London, UK: Thames and Hudson; 1986.

18. Hale J. *The Civilization of Europe in the Renaissance*. New York: Maxwell Macmillan International; 1994.

19. Matthews DO. *A Historical Study of the Aims, Contents, and Methods of Swedish, Danish,* *and German Gymnastics*. Proceedings of the National College Physical Education Association for Men; 1969.

20. Welch PD. *History of American Physical Education and Sport*, 2nd ed. Springfield, IL: Charles C. Thomas; 1996.

21. Karolides NJ, Karolides M. *Focus on Fitness*. Santa Barbara, CA: ABC-CLIO; 1993.

22. Barrow HM, Brown JP. *Man and Movement: Principles of Physical Education*, 4th ed. Philadelphia: Lea & Febiger; 1988.

23. Rice EA, Hutchinson JL, Lee M. *A Brief History of Physical Education*. New York: The Ronald Press; 1958.

24. Jenkins P. *A History of the United States*. New York: St. Martin's Press; 1997.

25. Nieman DC. *Fitness and Sports Medicine: An Introduction*. Palo Alto, CA: Bull Publishing; 1990.

26. Kraus H, Hirschland R. Minimum muscular fitness tests in school children. *Res Quart* 1954;25:178.

27. Morris JN, Heady JA, Raffle PA, et al. Coronary heart-disease and physical activity of work. *Lancet* 1953;265(6796):1111–1120.

28. Morris JN, Crawford MD. Coronary heart disease and physical activity of work; evidence of a national necropsy survey. *BMJ* 1958; 2(5111):1485–1496.

29. Kennedy JF. The soft American. *Sports Illustrated* 1960;13:15–17.

30. Kennedy JF. The vigor we need. *Sports Illustrated* 1962;17:12–15.

31. Cooper Aerobics Center, Kenneth H. Cooper, MD, MPH: Founder, President, and CEO—The Cooper Aerobics Center. Available at www.cooperaerobics.com. Accessed February 27, 2009.

32. United States Department of Health and Human Services. *Physical Activity and Health. A Report by the Surgeon General*. Centers for Disease Control and Prevention; 1996. Available at www.cdc.gov/nccdphp/sgr/sgr.htm. Accessed February 27, 2009.

33. Haskell WL, Lee IM, Pate RR, et al. Physical activity and public health: updated recommendation for adults from the American College of Sports Medicine and the American

Heart Association. *Circulation* 2007;116(9): 1081–1093.

34. Williams MA, Haskell WL, Ades PA, et al. Resistance exercise in individuals with and without cardiovascular disease: 2007 update: a scientific statement from the American Heart Association Council on Clinical Cardiology and Council on Nutrition, Physical Activity, and Metabolism. *Circulation* 2007; 116(5):572–584.

35. *Gymnastics and Tumbling*. Aviation Training Division, Office of the Chief of Naval Operations, US Navy; 1944.

36. Ogden CL, Carroll MD, Curtin LR, et al. Prevalence of overweight and obesity in the United States, 1999–2004. *JAMA* 2006;295(13): 1549–1555.

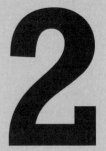
Defining Exercise and Fitness

■ FITNESS

The acquisition of fitness has been and continues to be a misunderstood concept for many individuals. This confusion stems from a lack of understanding of the basic principles that govern physical activity and exercise, and which has been perpetuated by self-proclaimed "fitness experts" who have greatly contributed to misinformation at the expense of public health.

We must always keep in mind that exercise is a double-edge sword. It can help but also harm (discussed in detail in Chapter 15). Only proper exercise can lead to fitness and health benefits. Indeed, appropriate exercise is the crux of the matter. However, defining the correct types of exercise is not a simple task. Proper exercise is dictated mostly by the age, current health status, and fitness of the individual, and for these reasons, exercise prescriptions must be tailored specifically to the individual or the population at hand.

In this chapter, the basic principles that govern physical activity and exercise are defined and discussed. Furthermore, the recent recommendations of the American College of Sports Medicine and the American Heart Association concerning physical activity and fitness for adults are presented.

Definition of Physical Activity and Exercise

Physical activity and exercise both describe a physiologic state that requires a degree of muscular effort that is beyond resting conditions. Although the terms can be used interchangeably in some instances, there are differences.

More specifically, **physical activity** is defined as movement that requires any form of skeletal muscle contraction and results in energy expenditure beyond resting levels.[1,2] This work can be performed as part of the daily requirements of the job or around the house (mowing the lawn, vacuuming, etc.), or leisure time (also known as recreational) activities. Accurate assessment of the level of physical activity in large populations becomes important in epidemiologic studies investigating associations between health benefits and a physically active lifestyle.

Exercise is best defined as a structured program designed to achieve a state of physical exertion of certain intensity, duration, and frequency.[2] Generally, exercise programs are designed with specific goals in mind. Such goals can range from improving athletic performance to improving or maintaining health. Unlike physical activity, exercise programs can be tailored to one individual. Furthermore, the intensity, duration, and frequency can be manipulated to produce the desired goals. For these reasons, exercise programs are implemented in interventional research studies to assess the effects of exercise on a specific physiologic parameter, such as blood pressure, body weight, blood lipids, etc.

Definition of Physical Fitness

The Centers for Disease Control and Prevention (CDC) and American College of Sports Medicine defines physical fitness as, "a set of physical attributes that people have or achieve that relates to the ability to perform physical activity."[2,3] These physical attributes and therefore the degree of physical fitness can be improved by engaging in appropriate physical training. For example, an individual endowed by certain physical attributes that allow him or her to run fast can improve that ability by engaging in appropriate training programs. Ultimately, how well one performs in these tasks is determined by several factors, some of which are controllable, such as training, diet, rest, and psychological factors, and others uncontrollable, such as genetics.

Physical activity is defined as movement that requires any form of skeletal muscle contraction and results in energy expenditure beyond resting levels.

Exercise is defined as a structured program designed to achieve a state of physical exertion of certain intensity, duration, and frequency.

Physical fitness is defined as a set of physical attributes that people have or achieve that relates to the ability to perform physical activity.

Aerobic and Anaerobic Fitness

To perform any task, we need energy. Because physical performance involves muscular work, the degree of performance of the task at hand (i.e., the degree of fitness) depends mainly on how the energy is made available and utilized by the muscles. To be more specific, it is not energy that is delivered to the muscles but the "raw materials." From these materials, the muscle cells extract the energy required for the task at hand. Cells can extract the necessary energy in one of two ways: with the use of oxygen and without oxygen. The utilization of oxygen to extract energy is referred to as **aerobic metabolism** (from the Greek word *aerobiosis*, meaning air-dependent living). Conversely, extracting energy without utilizing oxygen is referred to as **anaerobic** (air-independent living) metabolism.

The derivation of energy aerobically or anaerobically depends exclusively on the intensity of the activity. High-intensity activities derive their energy mainly without oxygen, while low intensity activities utilize oxygen to meet their energy requirements. Thus, activities that are referred to as **aerobic** or **anaerobic** meet most their energy requirements accordingly. Therefore, *aerobic fitness* refers to the degree or ability to provide the required energy for a specific task aerobically. Conversely, *anaerobic fitness* refers to the body's ability to provide the required energy for a specific task anaerobically.

Aerobic exercises or activities consist of repetitive, low resistance movements (walking or cycling) that last over a relatively long period of time (generally 5 minutes or more). Anaerobic exercises or activities on the other hand are characterized by bursts of intense activity lasting only a short time. Such activities include the lifting of a very heavy weight, jumping, sprinting, etc. These activities challenge the body to maximum or near maximum efforts. They require a great deal of energy within a short span of time and can only be sustained for a few seconds to minutes. The energy requirements are met predominately without the use of oxygen. For example, no oxygen is required to meet the energy necessary to run one hundred meters or lift a heavy weight.

It is important to point out that these two energy systems (aerobic and anaerobic) are almost always working together in a harmonious way, sharing the responsibility for providing the energy for the entire body. However, one is likely to be the predominant system to provide most of the energy for the particular activity at hand. The determining factors for which system will dominate in providing the energy for a particular task is discussed in more detail later in this chapter.

Aerobic fitness refers to the degree or ability to provide most of the required energy for a specific task aerobically or with the use of oxygen.

Anaerobic fitness refers to the degree or ability to provide the required energy for a specific task anaerobically or without oxygen.

Aerobic activities are of relatively low-intensity and long duration repetitive activities using large muscle groups.

Anaerobic activities are of relatively high-intensity and short duration.

Cardiovascular or Cardiorespiratory Fitness

As mentioned above, aerobic fitness refers to the ability to perform dynamic exercise utilizing large muscles for prolonged periods. Because long-lasting muscular work is by default low- to moderate-intensity work and therefore aerobic in nature, the energy requirements during such work are met by the constant supply of oxygen and nutrients to the working muscle. This is accomplished by a well-coordinated action of the cardiovascular system (heart and blood vessels) and the pulmonary system (lungs).

Thus, the degree of cardiorespiratory fitness depends on the coordinated functional state of three systems: (1) the respiratory system (lungs) to provide the necessary oxygen for the muscles, (2) the cardiovascular system (heart and vessels) to deliver the nutrients and oxygen requirements to the working muscles, and (3) the muscular system that utilizes the oxygen and nutrients delivered to meet the energy demands of the activity at hand. Naturally, the more efficiently these three systems become, the higher the performance will be.

Thus, aerobic fitness can be defined as the ability of the circulatory and the respiratory systems to supply the necessary oxygen for the muscle during prolonged work.[3] Consequently, aerobic fitness is referred to as **cardiovascular** or **cardiorespiratory fitness**. Because cardiovascular, cardiorespiratory, and aerobic fitness or aerobic capacity terms are so closely related, they can be used interchangeably.

Cardiovascular fitness or aerobic capacity can be assessed by a number of laboratory tests; however, such tests usually require expensive equipment and trained personnel. (These tests are detailed later in this chapter.) Because these tests are cost-prohibitive, cardiovascular fitness or aerobic capacity values are often estimated in large epidemiologic studies. In fact, our current knowledge of the health benefits related to physical activity is based mostly on cardiovascular fitness or exercise capacity. Relatively little information exists on the health benefits of anaerobic type of fitness such as weight or resistance training.

Generally, cardiovascular fitness is improved by habitual aerobic activities that involve large muscles and last for relatively long periods at specific intensities and frequency. Criteria recommended by the American College of Sports Medicine for the improvement of aerobic fitness are discussed in the next section.

Cardiorespiratory fitness is the ability to perform dynamic exercise utilizing large muscles for prolonged periods. Cardiorespiratory fitness depends on the coordinated functional state of the respiratory system to provide the necessary oxygen for the muscles, the cardiovascular system to deliver the nutrients and oxygen requirements to the working muscles, and the muscular system to utilize the oxygen and nutrients delivered and meet the energy demands of the activity.

Muscular Fitness

The American College of Sports Medicine defines **muscular fitness** as the ability of the muscle to perform tasks that require muscular strength or muscular endurance.

■ Muscular Strength

Muscular strength is defined as the ability of the muscle or muscle groups to exert force during a voluntary contraction.[2,4] Traditionally, the maximal force a muscle or group of muscles can exert is assessed by tests that require maximum effort against the greatest resistance one can move through the full range of motion once; this is known as *1-repetition maximum (1-RM)*. A percentage of this RM is then used to determine the number of repetitions one should perform to enhance the strength for a specific muscle. Generally, 8 to 12 repetitions at 40% to 60% of 1-RM are sufficient to enhance muscular strength. However, intensities as much as 80% and higher and relatively very

few repetitions (3 to 5) have been shown to be more effective for rapid strength gains.[3]

It is important to mention that the level of intensity for resistance exercises is not easy to determine and the 1-RM does not depict a true intensity. The number of repetitions and the percent of resistance based on 1-RM differ significantly between individuals and muscle groups. Thus, the 1-RM should only be used as a general guideline.[3]

■ Muscular Endurance

Muscular endurance is defined as the ability of the muscle or muscle groups to perform repetitive contractions over a period of time against a resistance, such as lifting a set amount of weight several times.[3] Muscular endurance is assessed by tests requiring more than 12 repetitions. A simple test of muscular endurance is the maximum number of push-ups or sit-ups one can execute without rest.[3]

Generally, muscular endurance is best developed with relatively high repetitions (12 to 20) and low resistance. However, more than 25 repetitions appear to have no further contribution to the development of muscular endurance.

■ Muscular Endurance Versus Aerobic Endurance

Muscular endurance often is confused with aerobic endurance. Some people claim that lifting a relatively light weight several times and quickly moving from exercise to exercise with no more than a few seconds of rest between sessions or stations, as is the case with circuit weight training, can increase aerobic performance. These claims are based on the substantial increase in heart rate observed during circuit weight training or resistance training in general. Although small gains in aerobic capacity with such training can occur,[6] it is not an efficient way to improve aerobic endurance for several reasons, which involve the following two principles.

Specificity Principle First, the body's response and adaptation to a specific type of exercise (stimulus) is very specific to that exercise. This is known as the **specificity principle** (discussed later in this chapter). Based on this principle, only exercises requiring increased oxygen consumption to meet their energy demand will enhance the aerobic capacity of the individual. The small gains in aerobic endurance reported by some scientists support this concept.[6] It is important to keep in mind that almost all physical activities have both an aerobic and an anaerobic component, and none is purely aerobic or purely anaerobic. The degree of involvement by each system depends mostly on the intensity of the activity. During circuit weight training, the resistance (intensity) used is relatively light and the number of repetitions high, which allows a certain degree of involvement of the aerobic system. Because this system is challenged, it responds by small improvements in its function.

Oxygen Consumption Link to Heart Rate Second, there is a linear relationship between oxygen consumption and heart rate during a graded aerobic activity. That is, as the intensity of the exercise increases, the oxygen consumption and heart rate increase in a linear fashion. Oxygen consumption reaches maximal levels when the maximal heart rate is achieved. Heart rate thus can be used as a surrogate for oxygen consumption and as an indicator of aerobic work *only if this linear relationship exists*. Indeed, exercise intensity is based on a percentage of maximal heart rate when aerobic activity is involved.

In resistance training, however, the increase in heart rate is the result of catecholamine surge and not oxygen demand. Thus, the heart rate increase is disproportionate to the increase in oxygen consumption.[5,6] Because the relationship between heart rate and oxygen consumption is no longer linear, the heart rate cannot be used as an indicator of aerobic work. The terms *muscular fitness* or *muscular endurance* therefore should be used to describe the ability of the muscle to perform mostly anaerobic work.

Muscular strength refers to the ability of the muscle or muscles to exert force.

Muscular endurance is the ability of the muscle or muscles to perform repetitive contractions over a period of time against a resistance.

■ ASSESSING EXERCISE AND PHYSICAL ACTIVITY

Exercise Components

For exercise or physical activity to yield health benefits, it must meet certain criteria and abide by specific principles. This section presents the components of exercise and the principles governing the physiologic changes and health benefits related to exercise.

Regardless of the type of exercise (aerobic or anaerobic), for changes to occur in any physiologic system as a result of exercise, a minimum amount (volume) of exercise or physical work is needed. The exercise volume is affected by four factors that are referred to as *exercise components*: intensity, frequency, duration, and length.[3]

Frequency refers to the number of exercise sessions per week. **Duration** refers to the length of each exercise session, and **intensity** refers to how hard one is working during the activity. **Length** refers to the weeks or months the particular activity sessions are sustained. All of the exercise components are important, and it is the interaction among all four that comprises the volume of exercise or work and produces the desired results.

Quantifying and Defining Exercise Components: Rationale

It is easy to understand why exercise needs to be defined and quantified. However, the need for quantifying or defining the exercise components may be less clear. To understand the significance of quantifying exercise components, an analogy is to view exercise as a type of medication. When a physician prescribes any type of medication, its dose, how often (frequency), and for how long (duration) it is taken must be considered to maximize its benefits and minimize its risks. Change any of these components and the efficacy of the medication is lowered, sometimes to the extent that it may cause harm and perhaps even death. In the same way, the intensity (dose), duration, and frequency of exercise all must be considered to maximize the beneficial effects of exercise and minimize the risks.

Determining Exercise Intensity

Of the four components of exercise, intensity is the most difficult to determine. This is especially true for aerobic type of work. Intensity can be viewed as to the degree by which exercise or the particular physical activity places a demand on the system (muscle, heart, or entire body) per unit of time. It can be described and quantified as a percentage of the maximum work a system or an individual is capable of performing. For certain types of work, intensity is easy to quantify. For example, if the maximum amount of weight one can lift at one time (1-RM) is known, the individual can choose any percentage of that amount (i.e., 50%), to perform repetitive lifts. The percentage chosen represents the intensity of exercise performed.

Determining Intensity for Aerobic Work

■ Direct Method

Determining the intensity for aerobic activities requires a similar approach. First, it is necessary to determine the maximum capacity of the aerobic system. The "true" maximum aerobic capacity is the maximum amount of oxygen (referred to as maximum oxygen uptake [$\dot{V}O_2$max]) the body can utilize during work. This can be established in laboratories by trained personnel using elaborate, expensive equipment. A brief description and rationale for this procedure, known as an exercise tolerance test (ETT) or graded exercise test (GXT), is as follows:

The individual breathes room air via a mouthpiece (with the nose occluded) that is connected by plastic tubes to an automated, computerized system called a metabolic cart. The mouthpiece is designed in such a way that it allows the expired air (or a sample of it) to enter the metabolic cart to be analyzed for its oxygen and carbon dioxide (CO_2) content. After resting samples are taken, the individual is subjected to a standardized exercise protocol on a treadmill or stationary bike (**Figure 2.1**). The exercise begins at a very low workload and increases every 2 to 3 minutes depending on the exercise protocol. The workload is determined by a standardized and progressive increase in the speed and/or elevation of the treadmill or (if a bike is used) the resistance. Heart rate and oxygen uptake are continuously monitored and recorded during the entire test. Blood pressure is assessed and recorded every 2 to 3 minutes.

Figure 2.1   Direct oxygen uptake is the most reliable method for assessing aerobic capacity.

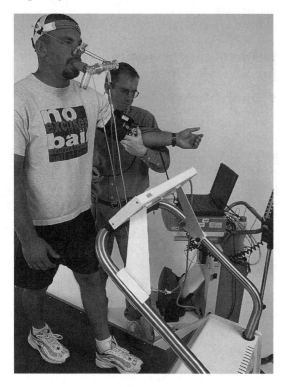

A linear relationship exists between workload and oxygen requirements. Thus, as the workload increases, the oxygen requirements also increase. At some point, the individual reaches fatigue (exercise protocols are designed to fatigue most people within 10 to 12 minutes) and the test is terminated. This level is referred to as the *maximal aerobic capacity* of the individuals. The oxygen utilized by the body at the point of fatigue is the individual's $\dot{V}O_2$max, which is expressed in liters per minute (L/min) or milliliters of oxygen per kilogram (kg) of body weight per minute (ml/kg/min).

The exercise intensities can now be based on the $\dot{V}O_2$max achieved. For example, let us assume that the $\dot{V}O_2$max of an individual is 50 ml/kg/min. Let us also assume that the exercise intensity is set between 60% and 80% of the maximum aerobic capacity or $\dot{V}O_2$max. Therefore, 60% of the individual's $\dot{V}O_2$max (50 ml/kg/min) is 30 ml/kg/min ([50 × 60]/100) and 80% is 40 ml/kg/min ([60 × 80]/100).

Obviously, this information is useful for research purposes. However, it is not practical for someone who wishes to know the exercise intensity during his or her training. For this purpose, the exercise intensity can be easily determined by the heart rate as it corresponds to the percentage of oxygen consumption. Because the heart rate and oxygen uptake are continuously recorded during a metabolic test, one can easily match a desired percentage of heart rate to the corresponding oxygen consumption. For the example above, the heart rate corresponding to the 30 ml of oxygen consumption per kg of body weight per minute and that corresponding to the 40 ml of oxygen per kg of body weight per minute can be used as the upper and lower exercise intensity criteria for this individual.

The advantage of the direct method is that it is highly accurate as it allows an assessment of the exercise intensity of an individual based on a measured—not estimated—aerobic capacity. Because it is cost- and time-prohibitive for large populations, the direct method is mostly used in patients with specific needs and for research purposes.

■ Percent of Maximum Heart Rate Method

The easiest and most straightforward method to establish the exercise intensity is to measure the percentage of the maximum heart rate (MHR). This method is based on the concept

Figure 2.2   Heart rate and oxygen consumption values of a 24-year-old female.

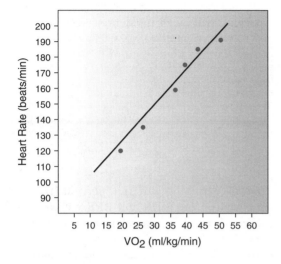

age of 70% to 85% corresponds fairly closely to the individual's 50% to 70% of $\dot{V}O_2$max. Keep in mind that this is a conservative and inaccurate method especially in low intensities.

■ Heart Rate Reserve Method (Karvonen Method)

Another way to determine the exercise heart rate is the heart rate reserve (HRR) method, which is also known as the Karvonen method.[7] It is more precise because it takes into account the individual's resting HR. The exercise intensity used for this method is 60% to 80% of MHR. To determine the exercise intensity based on the HRR method, the following steps should be followed:

Step 1: Calculate the MHR by subtracting the age of the individual from 220.

Step 2: Determine the resting HR after resting for 5 minutes.

Step 3: Subtract the resting HR from the maximum HR (MHR) to determine the heart rate reserve (HRR).

Step 4: Multiply the HRR by 0.6 or 60% and add the resting HR to that number. This will determine the lower limit of the exercise HR. Multiply the HRR by 0.80 or 80% and add the resting HR to determine the higher limit of the exercise HR.

that the HR increases in a linear fashion with the increase in workload and oxygen consumption (**Figure 2.2**). Theoretically, when the $\dot{V}O_2$max is achieved MHR is also achieved. Thus, a percentage of the individual's MHR can be used to establish the desired exercise intensity for that individual.

The question, of course, is how one can determine the MHR without actually measuring it by subjecting the individual to a maximal test. Interestingly, the MHR of an individual can be estimated with an acceptable degree of accuracy by subtracting the individual's age from 220.

$$HR = 220 - Age$$

For a 20 year old, the MHR will be 200 beats per minute (bpm; 220 – 20). and for a 50 year old, the MHR will be 170 bpm (220 – 50). A percent-

Example:
A 50 year old with a resting HR of 70 bpm.
MHR: 220 – 50 = 170 bpm
HRR: 170 – 70 = 100 (MHR – resting HR)
Exercise Heart Rate
Lower Limit:
(HRR × 0.60) + resting HR
(100 × 0.60) = 60 + 70 =130 bpm
Upper Limit:
(HRR × 0.80) + resting HR
(100 × 0.80) = 80 + 70 = 150 bpm

The 60% to 80% exercise heart rate values derived from the HRR method are associated with the heart rate corresponding to 60% to 80% of the directly measured $\dot{V}O_2$max for most physically fit individuals. However, the method overestimates the intensity for low-fit individuals.

■ $\dot{V}O_2$ Reserve Method

To correct for the intensity overestimation for low-fit individuals, Swain and Franklin[8] proposed to use the difference between $\dot{V}O_2$max and the resting O_2 uptake ($\dot{V}O_2$ reserve) as a more accurate method to estimate exercise intensity. This method is likely to be used in exercise interventional studies and not in epidemiologic research. However, a basic understanding of the rationale for the $\dot{V}O_2$ reserve method is important when the reader is faced with study information based on this method.

When the $\dot{V}O_2$ reserve method is applied, the association becomes stronger across all fitness levels. That is, 60% of HRR corresponds very closely to the HR at 60% of $\dot{V}O_2$ reserve. For example, let us assume that $\dot{V}O_2$max values of individual A is 40 ml/kg/min. Sixty percent of that value will be 24 ml/kg/min. According to the $\dot{V}O_2$ reserve method we will have:

$$\dot{V}O_2 \text{ reserve} = \dot{V}O_2\text{max} - 3.5$$
$$40 - 3.5 \text{ ml/kg/min} = 36.5 \text{ ml/kg/min}$$
Thus, 60% of $\dot{V}O_2$ reserve = (36.5 ml/kg/min × 0.60)
$$= 21.9 \text{ ml/kg/min}$$
$$+ 3.5 \text{ ml/kg/min (resting value)}$$
$$\overline{25.4 \text{ ml/kg/min}}$$

Table 2.1 presents different percent HR values based on the MHR and HRR methods. A resting HR of 70 is assumed to calculate the percentages for HRR. As one can see, the 50% of HRR value corresponds to approximately 70% of MHR and the 70% HRR values correspond to approximately 80% to 85% of the MHR values. **Table 2.2** presents actual data of a 24

		Percent of MHR			**Percent of HHR***	
Age (years)	**Maximum HR (bpm)**	**70%**	**80%**	**85%**	**50%**	**70%**
≤ 20	200	140	160	170	135	161
25	195	137	156	166	133	158
30	190	133	152	162	130	154
35	185	130	148	158	128	150
40	180	126	144	153	125	147
45	175	123	140	149	123	144
50	170	119	136	145	120	140
55	165	116	132	140	118	137
60	160	112	128	136	115	133
65	155	109	124	132	113	130
70	150	105	120	128	110	126
75	145	102	116	123	108	123
80	140	98	112	119	105	119

Table 2.1 Lower and Upper Exercise Heart Rate Limits for Different Ages

*A resting HR of 70 bpm is assumed. MHR = maximum heart rate; HHR = heart rate reserve.

Table 2.2 Data from a 24-year-old Woman with a Resting Heart Rate of 63 bpm and a Maximum Oxygen Uptake of 51.5 ml/kg/min

Percent of $\dot{V}O_2$max	$\dot{V}O_2$	HR Based on Max HR Method	Actual Heart Rate	HR Based on HR-Reserve Method
50	26	98	136	130
60	31	118	140	143
70	36	137	158	156
80	41	157	170	169
85	44	167	178	176
90	46	176	185	183
100	51.5	196	190	196

According to the data in Table 2.2, the percent HR derived from the HR-reserve method is relatively close to the heart rate achieved and the percent of VO_2max and VO_2 reserve achieved during the actual test. Note that 50% of the HR reserve corresponds to the 70% of the maximum HR and 70% to 80% of HRR corresponds to 80% to 85% of maximum HR.
VO_2max = maximum oxygen uptake; $\dot{V}O_2$ = oxygen uptake; HR = heart rate.

year old with a resting heart rate of 63 bpm and a $\dot{V}O_2$max value of 51.5 ml/kg/min.

Defining Exercise by Intensity

Exercise intensity is characterized by the American College of Sports Medicine and the American Heart Association as being either low, moderate, or high intensity. As mentioned earlier, the most practical way to determine exercise intensity is to base it on the percentage of the maximum heart rate that the individual achieves and maintains during exercise. A more elaborate classification of exercise intensities based on MHR and HRR are presented in **Table 2.3**.

Table 2.3 Classification of Exercise or Physical Activity Intensity

Exercise Intensity	HRR (%) or $\dot{V}O_2R$ (%)	MHR (%)	Activities
Very Light	< 20	< 50	Slow walk (25–30 min/mile), slow biking, yard work, dancing, etc.
Light	20–39	50–63	Walking the dog (20–25 min/mile)
Moderate	40–59	64–76	Brisk walk (16–18 min/mile), climbing stairs, mowing the lawn
Hard	60–84	77–93	Jogging at speeds of approximately 10–15 min/mile, tennis (singles), racquet ball, etc.
Very Hard	≥ 85	≥ 94	Running at speeds of less than 10 min/mile, basketball, soccer

The American College of Sports Medicine and other authorities recommend that the minimum exercise intensity for improvements in cardiovascular fitness is 40% to 49% of HRR or 64% to 70% of MHR. This is especially true for low-fit or sedentary individuals. For those who are relatively active and wish to improve their fitness level, the recommendation is that the exercise intensity is within the range of 60% to 80% of HRR or 77% to 90% of MHR.[3]

The American College of Sports Medicine and other authorities recommend that the minimum exercise intensity for improvements in cardiovascular fitness is 40% to 49% of HRR or 64% to 70% of MHR.

Exercise Duration

According to the American College of Sports Medicine's Position Stand, the duration of any aerobic activity necessary to promote aerobic capacity must be at least 20 continuous minutes.[3] In addition, several 10-minute bouts for a total 30 minutes duration have been shown to yield equivalent results as one 20-minute bout.[9,10]

Exercise duration is inversely related to intensity of the activity and, therefore, intensity and duration can interact to produce the desired results. It is also possible that a high-intensity, low duration activity can yield similar results if the intensity for the same activity is reduced and the duration increased. Accordingly, manipulations in duration and intensity can be applied in different populations to make exercise safe and yet still achieve the desired health benefits.

A daily accumulation of 20 to 60 minutes of continuous exercise is recommended in the general population. For those unable to sustain long exercise periods or for those who prefer it, intermittent bouts of exercise (10-minute minimum) can be performed several times throughout the day. This is also recommended strongly during the first few weeks of exercise. For example, one can exercise for 10 minutes in the morning and 10 minutes in the afternoon. Similar exercise benefits can be derived if the volume of exercise (continuous or intermittent) is equal.

Generally speaking, longer exercise durations offer added health and physical performance benefits (muscular and cardiovascular endurance). However, the rate of return for these benefits diminishes substantially beyond 60 minutes of continuous exercise. Thus, the small gain of benefits beyond 60 minutes of exercise and the increased risk for injury compel me to strongly recommend against exercising beyond 60 minutes.

It is also important to keep in mind the interaction between exercise intensity and duration. Generally speaking, the higher the exercise intensity, the lower the duration will be and vice versa. Thus, the cost of any given activity can be similar or identical with a different combination between exercise intensity and duration. For example, a 20-minute activity at 90% MHR theoretically will require a very similar caloric expenditure as a 40-minute activity at 45% of MHR. Thus, exercise duration and intensity must always be considered and manipulated to produce the desired results.

According to the American College of Sports Medicine Position Stand recommendations, the duration of any aerobic activity necessary to promote aerobic capacity must be at least 20 continuous minutes. In addition, several 10-minute bouts for a total 30 minutes have been shown to yield equivalent results as one 20-minute bout.

Exercise Frequency

The frequency of exercise is also important. Once a week is not enough and is perhaps counterproductive. Exercising every day is too much and also is counterproductive. Injuries ranging in severity from minor to fatal are more prone to occur with this type of training schedule. The American College of Sports Medicine and other health organizations recommend that exercise be performed three to five times per week. Some additional improvements in fitness may be realized if a sixth day a week is added, but exercising more than six times per week yields relatively small increases in fitness[3] and may even do more harm than good.

Cardiovascular fitness can also be improved by exercising only twice a week; this is especially true for de-conditioned individuals. This is strongly recommended as a start for sedentary individuals. A slow and progressive increase to three or four times per week should ensue when the individual feels comfortable. This usually occurs within the 4 to 6 weeks of appropriate training.

> The American College of Sports Medicine and other health organizations recommend that exercise be performed three to five times per week. Some additional improvements in fitness may be realized if a sixth day a week is added. Exercising more than six times per week yields relatively small increases in fitness and may even do more harm than good.

Length of Training Period

The length of the exercise training period has received the least attention of the four exercise components from researchers, yet it is important to recognize that exercise-related adaptations generally occur after several weeks of training.

The exact length of training for such adaptations is difficult to define for a number of factors, as some are known and others have yet to be considered. Naturally, the other exercise components (intensity, duration, and frequency) will strongly influence the length of training before changes are observed. Another important consideration is the particular system affected by exercise training. For example, measurable changes in blood pressure have been documented in just 2 weeks of exercise at three times per week, whereas lipoprotein changes are usually observed after 12 weeks.[11,12] Despite the uncertainty, it is safe to say that for most observable exercise-related chronic adaptations, the length of exercise training is about 8 weeks at three times per week. Changes continue beyond the 8 weeks and reach a plateau at about 12 months.

> Most research findings support that the length of exercise training for observable exercise-related chronic adaptations is about 8 weeks at three times per week. Changes continue beyond the 8 weeks and reach a plateau at about 12 months.

Exercise Volume

It has already been alluded that all chronic adaptations related to exercise for any physiologic system will only occur when a certain exercise volume is achieved. Exercise volume is the by-product of all exercise components. That is, exercise volume is the outcome of:

- Exercise intensity
- Exercise duration
- Frequency (times per week)
- Length of training (how many weeks)

For the desired results to occur, a certain "exercise volume threshold" must be achieved.

This *exercise volume threshold* is the result of the interaction of the intensity, duration of each exercise session, frequency, and length of training. In general, a long-duration and low-intensity exercise can yield similar benefits as those of short-duration and high-intensity if the exercise volumes are similar. Therefore, daily walks can be just as effective in yielding health benefits as jogging three times per week. Thus, it is imperative that when conducting exercise-related research, one must be mindful of the total volume of exercise achieved.

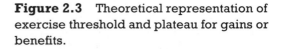

Exercise volume is the by-product of all exercise components: duration, intensity, frequency, and length of training.

Threshold and Plateau of Exercise

The exercise volume threshold exists for all individuals but can vary widely among individuals. This variability is due to many factors including age, genetics, and level of fitness. Small increases in physical work beyond this theoretical threshold tend to result in relatively large increases in benefits. To make things even more complicated, each exercise component has its own threshold.

There is also a maximum amount of work or exercise, beyond which the exercise-related health benefits are relatively small or nonexistent. This point is referred to as the *plateau*. An attempt to "push" the body beyond this point increases the risk of injury substantially, especially for older individuals.

A theoretical representation of the threshold and plateau is presented in **Figure 2.3**. Let us assume that one is lifting weights to get stronger. Let us also assume that the threshold is at 5 kg. As one can observe, there are no signifi-

cant strength gains if the amount lifted is below that threshold. However, when the weight lifted doubles the threshold weight (from 5 kg to 10 kg), the strength gains quadruple. If the weight lifted is three times the threshold weight (15 kg), then the strength gains are eight times higher, and at four times the threshold weight (20 kg), the strength gains are about 10 times higher. However, weight increases beyond this level result only in small gains in strength. Finally, a plateau is reached at approximately 30 kg with little or no additional gains in strength materialized beyond this level.

An argument can be made for the existence of two types of plateaus: an absolute plateau that cannot be manipulated and one that can be constantly reset by manipulating certain factors such as diet, training, and even ergogenic aids (that is, dietary substances or mechanical devices purporting to enhance physical performance, particularly in athletes).

Threshold and plateau levels for each component of exercise (intensity, duration, frequency, and length) also follow the same general rule just described. (This also was mentioned within the discussion of each exercise component.)

Figure 2.3 Theoretical representation of exercise threshold and plateau for gains or benefits.

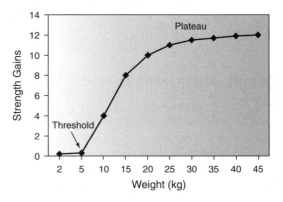

Dose-Response Association Between Physical Activity, Exercise, and Health

Exercise-related health benefits are also subject to an exercise threshold and plateau. In other words, no health benefits can be realized if the exercise volume does not meet and surpass a certain threshold. Benefits beyond this threshold appear to be related to the amount (dose) of exercise. Thus, the concept of a dose-response relationship between exercise volume as well as exercise components (duration, intensity, and frequency) and health benefits has been advocated. The basic question about the dose-response relationship between exercise and health benefits is whether it is linear or if it will reach a plateau at some point. More importantly, is there an increase in risk with higher exercise levels? Although this issue remains undecided, it is likely that a plateau in health benefits is reached and the risk of injury increases in a curvilinear fashion beyond a certain exercise volume.[13,14] A theoretical representation of this relationship is depicted in **Figure 2.4**. Although Figure 2.4 depicts a relationship with only exercise volume, similar relationships are believed to exist with exercise intensity and duration as well.

Assessing Exercise Volume

The true exercise or work volume performed can only be measured in the laboratory using a double-water labeling technique or respiratory chamber. However, such assessments are cost- and time-prohibitive and certainly not practical for large populations. For this reason, more practical and inexpensive methods have been developed over the years to assess relatively accurately the volume of physical activity, exercise, or work achieved by one individual or, more importantly, large cohorts. Certainly doing so has great significance in epidemiologic research as it attempts

Figure 2.4 Theoretical presentation of exercise benefits and risks.

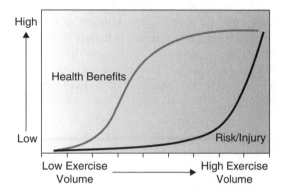

Source: Modified from: Dehn M, Mullins C. Physiologic effects and importance of exercise in patients with coronary heart disease. *Cardio Med* 1977;2:365. Haskell W. Dose-response issues from a biological perspective. In: Bouchard C, Shephard RJ, Stephens T, eds. *Physical activity, fitness and health: International proceedings and consensus statement.* Champaign, IL: Human Kinetics; 1994:1030–1039.

to understand the association between physical activity and health. A review of the available techniques and methods used to assess the physical are presented in the next sections.

Metabolic Equivalents

The need for a universal and more practical method to assess energy output in large populations during physical activity led scientists to develop a standardized exercise test and an estimate of the energy requirements for different workloads and eventually different activities.

The scientific basis for these estimates is the direct assessment of energy requirements (oxygen consumption). It is well established that the amount of oxygen used during resting conditions is 3.5 ml of oxygen per kg of body weight per minute (3.5 ml O_2/kg/min). This value was coined as *1 metabolic equivalent (1 MET).* Using this value as the baseline, over the years researchers have been able to quantify the MET level required for many occupational tasks and physical activities. Thus, tasks that require twice that amount (7 ml O_2/kg/min) require 2 METs and those triple the amount of oxygen require 3 METs, and so on. In addition, several standardized exercise protocols have been developed to assess the MET level and consequently exercise capacity of individuals for medical and other reasons.

---

1 MET = 3.5 ml of O_2/kg/min

- It is equivalent to the amount of energy expended per kg of body weight, during 1 minute of rest.
- Thus, a 70 kg individual requires 245 ml of oxygen per minute to sustain life at rest.
- Any activity above resting requires greater oxygen consumption and, therefore, has a higher MET level.
- MET levels can be used to define the intensity of an activity.

Thanks to the efforts of the American College of Sports Medicine and many investigators, we now have a vast database—the Compendium of Physical Activities—that contains the MET level of a wide variety of physical activities.[15] This information provides researchers and practitioners a standardized system for determining the amount of physical activity in large populations. A sample of select activities from this database is presented in Table 2.4.

Exercise Volume

Total exercise volume can be estimated by the number of times each activity is performed multiplied by the energy cost of that activity. This is expressed as MET-hours. For example, a brisk walk three times per week at 5 METs (intensity) for 60 minutes per session can be

Table 2.4 MET Level for Select Activities

Specific Activity	MET
Bicycling	4.0
< 10 mph	
10–11.9 mph	6.0
12–13.9 mph	8.0
14–15.9 mph	10.0
16–19 mph	12.0
> 19 mph	16.0
Bicycling stationary	7.0
General	
200–250 watts of resistance	10–12
Dancing	
Ballet, modern, twist, tap, jazz, jitterbug	4–5
Aerobic	6.5
Ballroom, fast	5.5
Stair-climber	9.0
Rowing (100–200 watts)	7–12
Weight lifting	3.3
Walking	
< 2 mph (level surface)	2.0
2 mph (level surface)	2.5
Walking the dog	3.0
2.5 mph (level surface)	3.0
3.0 mph (level surface)	3.3
3.5 mph (brisk)	3.8
4.0 mph (very brisk)	5.0
3.5 mph (uphill)	6.0
5 mph (fast)	8.0
Golf (general)	4.5
Football, baseball, softball	5–9
Basketball	6–8
Lacrosse	8.0
Soccer	7–10
Racquetball	7–10
Boxing	6–12
Roller skating	7.0
Skateboarding	5.0
Karate, Judo, kickboxing	10.0
Tennis	
General	7.0
Singles	8.0
Doubles	5–6
Volleyball	4–8
Track and field	6–10
Ice skating	7.0
Skiing	
General, 2.5 mph	7.0
Cross country 4–4.9 mph	8.0
Cross country 5–7 mph	9.0
Cross country > 8 mph	14.0

Source: Data from: Ainsworth BE, Haskell WL, Leon AS, et al. Compendium of physical activities: classification of energy costs of human physical activities. *Med Sci Sports Exerc* 1993;25(1):71–80.

expressed as 15 MET-hours per week (see formula).

> MET-hours = duration of activity (hr) ×
> energy cost (MET)
>
> in kilocalories (kcal)

Energy expenditure also can be expressed in kilocalories (kcal), where one kcal is the amount of energy (heat) required to raise the temperature of 1 kg of water by 1 degree Celsius. Because 1 MET is equivalent to 1 kcal/kg or body weight/hr, it is easy to calculate kcal spent in a certain activity if one knows the MET level, duration of the activity, and the weight of the individual. For example, the caloric expenditure a 70 kg individual exercising for 30 minutes at the intensity of 10 METs will be:

> kcal = (MET × kg of body weight ×
> exercise duration) / 60
>
> kcal = (10 × 70 × 30) / 60 = 350 kcal

As with METs, expressing energy expenditure in kcal is attractive because it provides a way to combine different activities to estimate the total volume of exercise by into one unifying measure.

> 1 MET= 3.5 ml of O_2/kg of body weight/minute
> 1 MET = ~1 kcal/kg of body weight/hour

Physical Activity Questionnaires

Epidemiologic studies rely on physical activity questionnaires to assess the physical activity of large populations. Several such questionnaires have been developed over the years. A collection of physical activity questionnaires was published in 1997 by the American College of Sports Medicine.[16] You can refer to this excellent resource for a more detailed description of physical activity questionnaires.

Because physical activity can be defined in several different ways, there is no single standard for measuring it. Thus, the most important factor in choosing a physical activity questionnaire is choosing the one that best fits the population to be studied. For example, when assessing the physical activity of children, it is wise to choose a questionnaire designed for children and if one is assessing the physical activity of women, then the questionnaire of choice should be the one that best reflect the physical activities and habits of women. Other factors to consider are time, culture, subjects' age, and prevalence of the activity in the population to be studied. For example, asking questions about participation in a sport such as ice hockey to those living in a warm climate is likely to yield very little valuable information.

Regardless of the questionnaire chosen, an assessment of physical activity volume requires gathering information about the following parameters:

1. Type of activity (walking, bike riding, tennis, basketball, etc.)
2. Frequency (how often is each activity performed per week?)
3. Duration (how long in minutes is each activity performed per session?)
4. Intensity (how hard is the subject working?)
5. Length of the activity (how many weeks, months, or years has a particular activity been performed?)
6. Weight of the individual

The information gathered from the questionnaires is then analyzed to determine the volume of physical activity. The volume is expressed in METs. An example of physical activity estimates is presented in **Figure 2.5**.

■ Reliability and Validity of Physical Activity Assessment

It is important to keep in mind that the information gathered by questionnaires is subjective. The information gathered by self-report methods (activity questionnaires) can be influenced by several factors, including the individual's ability to store and retrieve information, and by respondent and interviewer bias.

Reliability and validity studies have helped ensure the accuracy and quality of physical activity assessment based on questionnaires. A questionnaire is considered to have good reliability if it consistency provided the same results under the same circumstances. Validity refers to the ability of a questionnaire to measure what was designed to measure.[16]

Despite the drawbacks, self-report methods are simple to use, can be used in different populations, are relatively inexpensive, and provide a relatively accurate assessment of physical activity.

Devices Used to Assess Physical Activity

■ Accelerometers

The use of accelerometer devices to assess the physical activity of an individual is one of the most common methods in the past two decades. These devices are reliable, small, noninvasive, and relatively inexpensive. Because most units are small, light, durable, and can store a considerable amount of data, they can be worn for several days. In general, accelerometers provide reliable data of overall physical activity but have a less accurate prediction of caloric expenditure.[17] A list of the most popular accel-

Figure 2.5 Computation of energy expended during a week of physical activity.

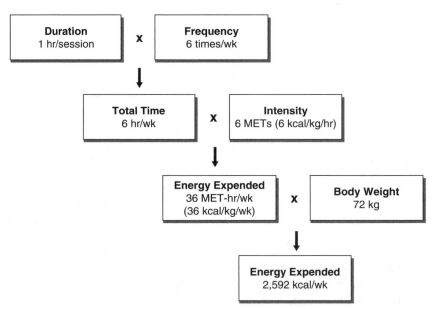

erometers and some of their unique features are presented in **Table 2.5**.

Accelerometry is based on movement, so factors that mask movement will influence the accelerometer's output. For example, the preferred body site for wearing the accelerometer is the hip. However, certain activities like biking or climbing stairs involve relatively little hip motion and, therefore, accurate assessment of activity or energy expenditure is not achieved. In addition, accelerometers cannot account for the increased energy cost required for uphill walking or carrying a weight during walking.

■ Pedometers

Pedometers are inexpensive, small, light, and provide accurate and objective measure of walking, which are certainly advantages over activity questionnaires that attempt to discern an individual's daily walking distance. These devices are capable of recording ambulatory activities that are in a horizontal motion, such as walking,

Table 2.5 Commonly Used Accelerometers and Their Characteristics

Accelerometer Manufacturer	Characteristics
ActiTrac Ver Med	• Developed by the same company as the Biotrainer. • Used mostly for sleep research. • Very small and light, and very sensitive to movement. • Adapted for physical activity research. • Preliminary results show strong predictive validity for estimating energy expenditure.
Biotrainer Pro Individual Monitoring Systems	• Bidirectional • Uses Windows-based software • Allows the user to define recording ranges from 15 seconds to 2 minutes. • Allows the user to define different sensitivity settings.
Caltrac Hemokinetics	• Does not allow data to be stored on a minute-by-minute basis. • Can only examine total activity accumulated over a specific period of time.
Computer Science and Applications (CSA)	• Smaller than most other monitors. • Continuous recording for 22 days at 1-minute intervals. • Expanded memory for longer recording durations. • Infrared computer interface.
Tritrac Professional Products	• Allows interfaces with computer for data storage. • Records data in three directions through the use of three separate accelerometers. • Provides an estimated activity and total energy expenditure.

jogging, or running, by counting the steps. They do not record upper body activities or vertical motion activities such as cycling or stair climbing.

The pedometer's accuracy can be influenced by a number of factors, including the walking speed, abdominal size, site of placement, and type of waistband. In general, pedometers are relatively accurate in counting steps at speeds of 2.5 mph or higher (24 minutes per mile). Significant underestimation of steps occurs when pedometers are attached to loose waistband, but abdominal size and waistband interferences can be minimized if the pedometer is attached to a firm waistband and in an upright position.

The popularity of pedometers increased following the reports by Hatano in 1993 and 1997,[18,19] who proposed that it took 10,000 steps per day—an estimated 333 kcal per day—to confer health benefits. Based on this concept, the activity level of an individual can be estimated (**Table 2.6**).

Pedometers appear to be an attractive motivational tool to increase physical activity in large populations. It provides instant feedback and a defined level of activity (a goal) in a simple and inexpensive way for most people. Although it does not measure all types of activities, the ease of walking with its documented health benefits[20,21] makes pedometers perhaps the most effective motivator to increase physical activity in individuals of all ages. This was supported by a recent meta-analysis of 26 studies of groups using pedometers. Bravata et al. reported that the use of pedometers was associated with a significant increase in physical activity and a significant decrease in blood pressure and body mass index.[22] However, some believe that a goal of 10,000 steps per day may not be sustainable for some populations, especially older adults and those living with chronic diseases.[23] The pedometer-based physical activity level for healthy adults proposed is described in Table 2.6.

■ Heart Rate Monitors

Use of the heart rate to estimate physical activity is based on the relationship between increased physical activity and heart rate. Heart rate increases beyond resting values upon the initiation of physical activity, an increase that is linear and directly proportional to the intensity of the activity.[3]

Modern heart rate monitors consist of a transmitter packaged in a small, lightweight unit attached to an elastic strap and a receiver designed as a wristwatch. The transmitter is strapped around the chest area. Beat-to-beat heart activity (electrocardiogram [ECG]) is sensed by the transmitter (chest unit) and the data are then transmitted wirelessly to the receiver (wristwatch), where the heart rate number is displayed (**Figure 2.6**). The average heart rate can be stored; the amount of data stored depends on the memory capacity of the

Table 2.6 Activity Level Based on Steps per Day

Steps per Day	Activity Level
< 5,000	Sedentary
5,000–7,499	Low activity
7,500–9,999	Moderately active
10,000–12,500	Active
> 12,500	Highly active

Source: data from: Tudor-Locke C, Bassett DR Jr. How many steps/day are enough? Preliminary pedometer indices for public health. *Sports Med* 2004;34(1):1–8.

Figure 2.6   Heart rate monitor.

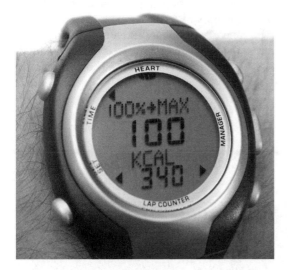

Because physical activity can be defined in several different ways, there is no single standard for measuring it. The method used can be influenced by a number of factors including the size of the population to be studied, age, gender, culture, and cost. Regardless of the method chosen, the ultimate goal is to attain reliable and accurate information.

Currently, there are several ways available for assessing physical activity. Applying multiple methods to access physical activity may yield more accurate results and, when possible, should be considered.

Emerging technologies provide progressively more accurate and at times relatively inexpensive ways to monitor physical activity under free-living conditions and will continue to do so.

receiver and the length of interval selected. Most are able to store approximately 3 to 4 days of exercise values at the length interval of 60-second epoch. Data can then be transferred to a personal computer. The estimated life for most heart monitors is approximately 2,500 hours of exercise or about 3 to 5 years.

Because the exercise intensity of aerobic activity depends on oxygen, heart rate monitors can be used to estimate energy expenditure. In addition, heart rate monitors offer the unique feature of programming lower and upper limits of exercise heart rate. The monitor beeps when heart rate is outside these criteria and the individuals can adjust exercise intensity accordingly.

The cost varies with the number and type of options offered by each unit. Cheaper models can start as low as 40 dollars and progressively increase to 500 dollars for the most elaborate units.

Defining Aerobic Fitness by Standardized Exercise Tests

As with exercise volume, the gold standard for defining the fitness of an individual or individuals is to directly assess the $\dot{V}O_2max$. However, as mentioned earlier, this method is cost- and time-prohibitive for large populations. Thus, population studies have relied on other methods of collecting information on the habitual physical activity of the population of interest: questionnaires, accelerometers, pedometers, and heart rate monitors. Using standardized methods, MET levels or kcal per week can be estimated as described earlier. Fitness then can be defined in a number of ways such as tertiles, quantiles, etc. For example, a cohort can be divided into three categories (low, moderate-fit, and high-fit) based on their MET levels.

There is also a more direct and objective method of defining the fitness level of an individual or individuals. This method is based on standardized exercise tests that follow the same principle with the direct assessment of $\dot{V}O_2$max with one exception. Oxygen consumption is not directly measured but is estimated based on equations derived from the actual assessment of $\dot{V}O_2$max.

The actual procedure is similar to that described for the assessment of $\dot{V}O_2$max, with the exception that the individual is not connected to a metabolic cart (that is, there is no breathing apparatus). However, the individual is connected to a heart rate monitor and subjected to a standardized exercise protocol on a treadmill or stationary bike. The most commonly used exercise protocols in the United States are described in **Table 2.7**. The exercise

Table 2.7 Commonly Used Treadmill and Bicycle Exercise Protocols

	Treadmill			
Stage	**Minutes**	**Speed (MPH)**	**% Grade**	**METS**
Bruce Protocol				
1	3	1.7	10	4.6
2	3	2.5	12	7.0
3	3	3.4	14	10.2
4	3	4.2	16	13.5
5	3	5.0	18	17.2
6	3	5.5	20	20.4
7	3	6.0	22	23.8
Modified Bruce Protocol				
1	3	1.7	0	2.3
2	3	1.7	5	3.5
3	3	1.7	10	4.6
4	3	2.5	12	7.0
5	3	3.4	14	10.2
6	3	4.2	16	13.5
7	3	5.0	18	17.2
8	3	5.5	20	20.4
9	3	6.0	22	23.8
Balke-Ware Protocol				
1	3	3.3	1	4.0
2	3	3.3	2	4.4
3	3	3.3	3	4.9
4	3	3.3	4	5.3
5	3	3.3	5	5.8
6	3	3.3	6	6.3
7	3	3.3	7	6.7
8	3	3.3	8	7.2
9	3	3.3	9	7.6
10	3	3.3	10	8.1
11	3	3.3	11	8.5

		Treadmill (continued)		
Stage	**Minutes**	**Speed (MPH)**	**% Grade**	**METS**
12	3	3.3	12	9.0
13	3	3.3	13	9.4
14	3	3.3	14	9.9
15	3	3.3	15	10.3
16	3	3.3	16	10.8
17	3	3.3	17	11.3
18	3	3.3	18	11.7
19	3	3.3	19	12.2
20	3	3.3	20	12.6
21	3	3.3	21	13.1
22	3	3.3	22	13.5
23	3	3.3	23	14.0
24	3	3.3	24	14.4
25	3	3.3	25	14.9
26	3	3.3	26	15.4
Balke Protocol				
1	2	3.0	2.5	4.3
2	2	3.0	5	5.4
3	2	3.0	7.5	6.4
4	2	3.0	10	7.4
5	2	3.0	12.5	8.5
6	2	3.0	15	9.5
7	2	3.0	17.5	10.5
Naughton Protocol				
1	2	1	0	1.8
2	2	2	0	2.5
3	2	2	3.5	3.5
4	2	2	7.0	4.5
5	2	2	10.5	5.4
6	2	2	14.0	6.4
7	2	2	17.5	7.4
8	2	2	21.0	8.3

		Standard Bicycle Protocol			
Stage	**Minutes**	**Revolutions per minute**	**Resistance (kg·m–min—1)**	**Resistance (Watts)**	**METS**
1	2 or 3	50	150	25	3.1
2	2 or 3	50	300	50	4.2
3	2 or 3	50	450	75	5.3
4	2 or 3	50	600	100	6.4
5	2 or 3	50	750	125	7.5
6	2 or 3	50	900	150	8.6

begins at a very low workload and increases every 2 to 3 minutes depending on the exercise protocol. The workload is determined by a standardized and progressive increase in the speed and/or elevation of the treadmill or (if bike if used) the resistance. Heart rate is continuously monitored and recorded during the entire test. Blood pressure is recorded every 2 to 3 minutes. The workload in METs is estimated for each exercise stage based on the speed and elevation of the treadmill. When the individual reaches volitional fatigue, the test is terminated. The MET level achieved at this level represents the maximal aerobic capacity of the individual. Because each MET is equal to 3.5 ml of O_2/kg/min, the $\dot{V}O_2$max can be estimated by multiplying the MET level achieved by 3.5.

Certainly, this is a more elaborate and expensive method compared to the methods described earlier. However, because it is used worldwide in hospitals and healthcare facilities for a number of cardiac and other clinical evaluations, several large databases contain much information. Several recent studies have used these databases as their standard when reporting fitness levels based on exercise capacity achieved during such exercise tests.[24,25]

It is important to mention that exercise capacity assessed by such exercise tests correlates well with physical activity status of the individual. However, the ability to perform aerobic work is also determined by a genetic component. Research currently estimates that the genetic effect on $\dot{V}O_2$max is about 25% to 40% and could be up to 70% for exercise capacity.[26-28] Physical activity questionnaires (when available) are a good adjunct to determine the association between MET level achieved and physical activity habits reported.

■ PRINCIPLES GOVERNING EXERCISE AND RELATED CHANGES

The positive effects that exercise or physical activity has on the human body will not occur unless exercise is implemented in such a way that stimulates (triggers) the body to respond. This response and consequent changes induced by exercise are specific to the type and amount of work. For example, leg work strengthens the legs but does nothing for the arms. Changes that occur in the heart with rowing, lifting weights, cycling, or jogging are different for each activity.

To understand the exercise-related adaptations, it is important to know the physiologic principles that govern the body, the types of exercise (work), exercise components, and the body's response when subjected to the different types of exercise.

Overload Principle

The legendary ancient Olympiad wrestler Milo ran the perimeter of the stadium every day carrying a newly born calf on his shoulder. As the calf grew, Milo had to work harder each day to complete the task. In doing so, Milo also became progressively stronger.

This story describes two important principles that apply to all physiologic changes in the body: the overload principle and the progressive resistance principle.

The **overload principle** states that any physiologic system (e.g., muscles, heart, brain, etc.) will improve (become more efficient) only if it is challenged beyond its present maximal capabilities. In other words, if one is training by lifting 30 pounds and no more, the muscles will only make the necessary changes (grow stronger) to lift 30 pounds. Additional changes will occur if the muscles are exposed to training with more weight. Similarly, the long distance runner will increase the distance running if the workload (distance) is gradually increased and/or the time to complete the distance is decreased.

Appropriate overload can be achieved by manipulating all exercise components (intensity, duration, and frequency).

Progressive Resistance Principle

The **progressive resistance principle** is similar to the overload principle. However, it expands on the first principle by stating that the association between the workload and physiologic adaptations behave in a dose-response fashion. That is, a progressive increase in the workload will yield progressive adaptations beyond the present level.

Specificity Principle

The **specificity principle** states that the body will make specific changes to accommodate the specific demand placed upon it. That is, if one is interested in being able to run for a long time, he or she must train by running long distances. On the other hand, if one is interested in improving speed, then he or she must train by running short distances at maximum speeds. An individual training for a marathon (running long distances) will never make a successful sprinter, nor will someone training for speed make a successful marathoner. To improve in a specific task (run, jump, shoot baskets), the best way to train is to perform the task itself over and over again.

It is important to recognize that the specificity principle is more complex than is implied by the aforementioned example. It affects all systems involved in a particular physical activ-ity in such a way that all systems become efficient in their own domain, so that ultimately they may contribute to enhance the task at hand. The precise changes that the body makes for the specific activity can be further appreciated by the following example. If we were to take an aerobic activity such as biking and running and measure the aerobic capacity of a runner on the bike and a biker on the treadmill, they will both be approximately 15% to 20% below their "true" fitness level.[29,30] The reason for this is that although biking and running are both aerobic activities and both use legs, the specific muscles, muscle fibers, and involvement of these muscles are different. These muscles will change precisely to meet the specific demand (biking or running) imposed upon them. Naturally, the more the two activities overlap, the higher is the transfer of benefits from one activity to the other.

The specificity principle has been simply and eloquently summarized by McArdle, Katch, and Katch as follows: ". . . specific exercise elicits specific adaptations creating specific training effects."[31]

Principle of Reversibility

According to the **principle of reversibility**, the level of fitness acquired through training will be lost if training is discontinued. It is estimated that once training ceases, a considerable amount of fitness gains are lost. In an early, very small observational study on wasting, aerobic capacity declined by 25% in five young men confined to bed rest for 20 consecutive days,[32] suggesting that the decline in aerobic capacity is approximately 1% per day of inactivity. Then, the same men followed a regimented exercise training program for 6 months, at which point almost all of the losses in aerobic capacity were regained.

In an effort to determine the degree of decline in cardiovascular fitness that is attributable to aging and de-conditioning, the same five individuals were reassessed 30 years later. The age-related decline in aerobic power among this group of now middle-aged men was 14%, substantially less than the 25% decline observed in the initial study. McGuire et al. concluded that physical inactivity accounts for as much as much as 40% of the age-related decline in aerobic capacity.[33] Their results suggest the following:

- Aging and de-conditioning are both detrimental to cardiorespiratory fitness. However, a few weeks of bed rest are more detrimental than 30 years of aging.
- Maintaining a physically active lifestyle can slow down the aging effects on the cardiorespiratory fitness.
- The exercise-related cardiorespiratory changes are similar in young and older individuals.

Others also have documented the complete loss of all cardiovascular fitness adaptations within 4 months of inactivity.[34]

Obviously, this has important implications for astronauts, hospitalized patients, stroke survivors, and for those who are injured and unable to walk. In such cases, some form of physical activity should be encouraged as soon as possible.

■ ACQUISITION OF CARDIORESPIRATORY AND MUSCULAR FITNESS

As mentioned in the introduction, the acquisition of fitness and health has been and continues to be a misunderstood concept for many. This confusion stems from a lack of understanding of the basic principles that govern physical activity and exercise, and perpetuated by self-proclaimed "fitness experts." To clarify the issue and to set the record straight, the American College of Sports Medicine (ACSM), Centers for Disease Control and Prevention (CDC), and the American Heart Association (AHA) over the years have constructed and published recommendations to help adults to achieve fitness and improve and maintain health in a safe and efficient way. The most recent recommendations were published in August 2007 by the AHA and the ACSM.[35–37] A summary of these recommendations is presented in **Tables 2.8** and **2.9**.

These recent guidelines are intended to upgrade and clarify some of the previous recommendations published in 1995 on the type, intensity, and amount of exercise needed by adults aged 18 to 65 years, and include separate guidelines for those 65 years of age and older. The central message and purpose of the recommendations is to provide a "clear, concise public health message that would encourage increased participation in physical activity by a largely sedentary U.S. population."[35–37] The recommendation is that both young and older adults should maintain an active lifestyle to promote and maintain good health.

Physical activity recommendations for adults aged 65 and older are similar to those for younger adults but have a few important differences. First, the individual's age is taken into account and the intensity of the activity is adjusted accordingly. Second, activities that promote muscle strength and flexibility, and especially balance exercises, are recommended to reduce the risk of falling.

In addition, the new recommendations aim to dispel the lingering assumptions by some on the issue of the exercise or physical activity intensity necessary to improve health. Some believe only vigorous or high-intensity physical

Table 2.8 Physical Activity Recommendations for Healthy Adults Aged 18 to 65 Years

Perform moderate-intensity aerobic (endurance) physical activity for a minimum of 30 min on 5 days each week or vigorous-intensity aerobic activity for a minimum of 20 min on 3 days each week.

Combinations of moderate and vigorous-intensity activity can be performed to meet this recommendation. For example, a person can meet the recommendation by walking briskly for 30 min twice during the week and then jogging for 20 min on two other days.

These moderate or vigorous intensity activities should be performed in addition to the light intensity activities frequently performed during daily life (e.g., self care, washing dishes, using light tools at a desk) or activities of very short duration (e.g., taking out trash, walking to the parking lot at store or office).

Moderate-intensity aerobic activity, which is generally equivalent to a brisk walk and noticeably accelerates the heart rate, can be accumulated toward the 30-min minimum by performing bouts each lasting 10 or more minutes.

Vigorous-intensity activity is exemplified by jogging, and causes rapid breathing and a substantial increase in heart rate.

In addition, at least twice each week, adults will benefit by performing activities using the major muscles of the body that maintain or increase muscular strength and endurance.

Because of the dose-response relation between physical activity and health, persons who wish to further improve their personal fitness, reduce their risk for chronic diseases and disabilities, or prevent unhealthy weight gain will likely benefit by exceeding the minimum recommended amount of physical activity.

Sources: Reprinted with permission. 1. Haskell WL, Lee IM, Pate RR, et al. Physical activity and public health: updated recommendation for adults from the American College of Sports Medicine and the American Heart Association. *Circulation* 2007;116(9):1081–1093. 2. Williams MA, Haskell WL, Ades PA, et al. Resistance exercise in individuals with and without cardiovascular disease: 2007 update: a scientific statement from the American Heart Association Council on Clinical Cardiology and Council on Nutrition, Physical Activity, and Metabolism. *Circulation* 2007;116(5):572–584.

activity will improve health, while others believe that light-intensity activity (house chores) is adequate. The recommendations state emphatically that only moderate-intensity aerobic activity and high-intensity activities promote health. These moderate or vigorous intensity activities should be in addition to the light intensity activities frequently performed frequently performed during daily life (e.g., self care, washing dishes, using light tools at a desk) or activities of very short duration (e.g., taking out trash, walking to the parking lot at a store or office). Light activities alone (although recommended) do not promote health. It is also important to emphasize that aerobic endurance training for fewer than 2 days per week and for less than 10 minutes each is not sufficient for maintaining or developing fitness.

Table 2.9 Physical Activity Recommendations for Healthy Adults Aged 65 Years and Older

Perform moderate-intensity aerobic (endurance) physical activity for a minimum of 30 min on 5 days each week or vigorous-intensity aerobic activity for a minimum of 20 min on 3 days each week. Moderate-intensity aerobic activity involves a moderate level of effort relative to an individual's aerobic fitness. On a 10-point scale, where sitting is 0 and all-out effort is 10, moderate-intensity activity is a 5 or 6 and produces noticeable increases in heart rate and breathing. On the same scale, vigorous-intensity activity is a 7 or 8 and produces large increases in heart rate and breathing. For example, given the heterogeneity of fitness levels in older adults, for some older adults a moderate-intensity walk is a slow walk, and for others it is a brisk walk.

Combinations of moderate and vigorous-intensity activity can be performed to meet this recommendation. These moderate or vigorous intensity activities are in addition to the light intensity activities frequently performed during daily life (e.g., self care, washing dishes) or moderate-intensity activities lasting 10 min or less (e.g., taking out trash, walking to the parking lot at store or office).

In addition, at least twice each week older adults should perform muscle strengthening activities using the major muscles of the body that maintain or increase muscular strength and endurance. It is recommended that 8–10 exercises be performed on at least two nonconsecutive days per week using the major muscle groups. To maximize strength development, a resistance (weight) should be used that allows 10–15 repetitions for each exercise. The level of effort for muscle-strengthening activities should be moderate to high.

Because of the dose-response relationship between physical activity and health, older persons who wish to further improve their personal fitness, reduce their risk for chronic diseases and disabilities, or prevent unhealthy weight gain will likely benefit by exceeding the minimum recommended amount of physical activity.

To maintain the flexibility necessary for regular physical activity and daily life, older adults should perform activities that maintain or increase flexibility on at least 2 days each week for at least 10 min each day.

To reduce risk of injury from falls, community-dwelling older adults with substantial risk of falls should perform exercises that maintain or improve balance.

Older adults with one or more medical conditions for which physical activity is therapeutic should perform physical activity in a manner that effectively and safely treats the condition(s).

Older adults should have a plan for obtaining sufficient physical activity that addresses each recommended type of activity.

Those with chronic conditions for which activity is therapeutic should have a single plan that integrates prevention and treatment. For older adults who are not active at recommended levels, plans should include a gradual (or stepwise) approach to increase physical activity over time. Many months of activity at less than recommended levels is appropriate for some older adults (e.g., those with low fitness) as they increase activity in a stepwise manner. Older adults should also be encouraged to self-monitor their physical activity on a regular basis and to reevaluate plans as their abilities improve or as their health status changes.

Sources: Reprinted with permission. 1. Nelson ME, Rejeski WJ, Blair SN, et al. Physical activity and public health in older adults: recommendation from the American College of Sports Medicine and the American Heart Association. *Med Sci Sports Exer* 2007;39(8):1435–1445. 2. Williams MA, Haskell WL, Ades PA, et al. Resistance exercise in individuals with and without cardiovascular disease: 2007 update: a scientific statement from the American Heart Association Council on Clinical Cardiology and Council on Nutrition, Physical Activity, and Metabolism. *Circulation* 2007;116(5):572–584.

Muscular Strength and Endurance, Body Composition, and Flexibility

■ Resistance Training or Weight Training

Resistance training was avoided for several decades partly because of the popularity of aerobic training and partly due to a few reports of individuals experiencing extremely high blood pressure levels when they were lifting heavy weights. Recently, resistance training has been recognized as an integral part of an adult fitness program when it is of a sufficient intensity to enhance strength, muscular endurance, and maintain fat-free mass.[37] To achieve this end, like other types of physical exercise, resistance training should be individualized, progressive in nature, and stimulate all of the major muscle groups. It is recommended that one should perform one set of eight to ten exercises that conditions the major muscle groups. These include the following:

Upper Body
    Chest
    Upper back
    Lower back
    Abdomen
    Shoulders
    Upper arm (biceps)
    Upper arm (triceps)
Lower Body
    Quadriceps (front of upper leg)
    Femoris (back of the leg)
    Gastrocnemius (lower leg)

One set of each exercise 2 to 3 days per week is recommended. Multiple-set regimens may provide greater benefits if time allows. Most persons should complete 8 to 12 repetitions of each exercise; however, for older and more frail persons (ages ~60 or more), 10 to 15 repetitions may be more appropriate. Twenty-five or more repetitions are usually not recommended.

■ Flexibility Training

Flexibility exercises should be part of the overall fitness program. The aim should be to develop and maintain range of motion. Stretching exercises should concentrate in the major muscle groups and be performed a minimum of two to three times per week. Stretching should include appropriate static and/or dynamic techniques.

■ SUMMARY

- Physical fitness is a set of physical attributes that people have or achieve that relates to the ability to perform physical activity. This endowed ability can be enhanced by the proper exercise training.
- Physical activities or exercise can be defined as aerobic or anaerobic. These definitions are based on the way the energy requirements for the specific activity are met.
- Aerobic exercises or activities consist of repetitive, low resistance movements (walking or cycling) that last over a relatively long period of time (generally 5 minutes or more).
- The energy requirements for aerobic activities are derived predominantly with the use of oxygen (aerobic metabolism).
- Anaerobic exercises or activities on the other hand, are characterized by bursts of intense activity lasting only a short time. Their energy requirements are derived predominantly without oxygen (anaerobic metabolism).
- Exercise components include intensity, frequency, and duration. Of the exercise

- components, intensity is the most difficult to determine.
- Exercise intensity can be described and quantified as a percentage of the maximum work a system or an individual is capable of performing.
- The most practical and widely used methods to assess aerobic exercise intensity are those based on a percentage of the individual's maximum heart rate.
- Exercise volume is the by-product of the exercise components. Assessing exercise volume (work) requires expensive equipment and trained personnel, making it impractical for large population studies.
- Thus, several methods have been advanced to estimate exercise volume. These methods are based on the premise that oxygen and energy output (kcal) are required for work and on the linear relationship between heart rate and oxygen consumption.
- Metabolic equivalent (MET) is a measure of energy output. One MET is equivalent to 3.5 ml of oxygen uptake per kilogram of body weight at rest or approximately 1 kilocalorie per kilogram of body weight per hour. An increase beyond one MET represents work.
- Standardized exercise treadmill and bike tests have been developed to assess the peak exercise capacity of an individual or individuals. Such methods are used extensively in hospitals, universities, and health facilities worldwide.
- Over the years, much data have been accumulated that have allowed researchers to estimate the MET level of an impressive number of activities. Based on these databases, the volume of work can be estimated for large populations.
- Other methods to estimate exercise volume are based on heart rate that is measured by portable heart rate monitors,

pedometers that measure the number of steps (horizontal distance) traveled, and accelerometers that detect movement.
- Exercise-related adaptations are governed by certain physiologic principles. The understanding of exercise-related changes requires a thorough knowledge of these principles.
- The ACSM and AHA recommend that all adults should maintain an active lifestyle to promote and maintain good health. This is defined as a minimum of 30 minutes on at least 5 days of each week or vigorous-intensity aerobic activity for a minimum of 20 minutes on 3 days of each week.
- Moderate-intensity aerobic activity, which is generally equivalent to a brisk walk and noticeably accelerates the heart rate, can be accumulated toward the 30-minute minimum by engaging in activity several times over the day, each lasting 10 or more minutes.
- Combinations of short bouts of moderate and vigorous-intensity activity (10 minutes per bout) can be performed to meet this daily recommendation.
- Aerobic endurance training **fewer** than 2 days per week, for less than 10 minutes, is not sufficient for maintaining or developing fitness.
- Older adults should perform muscle strengthening activities using the major muscles of the body. It is recommended that 8 to 10 exercises be performed on at least two nonconsecutive days per week using the major muscle groups. The recommended resistance (weight) to maximize strength development should allow for 10 to 15 repetitions for each exercise.
- Older persons who wish to improve their personal fitness further, reduce their risk for chronic diseases and disabilities, or prevent unhealthy weight gain will likely

benefit by exceeding the minimum recommended amount of physical activity.

■ REFERENCES

1. Public Health Service. Physical activity and health: a report by the Surgeon General. *MMWR Morbid Mortal Wkly Rep* 1996;45(Jul 12):591–592.
2. Caspersen CJ, Powell KE, Christenson GM. Physical activity, exercise, and physical fitness: definitions and distinctions for health-related research. *Public Health Rep* 1985; 100:126–131.
3. American College of Sports Medicine. *ACSM's Guidelines for Exercise Testing and Prescription*, 7th ed. New York: Lippincott Williams & Wilkins; 2006.
4. President's Council on Physical Fitness and Sports, Department of Health and Human Services. Definitions of health, fitness and physical activity. *PCPFS Research Digest*, 2000. Available at www.fitness.gov/digest_mar2000 .htm. Accessed February 9, 2009.
5. Wilmore JH, Parr RB, Ward P, et al. Energy cost of circuit weight training. *Med Sci Sports* 1978;10(2):75–78.
6. Beckham SG, Earnest CP. Metabolic cost of free weight circuit weight training. *J Sports Med Phys Fitness* 2000;40(2):118–125.
7. Karvonen M, Kentala E, Mustala O. The effects of training on heart rate: a longitudinal study. *Ann Med Exp Biol Fenn* 1957;35:307–315.
8. Swain DP, Franklin BA. $\dot{V}O_2$ reserve and the minimal intensity for improving cardiorespiratory fitness. *Med Sci Sports Exerc* 2002; 34(1):152–157.
9. DeBusk RF, Stenestrand U, Sheehan M, Haskell WL. Training effects of long versus short bouts of exercise in healthy subjects. *Am J Cardiol* 1990;65(15):1010–1013.
10. Murphy MH, Hardman AE. Training effects of short and long bouts of brisk walking in sedentary women. *Med Sci Sports Exerc* 1998;30(1):152–157.
11. Kokkinos PF, Narayan P, Colleran AJ, et al. Effects of moderate intensity exercise on serum lipids in African-American men with severe systemic hypertension. *Am J Cardiol* 1998;81(6):732–735.
12. Haskell WL, Superko R. Influence of exercise on plasma lipids and lipoproteins. In TR Horton, ed. *Exercise, Nutrition and Energy Metabolism*. New York: Macmillan; 1988: 213–227.
13. Dehn M, Mullins C. Physiologic effects and importance of exercise in patients with coronary heart disease. *J Cardiovasc Med* 1977; 2:365–387.
14. Haskell, W. Dose-response issues from a biological perspective. In C Bouchard, RJ Shephard, T Stephens, eds. *Physical Activity, Fitness and Health: International Proceedings and Consensus Statement*. Champaign, IL: Human Kinetics; 1994:1030–1039.
15. Ainsworth BE, Haskell WL, Leon AS, et al. Compendium of physical activities: classification of energy costs of human physical activities. *Med Sci Sports Exerc* 1993; 25(1):71–80.
16. Pereira MA, FitzerGerald SJ, Gregg EW, et al. A collection of physical activity questionnaires for health-related research. *Med Sci Sports Exerc* 1997;29(6 Suppl):S1–S205.
17. Welk GJ. Use of accelerometry-based activity monitors to assess physical activity. In GJ Welk, ed. *Physical Activity Assessments for Health-Related Research*. Champaign, IL: Human Kinetics; 2002:125–141.
18. Hatano J. Use of the pedometer for promoting daily walking exercise. *Int Counc Health Phys Activity Educ Recreation* 1993; 29:4–8.
19. Hatano J. Prevalence and use of pedometer. *Res J Walking*, 1997;1:45–54.
20. Manson JE, Greenland P, LaCroix AZ, et al. Walking compared with vigorous exercise for the prevention of cardiovascular events in women. *N Engl J Med* 2002;347(10): 716–725.
21. Manson JE, Hu FB, Rich-Edwards JW, et al. A prospective study of walking as compared with vigorous exercise in the prevention of coronary heart disease in women. *N Engl J Med* 1999;341(9):650–658.

22. Bravata DM, Smith-Spangler C, Sundaram V, et al. Using pedometers to increase physical activity and improve health: a systematic review. *JAMA* 2007;298(19):2296–2304.

23. Tudor-Locke C, Bassett DR Jr. How many steps/day are enough? Preliminary pedometer indices for public health. *Sports Med* 2004; 34(1):1–8.

24. Kokkinos P, Myers J, Kokkinos JP, et al. Exercise capacity and mortality in black and white men. *Circulation* 2008;117(5):614–622

25. Myers J, Prakash M, Froelicher V, et al. Exercise capacity and mortality among men referred for exercise testing. *N Engl J Med* 2002;346(11):793–801.

26. Bouchard C, Daw EW, Rice T, et al. Familial resemblance for V̇O₂max in the sedentary state: the HERITAGE family study. *Med Sci Sports Exerc* 1998;30(2):252–258.

27. Bouchard C, Dionne ET, Simoneau JA, Boulay MR. Genetics of aerobic and anaerobic performances. *Exerc Sport Sci Rev* 1992; 20:27–58.

28. Pérusse L, Tremblay A, Lablanc C, Bouchard C. Genetic and environmental influences on level of habitual physical activity and exercise participation. *Am J Epidemiol* 1989;129(5): 1012–1022.

29. Pechar GS, McArdle WD, Katch FI, et al. Specificity of cardiorespiratory adaptation to bicycle and treadmill training. *J Appl Physiol* 1974;36(6):753–756.

30. Gergley TJ, McArdle WD, DeJesus P, et al. Specificity of arm training on aerobic power during swimming and running. *Med Sci Sports Exerc* 1984;16(4):349–354.

31. McArdle WD, Katch FI, Katch VL. *Exercise Physiology*, 5th ed. Baltimore: Lippincott Williams & Wilkins; 2001.

32. Saltin B, Blomqvist G, Mitchell JH, et al. Response to exercise after bed rest and after training. *Circulation* 1968;38(5 Suppl): VII1–78.

33. McGuire DK, Levine BD, Williamson JW, et al. A 30-year follow-up of the Dallas Bedrest and Training Study: II. Effect of age on cardiovascular adaptation to exercise training. *Circulation* 2001;104(12):1358–1366.

34. Pickering GP, Fellmann N, Morio B, et al. Effects of endurance training on the cardiovascular system and water compartments in elderly subjects. *J Appl Physiol* 1997;83(4): 1300–1306.

35. Haskell WL, Lee IM, Pate RR, et al. Physical activity and public health: updated recommendation for adults from the American College of Sports Medicine and the American Heart Association. *Circulation* 2007;116(9): 1081–1093.

36. Nelson ME, Rejeski WJ, Blair SN, et al. Physical activity and public health in older adults: recommendation from the American College of Sports Medicine and the American Heart Association. *Med Sci Sports Exerc* 2007;39(8): 1435–1445.

37. Williams MA, Haskell WL, Ades PA, et al. Resistance exercise in individuals with and without cardiovascular disease: 2007 update: a scientific statement from the American Heart Association Council on Clinical Cardiology and Council on Nutrition, Physical Activity, and Metabolism. *Circulation* 2007; 116(5):572–584.

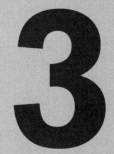

Dietary Concepts: The Essentials

---

*If we could give every individual the
right amount of nourishment and
exercise, not too little and not too much,
we would have found the safest way to
health.*

Hippocrates (460–370 BC)

I n recent years, we have come to realize the crucial role that improper diet plays in the development of chronic disease such as heart disease, cancer, osteoporosis, high blood pressure, diabetes, and obesity. More importantly, we now recognize that proper diets can prevent and even treat such diseases as well as benefit the individual by improving physical and mental performance, quality of life, and longevity. To achieve and maintain good health and to realize our potential in physical and mental performance, it is thus important that

we practice good nutritional habits. To do so, we need to understand basic nutritional principles.

Understanding basic nutritional principles is more imperative now than ever. The explosion of the Internet and Web sites brought by technology has made information and—unfortunately—misinformation on nutrition and diet readily available for almost everyone. Although the availability of information is generally beneficial, it is important to recognize that the benefits can only be realized if we can distinguish fact from fiction. This task becomes increasingly more difficult due to the following factors:

1. Most information is too scientific for the general public and requires simplification to be perceived accurately.
2. There is too much available information to the point that it has become overwhelming for most people.
3. Scientific information is often commercialized to promote profits.
4. Not all information is scientifically sound. A great deal of information that the public receives is based on hearsay and not backed by scientific research. Other information may be derived from poorly designed and poorly controlled pseudo-scientific studies.
5. Some well-intended information is just wrong due to a number of factors including wrong study design, mistakes made from bad science, or misinterpretation of findings.

An example of a possible misinterpretation of findings is the following. Several early epidemiologic studies reported that men and to a lesser extent women with blood cholesterol levels below 160 mg/dl exhibited an increase in mortality from cancer, stroke, respiratory and digestive disease, and suicide.[1–6] The question is: Does low cholesterol cause cancer or is it the cancer that causes blood cholesterol levels to decrease? This question cannot be answered by epidemiologic studies because this premise can be interpreted in three possible ways. First, low blood cholesterol causes cancer and the aforementioned diseases. Second, the diseases cause low blood cholesterol. A third possibility is that a number of unknown factors are related to both low cholesterol and mortality. As it turned out, later studies determined that the presence of disease caused blood cholesterol values to decrease and that the mortality seen in that cohort was due to the underlying disease and not to low blood cholesterol levels at all.[7,8]

The point is that, because of their design, epidemiologic studies can only show relationships and generate hypotheses that later can be evaluated by randomized clinical trials. Causal (cause and effect) relationships cannot be addressed directly by epidemiologic studies.

Another example of the misinterpretation of findings is the use of dietary supplements to promote health. The implication of oxidative stress found in most chronic diseases gave rise to the hypothesis that antioxidant supplements may decrease the potential damage of free radicals released during aerobic metabolism, known as reactive oxygen species. Consequently, hope, wishful thinking, and profits gave rise to the promotion of several antioxidant products as a way to combat premature cardiovascular disease and aging before appropriate studies were conducted and definitive answers were available. Unfortunately, thus far the research has not yielded convincing evidence that antioxidant vitamin supplements protect against premature cardiovascular disease.[9] Most disturbing is that some studies have shown that vitamin E and beta-carotene supplements increased the inci-

dence of stroke and death from cardiovascular disease and overall mortality in some populations.[10–23]

■ FOOD

Foods provide us with the materials necessary for growth and repair of body tissues and with components that make all body functions possible. In addition, foods provide us with energy required to sustain life and function.

All the foods are comprised of six basic elements:

1. Carbohydrates
2. Fats
3. Proteins
4. Vitamins
5. Minerals
6. Water

■ CARBOHYDRATES

Carbohydrates are generally starchy foods such as breads, pasta, rice, potatoes, corn, and sugars. All originate from plant sources except lactose, which is found in milk. They are formed when atoms of carbon, hydrogen, and oxygen combine in a certain way; the basic molecular formula is $C_nH_{2n}O_n$ or $(CH_2O)_n$. For example, blood sugar (glucose) contains 6 carbon, 12 hydrogen, and 6 oxygen atoms ($C_6H_{12}O_6$) (**Figure 3.1**).

Types and Functions

There are basically two kinds of carbohydrates: (1) monosaccharides or simple carbohydrates and (2) polysaccharides or complex carbohydrates. Their category is determined on the number of carbons present in each

Figure 3.1 Structure of the glucose molecule presented in the stick form (left) and ring form (right). The ring form is the structure of the molecule found in living cells.

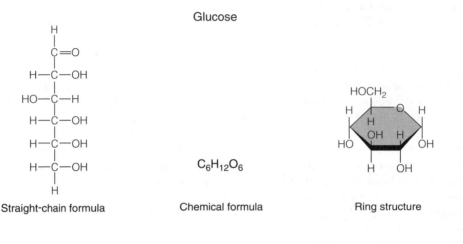

Glucose

$C_6H_{12}O_6$

Straight-chain formula   Chemical formula   Ring structure

carbohydrate molecule. Monosaccharides usually contain between three to seven carbon atoms.

Monosaccharides can be identified by their Greek prefix and suffix. The suffix is *ose*, the Greek word for sugars and the prefix indicates the number of carbons. For example triose is a sugar with three carbons (*tri*, Greek for three), pentose, a sugar with five carbons, and hexose, a sugar with six carbons. The most common simple carbohydrates are glucose (blood sugar), fructose (sugar found in fruits and honey), and galactose (sugar found in milk).

Polysaccharides are starches and fibers formed when a large number of monosaccharides are joined in a chain structure (**Figure 3.2**).

They usually contain more than 10 monosaccharide units. The most common complex carbohydrates in our diet are starches contained in corn, bread, cereal, pasta, beans, potatoes, seeds, and various grains.

The main function of carbohydrates is to provide the fuel for the energy requirements of the body. Carbohydrates also can combine with proteins to form glycoproteins, and with lipids to form glycolipids. Glycoproteins and glycolipids serve a number of functions in the cell membrane, one of which is to act as receptors for binding hormones such as insulin.[24]

Although the body can make fuel from other sources (fats and to a lesser extent proteins), the fuel carbohydrates provide is special for

Figure 3.2 Molecular structure of starch.

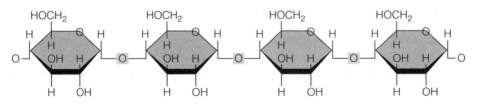

two important reasons: immediacy of fuel and brain fuel.

■ Required Fuel for Intense Work

Muscles have the capacity to use fat almost exclusively to meet their metabolic needs. However, the use of pure fat for fuel has unhealthy consequences. Therefore, the preferred fuel is a mixture of fat and glucose. The percent contribution of each to the energy requirements for muscular work depends largely on the intensity of the work. The glucose contribution ranges from about 50% for low-intensity activities to 100% for activities requiring maximal or near maximal effort. Glucose thus becomes essential especially during maximal or near maximal exercise or work intensities.

■ Preferred Fuel for the Brain

Under normal conditions, the brain uses blood glucose almost exclusively for its energy needs. Although the brain cells have the capacity to adapt and use fats for energy if necessary (during starvation or low carbohydrate intake), this is not a preferred condition and can only be a temporary solution. Mental and physical performance decreases when the availability of glucose is inadequate and the brain cells have to rely on excessive amounts of fats for their energy requirements.

There is also another health issue that results from excessive use of fat to meet the energy needs of the body in the absence of carbohydrates. By-products of carbohydrate metabolism are involved in the complete metabolism of fats. Inadequate carbohydrate metabolism leads to a deficiency of such products. Such conditions can occur either through inadequate glucose transport into the cell as is the case in uncontrolled diabetes mellitus, insufficient dietary intake of carbohydrates,

and/or severe exercise. Under such conditions, incomplete fat metabolism occurs. This leads to the formation and accumulation of a large amount of soluble chemicals called *ketone bodies* and their release in the bloodstream. Because these ketone bodies are acidic, their release into the bloodstream increases the acidity of body fluids, a condition that is harmful and possibly fatal if not reversed in time.[25]

Protein Sparing

As previously mentioned, the energy demands of the body are best met by a mixture of fats and carbohydrates (glucose). Energy deriving from glucose thus is so essential for a normal function that the body will resort to the synthesizing its own glucose when the amount in the diet is inadequate to maintain normal blood glucose levels. Under such conditions, glucose in synthesized from proteins (amino acids). However, using proteins to make glucose is not preferred because it normally is used for growth, tissue repair and maintenance, and to a lesser degree as a source of fuel. Protein breakdown means less protein available for those other important functions. Under some conditions, this protein conversion to glucose could reduce muscle protein and negatively affect strength.

> Protein breakdown for energy use increases when liver glycogen stores are depleted and carbohydrate availability for energy is inadequate.

Digestion and Absorption

Partial digestion of carbohydrates (approximately 3% to 5% of all carbohydrates) occurs in the mouth by the action of enzyme salivary amylase produced by the salivary glands. Digestion continues in the stomach where 30%

to 40% of carbohydrates are digested within about one hour.

As the stomach contents enter the small intestine, complete digestion of all carbohydrates takes place within 15 to 30 minutes by the powerful enzyme *pancreatic amylase*. As a result, the final products of all dietary carbohydrates are monosaccharides (glucose, fructose, or galactose), with glucose representing about 80% of the three. These simple carbohydrates are absorbed from the gastrointestinal track and enter the bloodstream. When these carbohydrates enter the liver, appropriate enzymes are available to convert fructose and galactose into **glucose**. The final product of almost all

dietary carbohydrates that enter the circulation after they pass through the liver is glucose (**Figure 3.3**).

Regulation of the Blood Glucose Concentration

All cells of the body need glucose for energy. In fact, the requirement of glucose for the body is about 200 g/day. This requirement is largely determined by the metabolic demands of the brain.[26,27] More than any other organ, the brain is most dependent upon glucose for its energy needs. If blood glucose falls below 40 mg/dl, the individual becomes severely confused.

Figure 3.3   Digestion and absorption of carbohydrates. Partial digestion of starches occurs in the mouth and continues in the stomach. Most of the digestion and absorption takes place in the small intestine. Simple sugars are then released into the portal circulation and enter the liver.

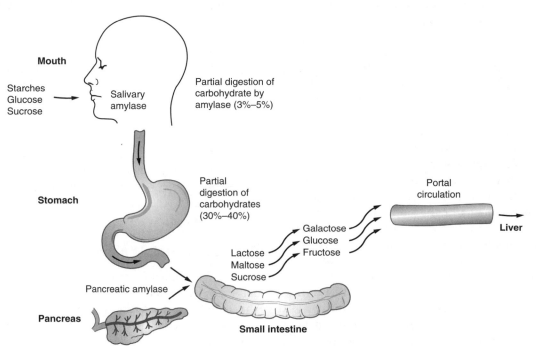

Seizures, coma, and even death may ensue.[26,27] Normal blood glucose levels therefore must be maintained tightly to guarantee a constant glucose supply to the brain.[25]

In the healthy individuals, the fasting concentration of blood glucose is between 70 and 90 mg of glucose per 100 ml of blood. Blood glucose levels are regulated tightly despite the blood glucose fluctuation following the ingestion of food or the absence of it. They serve to trigger the uptake or release of glucose from the liver. Control of blood glucose concentrations is accomplished by the delicate balance of two hormones, **insulin** and **glucagon**. This process is explained in the following sections.

■ Insulin and Glucose Uptake and Storage

About an hour following a carbohydrate-rich meal, blood glucose levels rise to about 150 mg/dl. It is important to emphasize that blood glucose is of no use to the body unless it enters into the cells. However, glucose cannot diffuse through the cell membrane. For it to enter the cell, it must be transported. Glucose does so through a mechanism referred to as **facilitated diffusion** or **carrier-mediated diffusion**. This simply means that glucose has to be bound into a protein carrier to be transported across the cell membrane. Such carriers are called **glucose transporters** and are abbreviated as GLUT. Muscle cells contain several forms of these proteins, but GLUT-4 is the most abundant. It is located within the cell and translocates to the cell membrane when necessary.

The rate of glucose transport into the cell is greatly influenced by the hormone insulin. It is released by specific cells in the pancreas (**beta-cells**) in response to the rise in blood glucose concentrations following a meal. Insulin is the key hormone that facilitates the entry of glucose into the cells. When large amounts of

insulin are present, the rate of glucose transport into the cell increases 15 to 20 times the rate of transport at normal insulin levels.

Insulin accomplishes this by binding to the cell membrane, making it more permeable to glucose by stimulating the translocation of the GLUT-4 transporters to the cell membrane (**Figure 3.4**). Insulin can be views as the "key" that "unlocks the door" to the cell for glucose to enter. In fact, with the exception of the brain and liver cells, the rate of glucose diffusion into cells without insulin is far from adequate to meet the glucose required for energy. An example of this deficiency is found in those with diabetes, as their insulin secretion by the pancreatic cells is inadequate or absent. Consequently, glucose transport into the cell is significantly reduced.

An increase in blood glucose concentrations of approximately two to three times the fasting level results in a dramatic increase in insulin secretion from the beta cells of the pancreas. Insulin concentrations in the blood then

Figure 3.4   Insulin-induced stimulation of glucose uptake by the cell.

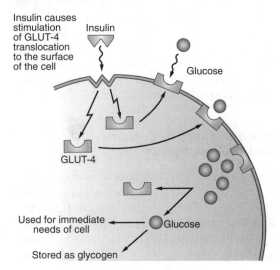

Insulin causes stimulation of GLUT-4 translocation to the surface of the cell

Insulin

Glucose

GLUT-4

Used for immediate needs of cell

Glucose

Stored as glycogen

increase to about 10 times the resting levels within 3 to 5 minutes. This level is maintained for about 10 minutes and then insulin levels decrease for the next 10 to 15 minutes to about half the level of the initial surge. A second increase in insulin follows that is even greater than the initial phase, and this increase reaches a plateau in 2 to 3 hours. As a result, blood glucose is removed from the bloodstream and now follows three possible routes.

1. It enters the liver where it is stored for later use.
2. It enters the muscle and other cells to be used for the immediate energy demands of the cell or is stored for later use.
3. After the liver and muscle stores are replenished, the remaining glucose is converted to fat and stored as body fat in the adipose tissue.

The glucose in the muscle and liver cells is stored in the form of glycogen. A well-nourished individual of average weight (about 175–180 lb) stores about 400 grams of glycogen in the muscles and 100 grams in the liver for a total of about 500 grams of glycogen. Each gram of carbohydrate contains 4 kilocalories. It follows that the 500 grams of glycogen stored by the average person releases approximately 2,000 kilocalories. It is important to emphasize here that after all liver and muscle depots have been replenished, any glucose that remains is stored as fat in the adipose tissue.

■ Significance of Exercise and Glucose Uptake

Increased physical activity or exercise requires a great deal of energy and glucose transport into the muscle cells is increased also. Indeed, exercise is a natural stimulus for increased glucose uptake by the working muscle cells. The mechanism by which physical activity stimulates

greater glucose transport into the cell is via the **GLUT-4 transporter** (**Figure 3.5**). What mediates the translocation of GLUT-4 transporters to the surface of the cell is not yet known. Several factors have been proposed as initiators of the translocation of GLUT-4 transporters to the surface of the cell. They include: changes in the pH (acidity) of the cell, bradykinin, calcium concentration that increases during activity, and other metabolites resulting from muscular contractions.[28,29] Consequently, glucose transport into the cell increases several fold.

The effects of exercise on GLUT-4 and ultimately glucose uptake are similar to those of insulin. However, three important factors are emphasized :

1. Glucose uptake stimulated by exercise is independent from that of insulin. That is, exercise will stimulate the translocation of GLUT-4 and facilitate glucose uptake by the cells to the same degree whether insulin is available or not.

Figure 3.5   Exercise-induced stimulation of glucose uptake by the cell.

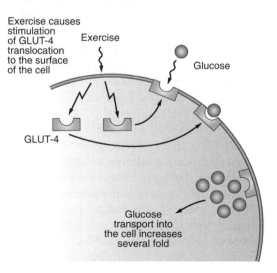

Exercise causes stimulation of GLUT-4 translocation to the surface of the cell

Exercise

Glucose

GLUT-4

Glucose transport into the cell increases several fold

2. Exercise will suppress insulin release from the pancreas but will not interfere with the insulin's ability to stimulate glucose uptake.
3. The effects of exercise and insulin on glucose uptake are additive.

The health implications associated with the exercise effects on glucose transport within the cell are certainly favorable to everyone, especially to those with diabetes. Insulin-induced glucose transport into the cell is compromised in diabetic patients. Exercise then becomes an important mechanism by which glucose uptake is enhanced. Indeed, when diabetic patients engage in exercise, the insulin requirements for the same amount of glucose transport into the cell are reduced. Accordingly, it is important to emphasize that the additive effects of exercise and insulin must be carefully considered for the diabetic patients who are taking insulin. When exercise takes place, diabetic patients who are on insulin must adjust their insulin intake (that is, take a lower dose) within the hour. Blood glucose can fall below normal levels (patients can develop hypoglycemia) during exercise if insulin intake is not properly adjusted. Because of this glucose reduction with exercise and the fact that the dose of insulin varies from patient to patient as well as the intensity and duration of exercise, the patient's physician should be consulted prior to any changes in insulin intake.

Glucagon and Glucose Release: Role of the Liver

Glucagon is a hormone secreted by the **alpha cells** of the pancreas. Its functions are the opposite of insulin. Most importantly, glucagon increases blood glucose concentrations by activating the breakdown of stored glycogen. Release of glucose from the liver meets the needs of the muscles, brain, and other organs.

This release of glucose from the liver is triggered by a fall of blood glucose below normal levels. This could be the result of food restriction or the increased uptake of glucose by the muscles during physical work. When alpha cells of the pancreas detect low blood glucose levels, they release glucagon into the bloodstream. When glucagon reaches the liver, it triggers the degradation of glycogen, so glycogen is now released in the form of glucose into the bloodstream and blood glucose levels rise. It is the balance of these two hormones—insulin and glucagon—that maintains blood glucose levels within the normal fasting limits of 70 to 90 mg/dl (**Figure 3.6**).

It is also important to note that the blood glucose concentration is the most potent factor controlling glucagon secretion. A blood glucose level below 70 mg/dl (hypoglycemic levels) can increase glucagon secretion by several folds. Conversely, glucagon secretion decreases when blood glucose levels increase to above 90 mg/dl.[24,26,27]

Glucagon and Exercise

Glucagon concentrations in the blood increase considerably during intense exercise. Although the mechanism or mechanisms for that increase are not well understood, the reason is obvious. Glucagon acts on the liver to slow down glycogen synthesis and foster glucose release by the liver. By doing so, it protects against hypoglycemic conditions that may occur during exercise. It is important to emphasize that glucagon acts only in the liver.

Glycogen Stores in Liver and Muscle

It should be emphasized that glucagon can only act on the liver and affect the glycogen stored in it. It cannot act on the muscles and therefore cannot trigger the release of glucose from the

Figure 3.6 **A.** Control of blood glucose by insulin and glucagon. **B.** Blood glucose concentrations.

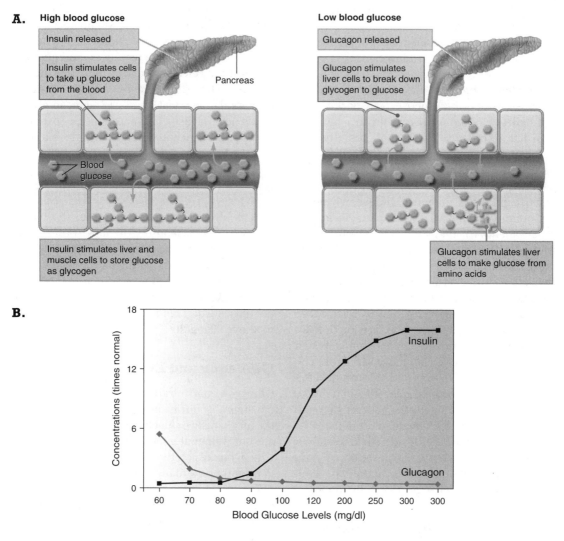

glycogen stored in the muscles. Once again, liver glycogen is used to meet the glucose needs of any cell in the body. That is, when the muscles or any other organ need glucose for energy, the liver releases part of the stored energy into the bloodstream as glucose. Blood then carries glucose to the muscles or other organs for conversion to energy.

However, the muscle behaves different from the liver. The stored glycogen in the muscle (about 400 grams) is only used to meet the glucose needs of that muscle tissue. Once glucose enters the muscle, it is chemically changed and cannot exit. In fact, at rest the muscles preserve glycogen stores for future strenuous physical work. Most metabolic needs of the muscle at rest are met by the metabolism of fat.

The reason for this is preservation. Although muscles can use fat for energy, they also need glucose to perform strenuous work. In fact, if glycogen stores decrease below a certain level, the individual is overcome by a sense of total fatigue and work becomes very difficult to continue. Because muscles must perform and their performance or lack of it can determine whether a human survives or perishes, energy requirements for the muscles are secured.

Glycemic Index

As mentioned previously, blood glucose levels increase after carbohydrate ingestion and digestion. However, the rate of carbohydrate digestion and therefore glucose entry into the bloodstream is not the same for all carbohydrates.

For years, the prevailing view was that carbohydrate digestion was determined by the chain length of the carbohydrate molecule. Complex carbohydrates thus would be digested relatively slowly whereas simple carbohydrates

would enter the bloodstream as glucose more quickly. However, this simplistic approach was challenged by a number of studies showing that the rate of carbohydrate metabolism depended on several factors including the carbohydrate category (simple vs. complex carbohydrate) and fiber, protein, and fat content of the food consumed.[27,30,31] In order to have an indicator as to the ability of an ingested carbohydrate to raise blood sugar levels, an index referred to as **glycemic index (GI)** was developed.[31] Specifically, the blood glucose levels were plotted over a period of 2 hours following the ingestion of a standard amount of pure glucose (50 grams) or white bread. The incremental area under the curve is now used as the baseline (or standard) to compare different foods. Levels of blood glucose plotted over 2 hours after eating any food containing 50 grams of carbohydrates (incremental area under the curve) are also plotted and compared against the standard. The GI of this food can now be calculated by dividing the incremental area under the curve by the area under the curve produced by the ingestion of pure glucose (standard) and divided by 100 (**Figure 3.7**).

Figure 3.7 Theoretical glycemic response after ingesting carbohydrates.

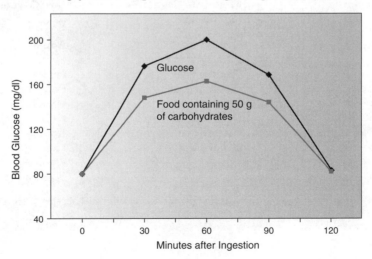

For example, a food with a GI of 70 indicates that the consumption of that food containing 50 grams of carbohydrates will raise blood sugar concentrations to the level that reaches 70% of that achieved during the ingestion of 50 grams of glucose. Foods have been classified based on how high a particular food raises blood glucose levels in a period of 2 hours: high (GI ≥ 70), moderate (GI: 56–69), or low (GI ≤ 55; **Table 3.1**).

What is the significance of GI? As you recall, a rise in blood sugar triggers the release of insulin and removal of sugar from the blood into the cells. The amount of insulin released into the bloodstream depends on the amount of sugar present in the blood. The higher the blood sugar levels, the greater the amount of insulin release and vice versa. Ideally, blood sugar levels should rise slowly rather than quickly and similarly, blood sugar should be removed slowly from the blood. Relatively normal blood sugar levels thus are maintained over an extended period of time. But when blood sugar rises quickly, it triggers an excessive amount of insulin release in the bloodstream, which results in a rapid removal of blood sugar from the blood. Consequently, this causes a drop in blood sugar below normal levels (hypoglycemia). Hypoglycemia in turn causes fatigue and triggers hunger, which may trigger the individual to eat more food to overcome hunger. This cycle may be repeated several times throughout the day.

The direct connection between dietary habits that promote excessive high and low swings in blood glucose and insulin and the development of diabetes has not yet been made. However, excessive consumption of calories leads to overweight, obesity, and diabetes. Foods that promote the slow release of glucose in the bloodstream thus should be preferred. Unfortunately, there is no simple rule that can be applied to distinguish carbohydrates with a high versus a low GI. For example, one may think that potatoes, a complex carbohydrate, are likely to have a low or at least moderate GI.

Table 3.1 Glycemic Index of Select Foods

High Glycemic (GI ≥ 70)	Moderate Glycemic (GI: 56–69)	Low Glycemic (GI ≤ 55)
Glucose	Corn	Apples
Carrots	Whole grain bread	Beans
Honey	White pasta	Lentils
White rice	Whole wheat pasta	Fructose
Potatoes	Oatmeal	Peanuts
White bread	Oranges	Peas
Instant rice	Grapes	Apples
Brown rice	Sweet potatoes	Figs
Raisins		Plums
Bananas		Milk, milk products

Source: Data from: Foster-Powell K, Holt SH, Brand-Miller JC. International table of glycemic index and glycemic load values: 2002. *Am J Clin Nutr* 2002;76(1):5–56.

It turns out that potatoes have a very high GI, even higher than table sugar.

Despite the complexity of the issue, some rules can be applied to make the right food choices. Keep in mind that the rise in blood sugar level depends on several factors including the carbohydrate category (simple vs. complex) as well as the fiber, protein, and fat content of the food consumed. As a general rule, foods that provide no nutritional value (other than sugar in candy, honey, or table sugar) are likely to raise blood glucose levels quickly and should be avoided. On the other hand, fruits and vegetables, foods rich in fiber, and those containing protein (beans, lentils, corn, apples, oranges, etc.) are less likely to cause a dramatic rise in blood sugar levels and should be preferred. The GI of select foods is presented in Table 3.1.[32]

It is important to keep in mind that foods should not be judged or qualified as healthy or unhealthy on the basis of their GI value alone. The GI was never intended for this purpose. Rather, all dietary information such as the amount and type of fat, cholesterol, salt, vitamins, and fiber content along with the information provided by the GI should be considered.

Foods should not be judged or qualified as healthy or unhealthy on the basis of their GI value alone. The GI was never intended for this purpose. Rather, all dietary information, including the amount and type of fat, cholesterol, salt, vitamins, and fiber content, should be considered with the GI value.

Carbohydrate Requirements

The 2005 Dietary Guidelines Advisory Committee recommends that the daily carbohydrate intake comprises 45 to 65 percent of total calories. Most of these carbohydrates should come from complex carbohydrates (starchy foods) and grains and natural sugars found in fresh fruits and vegetables, while products containing large amounts of added sugars should be avoided.[33]

Fiber

Dietary fiber is polysaccharides that cannot be digested. This term is used for several materials that make up the structural parts of plants. Fiber is classified as soluble or insoluble; soluble fiber partially dissolves in water while insoluble fiber does not. Evidence from a number of studies supports that fiber intake is important in maintaining good health. Diets high in complex carbohydrates and soluble fiber have been associated with reduced mortality rates from heart disease.[33-36] Heart health benefits provided by dietary fiber may be beyond those achieved by reductions in total and saturated fat alone. There is also evidence of an association between high fiber intake and lower risk of diseases such as diabetes, hypertension, and obesity; an improved glucose and lipid metabolism; and an improved constellation of factors that comprise the metabolic syndrome.[37-40] Some findings also support that high fiber intake may protect against colon cancer.[41]

The American Heart Association's (AHA) *Dietary Guidelines for Americans*[42] emphasizes the importance of consuming a variety of fiber sources to obtain the different types of fibers found in foods rather than supplements. Current recommendations suggest that adults consume 25 or more grams of dietary fiber per day. In addition, at least of half of the grain intake should come from whole grains.[43] The best sources are fresh fruits and vegetables, nuts, legumes, and whole-grain foods. Unfortunately, the average American eats only 14 to 15 grams of dietary fiber a day.

Carbohydrates have been blamed as the source of weight gain and obesity, diabetes, tooth decay, and a number of other diseases. Such claims gave rise to so-called "sugar-free" products and low-carbohydrate diets over the years. Although a few claims have some merit, it is important to emphasize that it is the excess consumption of the wrong carbohydrates that causes these health problems and not the proper carbohydrates consumed at appropriate amounts. I am referring here to *simple* and *complex* carbohydrates. Health problems have been associated with excessive consumption of simple sugars but not with complex carbohydrates.

■ LIPIDS AND LIPOPROTEINS

Lipids

Lipids (from the Greek word *lipos*, for fat) are comprised of a number of different chemical compounds formed by the same structural elements (carbon, hydrogen, and oxygen) as carbohydrates. However, they differ from carbohydrates in the way the atoms are linked together. They are not very soluble in water. Lipids are classified in three types:

1. **Simple lipids** or **neutral fats.** Fatty acids, triglycerides, waxes, and sterols.
2. **Compound lipids** or **phospholipids.** Triglycerides combined with other chemicals to form other compounds. For example, phospholipids are formed when triglycerides combine with a phosphorus-containing group and a nitrogenous base; glycolipids form when fatty acids are bound with carbohydrates and nitrogen; and lipoproteins form when proteins are joined with either phospholipids or triglycerides.

3. **Derived fats.** Fats formed from simple and compound fats (i.e., cholesterol, lipid-soluble vitamins, and hormones).

■ Triglycerides

Almost all dietary fats are triglycerides. A common feature of the triglycerides and phospholipids is their content of **fatty acids.** Fatty acids are long compounds with straight hydrocarbon chains. The number of carbon atoms in the chain is generally 16, 18, or 20. Three fatty acid molecules attached to a glycerol molecule form a **triglyceride** molecule (**Figure 3.8**). Triglycerides are mainly used to provide energy for the different metabolic functions. Cholesterol and phospholipids are used throughout the body primarily to maintain the integrity of cell membranes and a number of other cellular functions. Cholesterol is used to form the sex hormones.

■ Saturated Fatty Acids

Carbon atoms have four possible sites to which other atoms can be attached. Fatty acids that are comprised of all carbon atoms attached to each other by a single bond and hydrogen atoms attached to most of the remaining sites of the carbon are known as **saturated fatty acids** (**Figure 3.9**); that is, the fatty acid is fully saturated with hydrogen atoms. Saturated fatty acids abound in animal sources, such as beef, pork, and chicken, and are solid at room temperature. Exceptions to this rule are two saturated fats derived from plants: palm oil, which contains saturated and unsaturated fatty acids in equal amounts, and coconut oil, which contains over 90% saturated fatty acids.

■ Unsaturated Fatty Acids

Fatty acids that have at least one double bond between two carbon atoms along the carbon chain are referred to as **unsaturated fatty**

Figure 3.8   Triglyceride molecule. Note that three fatty acids are attached to glycerol backbone.

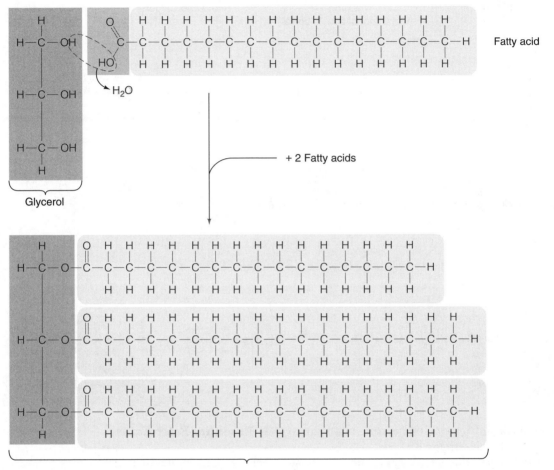

Formation of a triglyceride

Glycerol

Fatty acid

H_2O

+ 2 Fatty acids

Neutral fat or triglyceride

acids. Such a molecular arrangement leaves fewer sites available for hydrogen atoms to attach to carbon, so the particular fatty acid is not saturated with hydrogen atoms. They are derived from plants and, in room temperature, are usually in liquid form. Unsaturated fatty acids are further divided into the **monounsat-** **urated** and **polyunsaturated fatty acids** (see Figure 3.9).

Monounsaturated fatty acids are those that contain only one double bond along the carbon chain. Olive oil, canola oil, peanut oil, almond oil, and pecan oil all contain mainly monounsaturated fatty acids. Monounsaturated fats

Figure 3.9 Saturated (A), monounsaturated (B), and polyunsaturated (C) fatty acids. Note the single double bond between two carbon atoms along the carbon chain in the monounsaturated fatty acid (B) and the two double bonds in the polyunsaturated fatty acid (C).

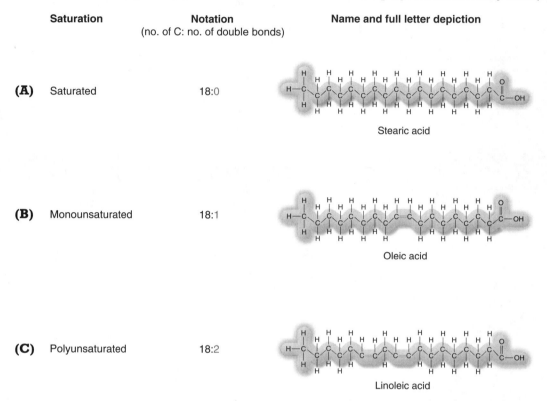

remain liquid at room temperature but begin to solidify in the refrigerator.

Polyunsaturated fatty acids include those with two or more double bonds along the carbon chain. Corn oil, safflower oil, sunflower oil, and soybean oil contain mainly polyunsaturated fatty acids. One important type, the **omega-3 fatty acids**, is found mostly in seafood. They are usually liquid at room temperature and in the refrigerator. There is general agreement that if used instead of saturated fats, monounsaturated and, to some extent, polyunsaturated fatty acids can lower the risk of developing heart disease and cancer.

■ Essential Fatty Acids

Humans and other mammals can synthesize their requirements for saturated and monounsaturated fatty acids. However, we lack the enzymes to synthesize certain long-chain polyunsaturated fatty acids such as omega-3 (linolenic acid) and omega-6 (linoleic acid). *Omega* (the last letter of the Greek alphabet) represents the last carbon of the chain and the number represents the position of the first double bond, counting from that carbon on the molecule.[44]

Such fatty acids, referred to as **essential fatty acids (EFAs)** are necessary for good health and must be obtained through diet. EFA are involved in maintaining the integrity of cell membranes, skin, cardiovascular, reproductive, immune, and nervous systems. They serve as precursors of important hormone-like substances, **prostaglandins**, which regulate body functions such as heart rate, blood pressure, blood clotting, immune function, and proper growth in children.[24] Select foods rich in EFA are presented in **Table 3.2**. Essential fatty acids are found in vegetable oils such as olive oil and safflower oil and must be obtained from the diet.

■ Trans Fatty Acids

Trans fatty acids (also referred to in commercial products as *partially hydrogenated oils*) are unsaturated fatty acids artificially formed by the partial hydrogenation of vegetable oils (solid shortening, hard stick margarine; most fried and processed foods). Chemically, trans fatty acids are made of the same building blocks as non-trans fatty acids but they differ in the way hydrogen atoms bond to a pair or pairs of double bonded carbon atoms. This different arrangement of hydrogen carbon bonding results in a straight configuration of the carbon chain of the trans fatty acid rather than the bent shape configuration of the naturally occurring unsaturated fatty acids (cis fatty acids; **Figure 3.10**).

Trans unsaturated fatty acids are produced commercially in large quantities by heating vegetable oils in the presence of metal catalysts and hydrogen to form shortening and margarine. Partially hydrogenated fats are attractive to the food industry because they have a long shelf life and can be sweetened to enhance the palatability of baked goods and sweets (i.e., cake icings).

Clinical studies have demonstrated that consumption of trans fatty acids or hydrogenated fats (saturated fatty acids) results in

Table 3.2 Foods Rich in Essential Fatty Acids

Omega-3 (Linolenic Acid)	Omega-6 (Linoleic Acid)
Flaxseed oil (highest linolenic content of any food)	Flaxseed oil
Walnuts	Grape seed oil
Pumpkin seeds	Pumpkin seeds
Brazil nuts	Pine nuts
Sesame seeds	Pistachio nuts
Avocados	Sunflower seeds (raw)
Some dark leafy green vegetables (kale, spinach, purslane, mustard greens, collards, etc.)	Olive oil
	Olives
Canola oil (cold-pressed and unrefined)	Corn
Soybean oil	Safflower
Wheat germ oil	Sunflower
Salmon	Soybean
Mackerel	Cottonseed
Sardines	
Anchovies	
Albacore tuna	

Figure 3.10 Trans and cis fatty acid configurations. Note that the hydrogen atoms bond the pair of the double bonded carbons on the opposite sides of the carbon chain in the trans configuration. Conversely, in the cis configuration, the hydrogen atoms bond on the same side of the carbon chain.

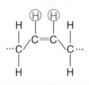

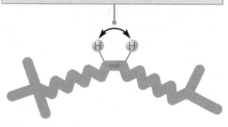

These two neighboring hydrogens repel each other, causing the carbon chain to bend

Cis form (bent)

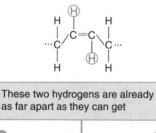

These two hydrogens are already as far apart as they can get

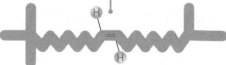

Trans form (straight)

higher blood cholesterol levels than consumption of naturally occurring oils. However, results from epidemiological studies on the association between trans fatty acid or hydro-genated fat intake and risk for cardiovascular disease are inconsistent. Difficulties inherent in estimating the population intake of trans fatty acids and several confounding factors associated with all dietary data, especially over long-term use, are some of the problems that need to be mastered before a definitive conclusion on the association can be made. However, despite the inconsistencies of the current data, it is prudent to avoid trans fatty acids when possible and instead use the naturally occurring non-hydrogenated oils. The AHA[43] and the 2005 Dietary Guidelines Advisory Committee[33] recommendation is that less that 1% of total energy is derived from trans fat.

Saturated fatty acids and trans unsaturated fatty acid consumption are associated with an increased risk of coronary heart disease. Monounsaturated fatty acids such as olive oil and polyunsaturated fatty acids (sunflower oil) without partially hydrogenated fatty acids (i.e., trans fatty acids) are protective against coronary heart disease. It is therefore strongly recommended that saturated and unsaturated trans fatty acids are avoided in diet and replaced by monounsaturated and polyunsaturated fatty acids. In addition, moderation in fat intake should always be practiced. The American Heart Association[43] and the 2005 Dietary Guidelines Advisory Committee[33] recommend that the daily overall fat consumption comprises 25% to 35% of the diet's daily energy content. Of this intake, less than 7% should come from saturated fats and the rest be divided equally between polyunsaturated and monounsaturated fats.

Monounsaturated and Polyunsaturated Fats

It is well accepted that diets high in monounsaturated and polyunsaturated fatty acids lower total cholesterol and LDL-cholesterol concentrations and the nutritional health benefits of both diets are well accepted and are recommended over saturated fats.[43]

However, there is evidence to support that diets rich in monounsaturated fats and more specifically olive oil, may be providing greater protection against heart disease.[45] This concept originated from the findings of the Seven Countries Study.[46,47] The consistent finding of these studies is that that much of Greece and southern Italy that followed a traditional dietary pattern had very low rates of coronary heart disease and certain types of cancer and had a long life expectancy, despite a high fat intake. The health benefits observed in these populations were attributed to the traditional diet they followed, the now well-known Mediterranean diet. Since olive oil is a key component of the traditional Mediterranean diet, the concept that olive oil may be mediating these health benefits has been under intensive investigation.

Evidence indicates that diets high in polyunsaturated fats tend to create a higher concentration of polyunsaturated fats within the LDL particles. Because polyunsaturated fats are more readily oxidized than monounsaturated due to the higher number of double bonds in their hydrocarbon chains, diets high in polyunsaturated fats enhance LDL oxidation.[48,49] On the contrary, a diet high in olive oil and other oils rich in monounsaturated fats such as oleic acid, not only lower LDL levels, but significantly decreased LDL oxidation.[49] This was also shown when an olive-oil–rich diet was compared to another monounsaturated oil diet (sunflower oil). The investigators concluded that although both monounsaturated fat diets lower cholesterol and LDL-cholesterol to similar levels, LDL oxidation was significantly lower in the olive-oil–rich diet when compared to the diet rich in sunflower oil.[50] Since the oxidation of LDL-cholesterol is a pivotal step in the process of atherosclerosis,[51] this finding suggest that olive oil provides a source of potent antioxidant properties superior to other polyunsaturated and monounsaturated oils. For these reasons and because olive oil (unlike other oils) has been safely used for thousands of years, the consumption of olive oil and products containing olive oil should be preferred when possible.

■ Role of Fats

Fats are essential for life. Fat typically provides approximately 20% to 40% of our daily calories. It is a most efficient way to store energy for two reasons. First, each gram fat yields 9 kilocalories of energy. This is more that two times the 4 kilocalories derived from carbohydrates. Second, fat is stored with relatively very little water, whereas each gram of glycogen is stored with about 3 grams of water. For these reasons, fat is a source of abundant stored energy for the body.

In addition to the energy fat provides, fat is involved in several other body functions essential for good health and survival. In fact, we cannot survive without fat. It is important to remember that adequate amount of fat in our diet is essential for good health. It is the wrong type of fat and excess fat in our diet that contributes to obesity, heart disease, and cancer. Moderation is the key to the consumption of all fat (saturated, unsaturated, and polyunsaturated). Here are some of the important functions of fat:

- It is the most abundant stored energy in the body and as such, it meets the necessary energy requirements of the body, especially long duration exercise.
- It is used in to structure the cell membrane and maintain its integrity.
- It is used to make several hormones.

- It serves as a carrier of fat-soluble vitamins.
- It is a good insulator against extreme heat or cold.
- It cushions body organs and protects them from injury.

■ Digestion and Absorption

Almost all dietary fats are digested and absorbed in the small intestine. From there, they are transported into the lymph vessels and hence to the blood.

The first step involves the breakdown of fats into smaller fat droplets, a process called **emulsification**. This is accomplished by **bile** secreted from the liver. Then, the pancreatic enzyme (pancreatic lipase) splits most of the triglycerides into free fatty acids (FFA) and monoglycerides, a process called **hydrolysis**. FFA and monoglycerides mix with bile salts and cholesterol to form small particles (smaller than those formed by emulsification) called micelles. These micelles act as a transport medium to carry the FFA and monoglycerides into the mucosal cells. There, the fats are re-formed, coated with a thin layer of protein and secreted into the bloodstream as **chylomicrons** (Figure 3.11).

■ Chylomicron Metabolism

As the triglyceride-laden chylomicrons enter the peripheral circulation, they come in contact with the enzyme **lipoprotein lipase**, found on the inner surface of capillaries. The enzyme hydrolyzes the triglycerides to FFA and the proteins are removed from the chylomicrons. The chylomicron remnants, now rich in cholesterol, are taken up by the liver (**Figure 3.12**).[44,53]

The released fatty acids can be used by the muscles for energy or taken up by the liver. What remains is deposited as fat.

■ Fatty Acid Oxidation

Fatty acids constitute the most compact fuel available to the body. As mentioned earlier, the energy yield from 1 gram of fat is 9 kilocalories versus 4 kilocalories from 1 gram of glucose. The energy from fat supplies more than 50% of the energy during rest and up to 80% during prolonged exercise.

The degradation and oxidation of fatty acids is strictly confined to the mitochondria via a process known as **beta-oxidation** (**Figure 3.13**). It can proceed only under aerobic conditions (requires oxygen) and fat metabolism is halted during anaerobic conditions.

Fatty acids are released in the bloodstream from adipose tissue (body fat) and are carried to the cells. They are then transported by a carrier substrate **carnitine** into the mitochondria, where oxidation occurs and energy is released. During beta-oxidation, the fatty acid molecule is progressively degraded by the reaction that is repeated several times. Each time the reaction goes through a complete cycle, two carbon segments and four hydrogen atoms are released and acetyl coenzyme A (acetyl-CoA) is formed. The process is repeated over and over until the entire fatty acid molecule is split into acetyl-CoA.[44,53,54] The complete oxidation of each 18-carbon acid molecule generates 147 molecules of **adenosine triphosphate (ATP)**, a form of energy used by cells (discussed in Chapter 6). This is four times more than the 36 ATP molecules generated from glucose metabolism.[54]

■ Fatty Acid Formation from Glucose and Proteins

It is important to emphasize that, once dietary carbohydrates are digested and absorbed, the glucose released is either used for the immediate energy needs of the cells or stored in the liver and muscles as glycogen for later use.

Figure 3.11   Digestion and absorption of fats. The dietary fats are emulsified by the liver-secreted bile. Then triglycerides are hydrolyzed by the enzyme, lipase, secreted by the pancreas, and free fatty acids are released. In turn, fatty acids are absorbed by mucosal cells, repackaged as chylomicrons, and released into the bloodstream.

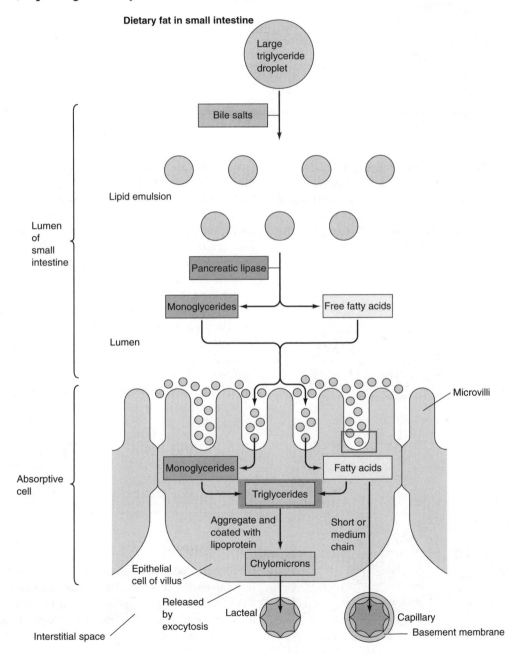

Figure 3.12 Chylomicron metabolism. Fatty acids and proteins are removed from the circulating chylomicrons by the lipoprotein lipase. Chylomicron remnants are taken up by the liver.

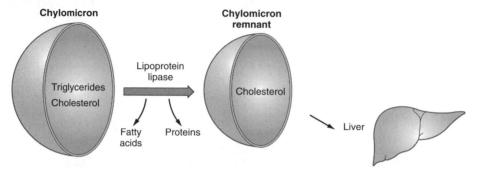

Figure 3.13 Beta oxidation. Fat metabolism occurs in the mitochondria. Activated fatty acids combine with carnitine to enter the mitochondria. Within the mitochondria, fatty acyl-CoA then enters the Krebs cycle through beta-oxidation.

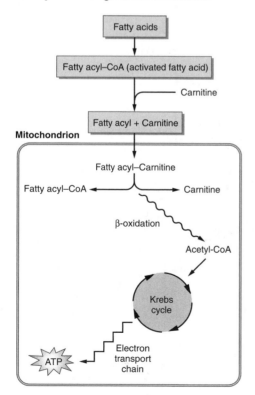

Once these needs are satisfied, any remaining glucose is converted to fatty acids and is eventually stored as fat.[24,44,53,55,56] It is important to keep in mind that the conversion of glucose to fat is "one-way street." That is, fats cannot be converted to glucose. This should not discourage adequate carbohydrate consumption. Keep in mind that adequate carbohydrate consumption is essential for good health.[44,53,54]

We also have the capacity to convert proteins into fatty acids and eventually store them as fat. Therefore, excess protein (more than can be utilized for tissues' integrity and energy) is converted to fat. This is important to keep in mind for those who consume excessive amounts of protein for muscle building or follow high-protein diets.

Glucose and protein can be converted to fatty acids and eventually stored as fat. However, fatty acids cannot be converted back to glucose or proteins.

■ Cholesterol

Cholesterol is a water-insoluble white crystalline substance. It is found in a number of animal foods we consume. Despite its bad reputation, it is important to note that cholesterol is an essential component of cell membranes and a precursor to certain hormones and bile acids, functions necessary for maintaining good health. For these reasons, not only do we depend on dietary cholesterol, but also cells have the capacity to synthesize it. In fact, the average daily cholesterol from dietary sources meets about 25% of the cholesterol needs of the body. The remaining 75% is synthesized by the cells.[57,58]

> The average daily cholesterol from dietary sources meets about 25% of the cholesterol needs of the body. The remaining 75% is synthesized by the cells.

The liver plays an important role in cholesterol metabolism. Cholesterol in the liver comes from three sources.[57] First, dietary cholesterol from the foods consumed is incorporated into chylomicrons (large lipoprotein particles) and enters the circulation. After the removal of triglycerides and proteins, the cholesterol-rich chylomicron remnants are taken up by the liver and cholesterol is removed. Second, cholesterol is brought to the liver from other cells of the body via lipoproteins. Third, if cholesterol supplies are inadequate via the two sources mentioned, the liver can synthesize it. The rate of synthesis is controlled by the concentrations of cholesterol in the liver.[53,57]

> Despite its bad reputation, it is important to note that cholesterol is an essential component of cell membranes and a precursor to certain hormones and bile acids, functions necessary for maintaining good health.

Lipoproteins

Cholesterol, like any other fat, does not dissolve in water or blood, so it cannot be transported outside the artery wall. In order to transport cholesterol out of the artery and to the cells, it must be bound to special "transporters" made from proteins and fats called **lipoproteins**. The major role of lipoproteins is to transport lipids in the blood.

Lipoproteins are spherical particles. The outer layer contains *apolipoprotein*, the main structural component, and *phospholipids* with their polar heads oriented towards the aqueous environment of plasma. Free cholesterol is also inserted within the phospholipid layer. The core of the lipoprotein contains the hydrophobic cholesterol esters and triglycerides.

Lipoproteins vary in size and density, lipid, and apolipoprotein content. Four different lipoproteins have a role in the transport and metabolism of lipids. The nomenclature of the lipoproteins, with the exception of chylomicrons, is based on their hydrated density (**Figure 3.14**). These are: (1) chylomicrons, already discussed in this chapter, (2) very low density lipoproteins (VLDL), (3) low density lipoproteins (LDL), and (4) high density lipoproteins (HDL).

Figure 3.14 Relative size and density of lipoproteins.

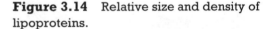

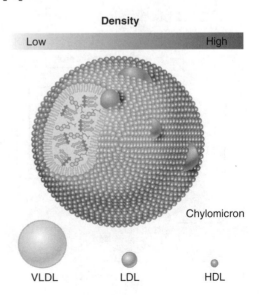

■ Very Low Density Lipoprotein

Very low density lipoprotein (VLDL) is a triglyceride-rich particle produced by the liver and the gut. VLDL enters the circulation as premature particles (nascent VLDL). They interact with other lipoproteins (HDL) and acquire cholesterol, and are transformed to mature VLDL. Subsequently, they come in contact with the enzyme lipoprotein lipase and the FFA are removed. What remains is referred to as *VLDL remnant.* Some of these VLDL remnants are taken up by the liver and are recycled or transformed. Others shed more of their triglyceride load, a process involving the enzyme **hepatic triglyceride lipase**, and are transformed to LDL particles (**Figure 3.15**).[59]

Figure 3.15 VLDL metabolism.

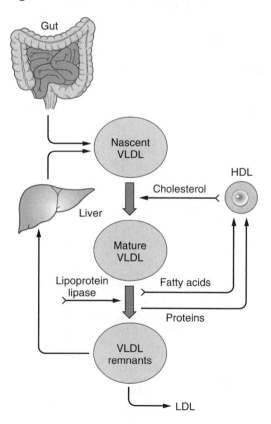

■ Low Density Lipoprotein

Low density lipoprotein (LDL) can be generated by three different sources: the liver, the gut, and triglyceride-rich lipoproteins (VLDL and chylomicrons) after triglyceride hydrolysis. It is the major carrier of cholesterol, carrying about 60% to 80% of all cholesterol in the blood. It is the lipoprotein responsible for carrying cholesterol to the cells.

The mechanism by which cholesterol carried by LDL (LDL-cholesterol) is delivered to the cells was described by Brown and Goldstein.[60–62] In 1985, these two scientists received the Nobel prize in medicine for their contribution to science. Their discoveries also led to the development of the current cholesterol-lowering agents known as **statins**.

Briefly, liver and other cells generate LDL receptors that aggregate at the cell surface. The cholesterol-laden LDL particles come in contact with these receptors and bind with them. Then the receptor-bound LDL is carried into the cell. There, the protein and cholesterol are removed from LDL and used for the needs of the cell (**Figure 3.16**).

In addition to meeting the needs of the cell, the cholesterol delivered to the cell serves to regulate and maintain a constant level of cholesterol within the cell in the following ways. First, as previously discussed, cells have the capacity to synthesize cholesterol when their requirements are not met from dietary sources. This process is regulated by the amount of free cholesterol within the cell. When the incoming cholesterol is adequate to meet the cell's demands, free cholesterol within the cell builds up. Consequently, three processes occur:

1. The key enzyme responsible for cholesterol formation, 3-hydroxy-3-methyl-glutaryl coenzyme A reductase (HMG CoA reductase), is down-regulated

Figure 3.16 LDL-cholesterol metabolism under normal conditions.

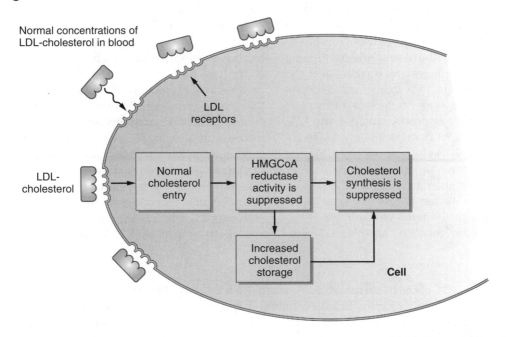

and cholesterol synthesis by the cell is suppressed.

2. LDL receptor synthesis is suppressed, thereby suppressing the cholesterol influx into the cell.

3. The mechanism for cholesterol storage within the cell is enhanced.

Conversely, when cholesterol deliveries within the cell are inadequate to meet the cell's demands because of dietary or other reasons, synthesis of LDL receptors and cholesterol by the cell is enhanced (see Figure 3.16). Collectively, these processes regulate cholesterol formation and use by the cells.[63]

The action of the cholesterol-lowering agents known as statins is based on the processes described above. Statins suppress the activity of the enzyme HMG CoA reductase, which is responsible for cholesterol synthesis.

Consequently, cholesterol synthesis by the cell is reduced. The cell then forms more LDL receptors on its surface. As a result, more of the circulating LDL-cholesterol binds with the receptors and is brought into the cell, ultimately lowering the blood cholesterol levels.

Low density lipoprotein is the major carrier of cholesterol, as it can transport about 60% to 80% of all cholesterol in the blood. It is the lipoprotein responsible for carrying cholesterol to the cells.

The important role LDL receptors play in blood cholesterol concentrations can be appreciated in individuals with a genetic disease known as *familial hypercholesterolemia (FH)*. Individuals with the heterozygous form of FH (those who inherit the mutant gene from only one parent; a milder form of the disease) have about half of the number of LDL receptors on the surface of their cells than individuals without FH. Thus, relatively less blood LDL-cholesterol binds to the receptors and is brought into the cell, and cholesterol removal from the blood is inadequate. In response, the cells synthesize large amounts of cholesterol to meet their needs, further down-regulating the LDL receptors (**Figure 3.17**). Consequently, the blood LDL-cholesterol levels of those with FH are about two to three times above normal. They usually suffer a heart attack or have advanced coronary heart disease before reaching age 50. Individuals with the more severe form of the disorder (homozygous FH) have LDL-C levels

six to eight times above normal and are likely to have heart attack before age 20.[63]

Naturally, most Americans do not have FH, yet we do have elevated blood LDL-cholesterol levels and suffer premature heart attacks. Why do we have high cholesterol levels? In addition to genetic abnormalities, studies have shown that the consumption of diets containing high concentrations of saturated fats is more likely to result in high blood cholesterol than diets containing polyunsaturated fats.[64,65] Although the mechanism or mechanisms by which consumption of high monosaturated and saturated fats affect cholesterol metabolism are not fully understood, suppression of LDL receptors appears to be involved.[65,66] When high fat diets

Figure 3.17   LDL-cholesterol metabolism when the number of LDL receptors is lower than normal (i.e., familiar hypercholesterolemia) or the receptors are defective. As the cell receives less cholesterol from the blood, it is forced to synthesize its own. This down-regulates the LDL receptors, leading to even less cholesterol entering the cell. A vicious cycle thus is created resulting in elevated blood cholesterol levels.

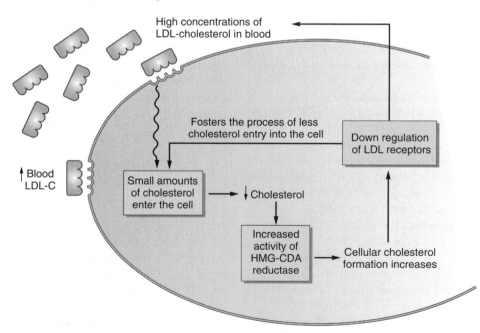

are consumed, the ingested cholesterol builds up in liver membranes. This blocks certain receptor proteins involved in cell signaling of the formation of LDL receptors. As a result, the liver cells produce fewer LDL receptors. In turn, LDL-cholesterol clearance by the liver is reduced and LDL-cholesterol accumulates in blood.

■ High Density Lipoprotein

The **high density lipoprotein (HDL)** is the smallest of the lipoproteins. It is secreted by the liver and gut as an immature, disk-shaped particle referred to as *nascent HDL*.[67] As these particles circulate, they acquire unesterified (free) cholesterol. With the action of the enzyme lecithin-cholesterol acyl transferase (LCAT), the cholesterol is esterified.[68] This esterified cholesterol then enters the core of the nascent HDL particles. As cholesterol within the core of the nascent HDL accumulates, the particles become spherical and are now called HDL_3.

As more cholesterol is acquired, the HDL_3 particles are transformed to HDL_{2a}. The HDL_{2a} particles undergo more transformations as they interact with other lipoproteins and exchange properties. In this process, cholesterol esters are transferred to VLDL and triglycerides are acquired. The particles are now transformed into HDL_{2b}. Subsequently, the HDL_{2b} particles are hydrolyzed by the enzyme hepatic lipase and triglycerides are released to form HDL-3. The process is known as the *HDL cycle* (**Figure 3.18**).[69]

■ Reverse Cholesterol Transport

The role of the HDL cycle is to assure the transportation of cholesterol from the peripheral tissues to the liver. This process is either

Figure 3.18 HDL cycle.

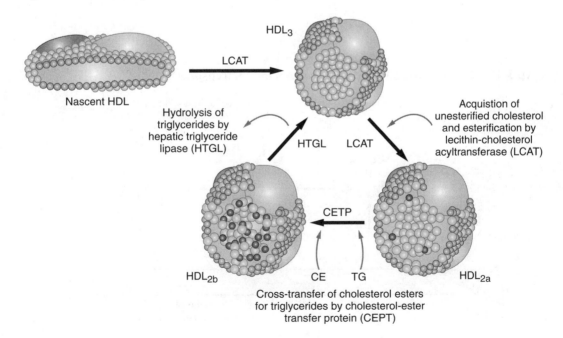

accomplished by the liver taking up the HDL-cholesterol via special HDL-cholesterol receptors or the transfer of cholesterol from the HDL particle to VLDL and subsequent uptake of VLDL by the liver. The process, first proposed by Glomset,[68] is known as **reverse cholesterol transport** (Figure 3.19).

The role of the HDL is to transport cholesterol from the peripheral tissues to the liver. The process is known as reverse cholesterol transport.

The reverse cholesterol transport is essential for protection against *atherosclerosis* (hardening of the arteries) as will be discussed in Chapter 8. Briefly, the mechanism proposed is that the removal of HDL-cholesterol from the periphery to the liver for catabolism lowers blood cholesterol concentrations, thereby preventing cholesterol accumulation within the arterial wall.

■ Apolipoproteins

Apolipoproteins are found in the outer layer of lipoproteins and are the main structural component of the lipoproteins. Apolipoproteins are involved in four major functions: (1) assembly and secretion of the lipoprotein, (2) providing structural integrity of the lipoprotein, (3) acting as cofactors for enzymes, and (4) binding to specific receptors and proteins for cellular uptake or exchange of lipid components. Apolipoproteins direct the lipoprotein to the various receptors.

Apolipoproteins are abbreviated as Apo followed by a capital letter that may have a Roman letter or Arabic number suffix. The major classes of apolipoproteins and their roles are presented in **Table 3.3**. Studies suggest that Apo A-I and Apo B may be better predictors of an increased risk for heart disease than levels of cholesterol and other lipoproteins.[70–73] The role of apolipoproteins D and J is not well understood.

Figure 3.19   HDL metabolism and reverse cholesterol transport.

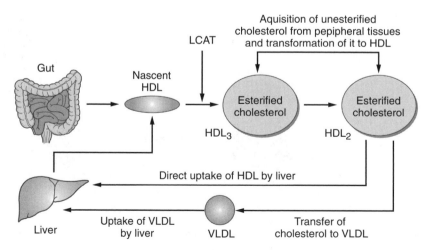

Table 3.3 Apolipoproteins

Name	Predominant Lipoprotein	Role
Apo A-I	HDL	Structural, enzyme activation
Apo A-II	HDL	Structural
Apo B100	LDL, VLDL	Structural, LDL receptor binding
Apo B48	Chylomicrons	Structural
Apo CI, CII, CIII	Chylomicrons, VLDL	VLDL catabolism, LPL activation and inhibition
Apo D	HDL	Enzyme activation
Apo E	Chylomicron remnants	Chylomicron metabolism, LDL receptor binding
Apo J	HDL	?

■ Proteins

Proteins, from the Greek word *proto*, meaning "first" or "of primary importance," are a class of large organic compounds that are present in and vital to every living cell. Like carbohydrates and fats, proteins contain atoms of carbon, oxygen, and hydrogen. In addition, they contain nitrogen. Proteins are comprised of building blocks known as **amino acids**. There are 20 different amino acids present in proteins.

Proteins are found in meats, fish, poultry, eggs, and dairy products as well as some plants such as peanuts, beans, chick peas, lentils, and almonds. The end product of almost all proteins consumed and digested are amino acids. The body reconstructs its own proteins by arranging the amino acids to its own specifications.

When the appropriate amino acids are present, the cell then can proceed to synthesize complete proteins. Amino acids are assigned and strung together by **peptide linkages** to form long *peptide chains*. Peptides containing hundreds of amino acids are usually referred to as **polypeptides**. Proteins are comprised of one or more polypeptide chains. Its function is in control of the DNA-RNA system of each individual cell.[24] The specific sequence of the amino acid chain gives the protein its specific properties. Protein synthesis requires a great amount of energy. In it is one of the most energy consuming processes of the cell.[24]

■ Essential Amino Acids

As previously mentioned, there are 20 different amino acids present in our proteins. We can synthesize most of the amino acids, but humans and higher animals cannot synthesize nine of them.[74] These nine amino acids, known as **essential amino acids**, must be obtained through diet. They are significant because complete proteins can only be structured if these amino acids are present. In other words, a chain of amino acids cannot form a **complete protein** until essential amino acids become part of that chain.

> Essential amino acids are required to form a complete protein.

> The primary function of proteins is to form or rebuild body tissue. In some instances, proteins can be used to form glucose for energy.

Proteins from animal sources are high quality whereas those from vegetables are usually incomplete. Purely vegetarian diets thus have the potential of not providing the necessary amino acids needed to form complete proteins and eventually this may lead to protein malnutrition. Malnutrition can be remedied by combining a variety of vegetables rich in amino acids, which is likely to provide all of the essential amino acids to form complete proteins.

■ Role of Proteins

The major function of proteins is to form or rebuild body tissue—such as skin, hair, cartilage, muscles, tendons, and ligaments—and provide structure to the body. In addition, they are used in muscle contractions, blood clotting, enzyme and antibody formation, and in transporting oxygen and nutrients throughout the body.

Proteins are not usually used for energy except under extreme conditions like starvation, certain diseases, and excess proteins in diet. About 3% to 6% of the energy fuel required during prolonged exercise comes from proteins. A notion that protein provides most of the energy for activities when energy stores are depleted is not true. Under normal conditions, energy stores are never depleted due to the large energy stored in body fat. The use of protein for energy during exercise becomes pronounced only when carbohydrate reserves are depleted. However, a well-nourished individual has enough energy stored in the form of glycogen to last for approximately a 20-mile walk.[54] The formation of glucose from proteins is known as **gluconeogenesis** (Greek for formation of new glucose).

■ Protein Requirements

Contrary to popular belief, we only need relatively small amounts of protein to maintain good health. Adults require as little as 0.8 grams per kilogram of body weight. A person weighing 82 kg (about 180 lbs) thus will require about 66 grams of protein in his or her daily diet ($82 \times 0.8 = 65.6$).

An even bigger misconception about protein requirements is with athletes and those who are physically active. Coaches, trainers, and athletes (along with profiteers) have perpetuated the myth that protein intake is linked to performance and muscle strength. For decades, high protein diets have been advocated and protein supplements are now part of the athlete's daily diet.

Research supports that athletes or highly active people (heavy labor) may require more protein than non-athletes. It is recommended that athletes participating in heavy training (weight training, aerobic training) consume between 1.2 to 1.8 grams of protein per kilogram of body weight which can be met by the average diet.[47] In addition, athletes get the extra protein simply by eating greater amounts of food. In other words, a sensible diet will meet the protein requirements even for the avid runner or weight lifter, with no need to consume protein supplements. When it comes to protein intake, the following factors should be kept in mind:

1. When protein intake is adequate, extra protein does not increase performance. There is no connection between high protein intake and performance or muscle mass.

2. High protein intake places strain in the liver and kidney and the overall digestion of food. This is bound to have an adverse effect on performance.
3. Protein intake of greater than 3 grams per kilogram of body weight may interfere with the body's ability to utilize protein. Under such condition, protein synthesis may actually be hampered. Eventually, muscle mass can be adversely affected.
4. High protein intake interferes with calcium absorption. This decreases bone mass and consequently increases the risk for osteoporosis.
5. Once the protein requirements of the body are met, the excess is either used for energy or stored as fat.

It is not wise to consume amounts of protein greater than 1.5 g/kg body weight/day, whether it comes from the foods you eat or as a powder sold in stores.

■ SUMMARY

- Foods are comprised of carbohydrates, proteins, fats, vitamins, minerals, and water. Foods provide the materials necessary all body functions possible and the required energy to sustain life and function.
- There are basically two kinds of carbohydrates: monosaccharides or simple carbohydrates, and polysaccharides or complex carbohydrates. The main function of carbohydrates is to provide the fuel for the energy requirements of the body.
- All carbohydrates (complex or simple) are ultimately converted to glucose, the simplest sugar. Glucose is then released in the blood and carried to the tissues to meet the immediate energy needs of the

cell. What remains is stored in the liver and muscle in the form of glycogen for later use or as fat in the adipose tissue.
- Control of blood glucose concentrations is accomplished by the delicate balance of two hormones, insulin and glucagon.
- The 2005 Dietary Guidelines Advisory Committee recommends that the daily carbohydrate intake comprises 45 to 65 percent of total calories. Most of these carbohydrates should come from complex carbohydrates (starchy foods) and grains and natural sugars found in fresh fruits and vegetables, while products containing large amounts of added sugars should be avoided.
- Lipids (fats) are classified as triglycerides or neutral fats, phospholipids or compound lipids, and cholesterol. Lipids are not very soluble in water.
- Almost all dietary fats are triglycerides. A common feature of triglycerides and phospholipids is their content of fatty acids. Three fatty acid molecules attached to a glycerol molecule form a triglyceride molecule.
- Fatty acids can be unsaturated or saturated. Unsaturated fatty acids can further be classified as monounsaturated and polyunsaturated. Generally, unsaturated fatty acids are vegetable oils whereas saturated fatty acids come from animal fats.
- Another classification based on their chemical configuration is known as trans fatty acids and cis fatty acids.
- Unsaturated or partially hydrogenated trans fatty acids are produced commercially in large quantities by heating vegetable oils in the presence of metal catalysts and hydrogen to form shortening and solid margarine.
- Overconsumption of trans fatty acids or hydrogenated fats results in higher blood

cholesterol levels than consumption of naturally occurring oils.

- Triglycerides are mainly used to provide energy for the different metabolic functions. Cholesterol and phospholipids are mainly used throughout the body for the integrity of cell membranes and a number of other cellular functions.
- The degradation and oxidation of fatty acids is strictly confined to the mitochondria via a process known as beta-oxidation.
- Cholesterol is a water-insoluble white crystalline substance and is found in a number of animal-based foods.
- Cholesterol is an essential for a number of bodily functions necessary for maintaining good health. For this reason, not only do we depend on dietary cholesterol, but our cells have the capacity to synthesize it.
- Cholesterol delivery to the cells and its metabolism is accomplished by special transporters made from proteins and lipids, known as lipoproteins. These lipoproteins are: chylomicrons, very low density lipoproteins (VLDL), low density lipoproteins (LDL), and high density lipoproteins (HDL).
- Cholesterol bound with LDL (LDL-cholesterol) is delivered to the cells, while cholesterol bound with the HDL (HDL-cholesterol) is carried to the liver for catabolism. Low blood LDL-cholesterol and high HDL-cholesterol concentrations are desirable.
- Proteins are found in meats, fish, poultry, eggs, and dairy products as well as some plants such as peanuts, beans, chick peas, lentils, and almonds. The end product of almost all proteins consumed and digested are amino acids.
- The body reconstructs its own proteins by arranging the amino acids to its own specifications. When the appropriate amino acids are present, the cell can then proceed to synthesize complete proteins.
- Amino acids are assigned and strung together by peptide linkages to form long peptide chains. The specific sequence of the amino acid chain gives the protein its specific properties.
- The major function of proteins is to form or rebuild body tissue. In addition, they are used in muscle contractions, blood clotting, enzyme and antibody formation, and in transporting oxygen and nutrients throughout the body. Proteins are not usually used for energy except under extreme conditions (starvation, certain diseases, excess proteins in diet).
- Protein requirements for adults are 0.8 grams per kilogram of body weight.
- It is recommended that athletes participating in heavy training (weight training, aerobic training) or highly active people (heavy labor) consume between 1.2 to 1.8 grams of protein per kilogram of body weight.

■ REFERENCES

1. Cowan LD, O'Connell DL, Criqui MH, et al. Cancer mortality and lipid and lipoprotein levels. Lipid Research Clinics Program Mortality Follow-up Study. *Am J Epidemiol* 1990; 131:468–482.
2. Garcia-Palmieri MR, Sorlie PD, Costas R Jr, Havlik RJ. An apparent inverse relationship between serum cholesterol and cancer mortality in Puerto Rico. *Am J Epidemiol* 1981; 114:29–40.
3. Keys A, Aravantis C, Blackburn H, et al. Serum cholesterol and cancer mortality in the Seven Countries Study. *Am J Epidemiol* 1985;121: 870–883.
4. Sherwin RW, Wentworth DN, Cutler JA, et al. Serum cholesterol levels and cancer mortality

in 361,662 men screened for the Multiple Risk Factor Intervention Trial. *JAMA* 1987;257: 943–948.

5. Sorlie PD, Fienleib M. The serum cholesterol-cancer relationship: an analysis of time trends in the Framingham Study. *J Natl Cancer Inst* 1982;69:989–996.

6. Jacobs D, Blackburn H, Higgins M, et al. Report of the Conference on Low Blood Cholesterol: mortality associations. *Circulation* 1992;86:1046–1060.

7. Iribarren C, Reed DM, Chen R, et al. Low serum cholesterol and mortality. Which is the cause and which is the effect? *Circulation* 1995;92:2396–2403.

8. Meilahn EN. Low serum cholesterol. Hazardous to health? *Circulation* 1995;92: 2365–2366.

9. Kris-Etherton PM, Lichtenstein AH, Howard BV. Antioxidant vitamin supplements and cardiovascular disease. *Circulation* 2004;110: 637–641.

10. The effect of vitamin E and beta carotene on the incidence of lung cancer and other cancers in male smokers. The Alpha-Tocopherol, Beta Carotene Cancer Prevention Study Group. *N Engl J Med* 1994;330:1029–1035. (see comments)

11. Ballmer PE, Stahelin HB. Beta carotene, vitamin E, and lung cancer. *N Engl J Med* 1994; 331:612–613.

12. Brown BG, Zhao XQ, Chait A, et al. Simvastatin and niacin, antioxidant vitamins, or the combination for the prevention of coronary disease. *N Engl J Med* 2001;345:1583–1592.

13. Goldstein MR. Beta carotene, vitamin E, and lung cancer. *N Engl J Med* 1994;331:612. (see comments)

14. Grady D, Herrington D, Billner V, et al. Cardiovascular disease outcomes during 6.8 years of hormone therapy: heart and estrogen/progestin replacement study follow-up (HERS II). *JAMA* 2002;288:49–57.

15. Greenberg ER, Baron JA, Tosteson TD, et al. A clinical trial of antioxidant vitamins to prevent colorectal adenoma. Polyp Prevention Study Group. *N Engl J Med* 1994;331:141–147. (see comments)

16. Hennekens CH, Buring JE, Peto R. Antioxidant vitamins: benefits not yet proved. *N Engl J Med* 1994;330:1080–1081.

17. Kritchevsky D. Beta carotene, vitamin E, and lung cancer. *N Engl J Med* 1994;331:611–612. (see comments)

18. Leo MA, Lieber CS. Beta carotene, vitamin E, and lung cancer. *N Engl J Med* 1994;331:612. (see comments)

19. Marantz PR. Beta carotene, vitamin E, and lung cancer. *N Engl J Med* 1994;331:611. (see comments)

20. Omenn GS, Goodman GE, Thornquist MD, et al. Effects of a combination of beta carotene and vitamin A on lung cancer and cardiovascular disease. *N Engl J Med* 1996;334: 1150–1155.

21. Pryor WA. Beta carotene, vitamin E, and lung cancer. *N Engl J Med* 1994;331:612.

22. Waters DD, Alderman EL, Hsia J, et al. Effects of hormone replacement therapy and antioxidant vitamin supplements on coronary atherosclerosis in postmenopausal women: a randomized controlled trial. *JAMA* 2002; 288:2432–2440.

23. Bjelakovic G, Nikolova D, Gluud LL, et al. Mortality in randomized trials of antioxidant supplements for primary and secondary prevention: systematic review and meta-analysis. *JAMA* 2007;297:842–857. (see comments)

24. Guyton AC. *Textbook of Medical Physiology.* Philadelphia: W.B. Saunders; 1991.

25. Guyton AC, Hall J. *Human Physiology and Mechanisms of Disease.* Philadelphia: W.B. Saunders; 1997.

26. Cahill GF Jr, Starvation in man. *N Engl J Med* 1970;282:668–675.

27. Ludwig DS. The glycemic index: physiological mechanisms relating to obesity, diabetes, and cardiovascular disease. *JAMA* 2002;287: 2414–2423.

28. Hayashi T, Hirshman MF, Kurth EJ, et al. Evidence for 5' AMP-activated protein kinase mediation of the effect of muscle contraction on glucose transport. *Diabetes* 1998;47: 1369–1373.

29. Kishi K, Morimoto N, Nakaya Y, et al. Bradykinin directly triggers GLUT-4 translocation via

an insulin-independent pathway. *Diabetes* 1998;47:550–558.

30. Bantle JP, Laine DC, Castle GW, et al. Postprandial glucose and insulin responses to meals containing different carbohydrates in normal and diabetic subjects. *N Engl J Med* 1983;309:7–12.

31. Jenkins DJ, Wolevar TM, Taylor RH, et al. Glycemic index of foods: a physiological basis for carbohydrate exchange. *Am J Clin Nutr* 1981;34:362–366.

32. Foster-Powell K, Holt SH, Brand-Miller JC. International table of glycemic index and glycemic load values: 2002. *Am J Clin Nutr* 2002;76(1):5–56.

33. US Department of Health and Human Services; US Department of Agriculture. *Dietary Guidelines for Americans, 2005*, 6th ed. Washington, DC: US Government Printing Office; 2005.

34. Brown L, Rosner B, Willett WW, Sacks FM. Cholesterol-lowering effects of dietary fiber: a meta-analysis. *Am J Clin Nutr* 1999;69:30–42. (see comments)

35. Pereira MA, O'Reilly E, Augustsson K, et al. Dietary fiber and risk of coronary heart disease: a pooled analysis of cohort studies. *Arch Intern Med* 2004;164:370–376.

36. Rimm EB, Ascherio A, Giovannucci E, et al. Vegetable, fruit, and cereal fiber intake and risk of coronary heart disease among men. *JAMA* 1996;275:447–451.

37. McKeown NM, Meigs JB, Liu S, et al. Carbohydrate nutrition, insulin resistance, and the prevalence of the metabolic syndrome in the Framingham Offspring Cohort. *Diabetes Care* 2004;27:538–546. (see comments)

38. McKeown NM, Meigs JB, Liu S, et al. Whole-grain intake is favorably associated with metabolic risk factors for type 2 diabetes and cardiovascular disease in the Framingham Offspring Study. *Am J Clin Nutr* 2002;76: 390–398.

39. Fung TT, Hu FB, Pereira MA, et al. Whole-grain intake and the risk of type 2 diabetes: a prospective study in men. *Am J Clin Nutr* 2002;76:535–540.

40. Schulze MB, Liu S, Rimm EB, et al. Glycemic index, glycemic load, and dietary fiber intake and incidence of type 2 diabetes in younger and middle-aged women. *Am J Clin Nutr* 2004;80:348–356.

41. Fuchs CS, Giovannucci EL, Colditz GA, et al. Dietary fiber and the risk of colorectal cancer and adenoma in women. *N Engl J Med* 1999;340:169–176. (see comments)

42. Krauss RM, Eckel RH, Howard B, et al. AHA Dietary Guidelines: revision 2000: A statement for healthcare professionals from the Nutrition Committee of the American Heart Association. *Circulation* 2000;102(18):2284–2299.

43. Lichtenstein AH, Appel LJ, Brands M, et al. Diet and lifestyle recommendations revision 2006: a scientific statement from the American Heart Association Nutrition Committee. *Circulation* 2006;114(1):82–96.

44. Mougios V. *Exercise Biochemistry*. Champaign, IL: Human Kinetics; 2006.

45. Kris-Etherton PM. AHA Science Advisory. Monounsaturated fatty acids and risk of cardiovascular disease. American Heart Association. Nutrition Committee. *Circulation* 1999; 100(11):1253–1258.

46. Keys A. Coronary heart disease in seven countries. *Circulation*. 1970;41(suppl I):I-1–I-211.

47. Panagiotakos DB, Pitsavos C, et al. The role of traditional mediterranean type of diet and lifestyle, in the development of acute coronary syndromes: preliminary results from CARDIO 2000 study. *Cent Eur J Public Health* 2002;10(1-2):11–15.

48. Bonanome A, Pagnan A, et al. Effect of dietary monounsaturated and polyunsaturated fatty acids on the susceptibility of plasma low density lipoproteins to oxidative modification. *Arterioscler Thromb* 1992;12(4):529–533.

49. Fito M, Covas MI, et al. Protective effect of olive oil and its phenolic compounds against low density lipoprotein oxidation. *Lipids* 2000; 35(6):633–638.

50. Oubina P, Sanchez-Muniz FJ, et al. Eicosanoid production, thrombogenic ratio, and serum and LDL peroxides in normo- and hypercholesterolaemic post-menopausal women

consuming two oleic acid-rich diets with different content of minor components. *Br J Nutr* 2001;85(1):41–47.

51. Chisolm GM, Steinberg D. The oxidative modification hypothesis of atherogenesis: an overview. *Free Radic Biol Med* 2000;28(12): 1815–1826.

52. Summary of the second report of the National Cholesterol Education Program (NCEP) Expert Panel on Detection, Evaluation, and Treatment of High Blood Cholesterol in Adults (Adult Treatment Panel II). *JAMA* 1993; 269:3015–3023.

53. McMurray WC. *Essentials of Human Metabolism*. Philadelphia: Harper & Row; 1983.

54. McArdle WD, Katch FI, Katch VL. *Exercise Physiology*, 5th ed. Baltimore: Lippincott Williams & Wilkins; 2001.

55. Borer KT. *Exercise Endocrinology*. Champaign, IL: Human Kinetics; 2003.

56. Hargreaves M, Spriet L. *Exercise Metabolism*, 2nd ed. Champaign, IL: Human Kinetics; 2006.

57. Grundy SM. Cholesterol metabolism in man. *West J Med* 1978;128:13–25.

58. Grundy SM, Ahrens EH Jr. Measurements of cholesterol turnover, synthesis, and absorption in man, carried out by isotope kinetic and sterol balance methods. *J Lipid Res* 1969; 10:91–107.

59. Havel RJ. Lipoprotein biosynthesis and metabolism. *Ann NY Acad Sci* 1980;348:16–29.

60. Brown MS, Kovanen PT, Goldstein JL. Regulation of plasma cholesterol by lipoprotein receptors. *Science* 1981;212:628–635.

61. Brown MS, Goldstein JL. A receptor-mediated pathway for cholesterol homeostasis. *Science* 1986;232:34–47.

62. Brown MS, Goldstein JL. How LDL receptors influence cholesterol and atherosclerosis. *Sci Am* 1984;251:58–66.

63. Goldstein JL, Brown MS. Insights into the pathogenesis of atherosclerosis derived from studies of familial hypercholesterolemia. In LA Carlson, B Pernow, eds. *Metabolic Risk Factors in Ischemic Cardiovascular Disease*, New York: Raven Press; 1982.

64. Mazier MJ, Jones PJ. Dietary fat quality and circulating cholesterol levels in humans: a review of actions and mechanisms. *Prog Food Nutr Sci* 1991;15:21–41.

65. Stucchi AF, Terpstra AH, Nicolosi RH. LDL receptor activity is down-regulated similarly by a cholesterol-containing diet high in palmitic acid or high in lauric and myristic acids in cynomolgus monkeys. *J Nutr* 1995;125: 2055–2063.

66. Anderson RG, Goldstein J, Brown M. From cholesterol homeostasis to new paradigms in membrane biology. *Trends Cell Biol* 2003; 13:534–539.

67. Hamilton RL, Williams MC, Fielding CJ, Havel RJ. Discoidal bilayer structure of nascent high density lipoproteins from perfused rat liver. *J Clin Invest* 1976;58:667–680.

68. Glomset JA. The plasma lecithins: cholesterol acyltransferase reaction. *J Lipid Res* 1968;9: 155–167.

69. Grundy SM, Vega GL. Fibric acids: effects on lipids and lipoprotein metabolism. *Am J Med* 1987;83:9–20.

70. Genest JJ Jr, Bard JM, Fruchart JC, et al. Plasma apolipoprotein A-I, A-II, B, E and C-III containing particles in men with premature coronary artery disease. *Atherosclerosis* 1991; 90:149–157.

71. Gotto AM Jr, Whitney E, Stein EA, et al. Relation between baseline and on-treatment lipid parameters and first acute major coronary events in the Air Force/Texas Coronary Atherosclerosis Prevention Study (AFCAPS/TexCAPS). *Circulation* 2000;101:477–484.

72. Raiha H, Lehtonen L, Korhonen T, Korvenranta H. Family functioning 3 years after infantile colic. *J Dev Behav Pediatr* 1997;18: 290–294.

73. Raiha I, Marniemi P, Puuka T, et al. Effect of serum lipids, lipoproteins, and apolipoproteins on vascular and nonvascular mortality in the elderly. *Arterioscler Thromb Vasc Biol* 1997;17:1224–1232.

74. Murray RK, Granner DK, Peter A, Mayes VRW. *Harpers' Biochemistry*, 24th ed. Stamford, CT: Simon & Schuster; 1996.

CHAPTER

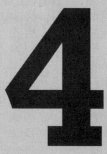

Vitamins, Minerals, and Water

Vitamins, minerals, and water are essential to maintain life.

All living beings require nutrients. Plants absorb them from the soil, air, and sunlight, and some carnivorous plants (like the Venus flytrap) can gain them through capturing and digesting insects and animals. Classified as macronutrients (needed in large quantities) and micronutrients (needed in tiny quantities), nutrients help plants to build their structure and undergo all of the processes of life and death. Animals and humans must garner nutrients from sunlight and a nutrient-rich diet of plants and other animals.

From 75% to 85% of any single tissue in the human body is comprised of water. It is easy to see that for us to live, we must drink water. Water is the solvent for every chemical of life that maintains our metabolism. Dangerous toxins from the air we breathe, food we eat, and chemicals infused through our skin are transported out of the cells and released from the body by the water found in our lymphatic, blood, and digestive systems. Water cushions our joints, maintains our blood pressure, regulates body temperature, and floats nutrients into and wastes out of our cells. Cold water and ice can combat inflammation and reduce fever; hot water and steam can soothe stress and stimulate the immune system.

Chapter 3 discussed our physical necessity for macronutrients (carbohydrates, fats, and protein). Here, we examine the micronutrients—vitamins and minerals—focusing on their importance in health and disease. This chapter also takes a close look at the crucial role of water in cardiovascular health and the destructive effects of dehydration and heat-related illness.

■ VITAMINS

Vitamins are organic substances found only in living things. More specifically, vitamins are found in the green leaves and roots of plants, except Vitamin B_{12}, which is found only in animal foods and products.

Vitamins are essential to the normal functioning of the body. They are necessary for growth, vitality, health, general well-being, and for the prevention and cure of many health problems and diseases. Vitamins also are involved in metabolic reactions that release energy from food, the regulation of tissue synthesis, and the integrity of cell membrane. With the exception of vitamin D, the body cannot manufacture vitamins and therefore they must be supplied through diet.

There are two types of vitamins: fat soluble and water soluble. Fat soluble vitamins are A, D, E, and K. These vitamins are stored in fat within the body. Water soluble vitamins are C and the B complex, which include: B_1 (thiamin), B_2 (riboflavin), B_3 (niacin), B_5 (pantothenic acid), B_6 (pyroxene), B_7 (biotin), B_9 (folic acid, folacin, folate), and B_{12} (cobalamin). Because these vitamins are not stored in the body, they must be consumed in the daily diet to prevent vitamin deficiency. Vitamin sources and their function are presented in **Table 4.1**.

Supplements

It is a fact that vitamin deficiency leads to poor health and even death. This fact has led to the persistent notion that vitamin supplements are necessary to maintain health and vigor. Thus, vitamin supplements have evolved into a big business with an estimated 50% of adult Americans taking them daily.

Keep in mind that fat soluble vitamins are stored in the body and, therefore, high doses of these vitamins can cause vitamin toxicity and lead to undesirable side effects. For example, excessive amounts of vitamin A can cause headache, nausea, vomiting, hair loss, and loss of calcium from bones. Excessive amounts of

Table 4.1 Vitamin Sources and Functions

	Dietary Sources	Functions
Water-Soluble Vitamins		
B_1 Thiamin	Pork, whole grains, legumes	Involved in the removal of carbon dioxide
B_2 Riboflavin	Generously distributed in all foods	Involved in energy metabolism
B_3 Niacin	Liver, lean meats, grains, legumes	Involved in metabolism
B_6 Pyroxine	Meats, vegetables, whole-grain cereals	Involved in metabolism
B_{12} Cobalamin	Meats, eggs, dairy products	Involved in metabolism
B_7 Biotin	Legumes, vegetables, meats	Involved in metabolism
B_9 Folic acid	Legumes, green vegetables, whole-wheat products	Protein metabolism
B_5 Pantothenic acid	Generously distributed distributed in all foods	Involved in metabolism
C	Citrus fruits, tomatoes, green peppers, salads	• Maintains healthy bones cartilage and collagen synthesis • Actively removes reactive oxygen species (ROS) • Reduces muscle soreness and improves recovery
Fat-Soluble Vitamins		
A (Beta-carotene)	Green vegetables, dairy products	Involved in: • Vision • Development • Testicular function • Bone growth
D	Eggs, dairy products, cod-liver oil, margarine	Bone growth
E (alpha, beta, delta, and gamma tocopherol)	Green leafy vegetables, seeds, margarine	• Strong antioxidant • Protects cells from damage and aging • Protects against heart disease, cancer
K	Green leafy vegetables, small amount in cereals, fruits, meats	Important in blood clotting

vitamin D can cause hypercalcemia (a blood disorder that can mimic hyperparathyroidism), calcification of soft tissue, and kidney damage.[1] Conversely, vitamin D deficiency is associated with increased incidence of cardiovascular disease.[2]

Water soluble vitamins are not stored in the body and are less likely to cause health problems. However, mega-doses of water soluble vitamins such as B_3 and B_6 can be toxic.

In general, vitamin supplements may be useful for people with unusual lifestyles or modified diets, including certain weight reduction regimens and strict vegetarian diets, women who are pregnant or lactating, and infants. Vitamins in therapeutic amounts may be indicated for the treatment of certain conditions in which absorption and utilization of vitamins are reduced or requirements for them are increased, and for certain disease processes. The decision to employ vitamin preparations in therapeutic amounts clearly rests with the physician. A healthy adult who consumes a usual, varied diet does not need to take vitamin supplements.[1]

Fat soluble vitamins are stored in the body. High doses of these vitamins can cause vitamin toxicity and lead to undesirable side effects. Water soluble vitamins are not stored in the body and high doses of them are less likely to cause health problems.

Antioxidants, Supplements, and Disease Prevention

As discussed in Chapter 3 in the fatty acid oxidation section, generation of adenosine triphosphate (ATP) via the aerobic pathways requires oxygen. Most of this oxygen combines with hydrogen to form water. However, a small fraction of the oxygen molecules have an uneven number of electrons in their outer shells (most ions have their electrons in pairs) during the final steps of aerobic metabolism (i.e., the electron transport chain). This gives rise to the superoxide, which are highly chemically reactive molecules known as **free radicals** or **reactive oxygen species (ROS)**. The ROS tend to take electrons from nearby compounds in order to attach them to the unpaired electrons in their outer layer. An excessive accumulation of free radicals increases the potential for cell damage that may eventually lead to chronic diseases such as cancer and cardiovascular disease.[3–5]

To buffer the deleterious effects of ROS the body possesses an antioxidant defense mechanism. However, the delicate balance between formation of ROS and antioxidants may be disturbed either by an increased production of ROS or a reduction in antioxidant species. This leads to the excessive accumulation of free radicals, a condition regarded as **oxidative stress**.[3,4]

The implication of oxidative stress in most chronic diseases gave rise to the hypothesis that antioxidant supplements may decrease the potential damage of ROS. Consequently, antioxidants in pill form have emerged as a way for many people to combat premature disease and aging. The potential health-promoting properties of the antioxidants vitamins E, C, and a form of vitamin A (beta carotene) have been investigated extensively. Unfortunately, to date the research has not yielded convincing evidence that antioxidant vitamin supplements can protect against premature cardiovascular disease.[6–9] Most disturbing is that some studies have shown that Vitamin E and beta carotene supplements increased the incidence of stroke and death from cardiovascular disease and overall mortality.[10]

The potential of harm with vitamin supplements has been reinforced by a meta-analysis published recently in the *Journal of the American Medical Association*.[11] A meta-analysis is a statistical procedure that allows the findings of a number of studies addressing the same issue (in this case vitamin supplements and disease) to be combined. As a result, the number of the subjects investigated increases and a more comprehensive picture of the relationship between factors of interest (vitamin consumption and disease or death) emerges. In this study, the effects of antioxidant supplements that included beta carotene; vitamins A, E, and C; and selenium on mortality were assessed. After analyzing 68 randomized controlled trials with 232,606 participants, the authors found no convincing evidence that antioxidant supplements decreased mortality. On the contrary, they found that beta carotene and vitamins A and E seem to increase the risk of death, while the effects of vitamin C and selenium could not be established.[11] Although this study may not definitively settle the issue, it should raise concern and skepticism about the value of vitamin supplements.

Currently, there is no consistent and strong evidence to support the notion that consuming vitamins at levels that exceed those provided by a dietary pattern consistent with American Heart Association (AHA) Dietary Guidelines will confer additional benefit with regard to cardiovascular disease (CVD) risk reduction.[12] Based on this evidence, the AHA and the American College of Cardiology do not currently recommend using antioxidant vitamin supplements for the prevention of CVD in women[13] and patients with chronic stable angina[12] until more complete data are available. Instead, their recommendation is that people eat a variety of nutrient-rich foods daily from all of the basic food groups that are low in saturated fat, trans fat, and cholesterol. Such foods provide a natural source of these vitamins, minerals, and fiber. The scientific evidence supports that a reduced risk of CVD is more likely to occur from diets that are high in food sources of antioxidants and other heart-protecting nutrients, such as fruits, vegetables, whole grains, and nuts instead of antioxidant supplements.

Do Active People Need Vitamin Supplements?

It sounds logical that if one participates in heavy physical activity or leads a busy, demanding lifestyle, he or she may need more vitamins. Some even go further by claiming that vitamin supplements enhance physical and mental performance.

In fact, severe vitamin deficiencies—particularly vitamin B deficiencies—are likely to decrease physical performance just as any other nutritional deficiencies. General fatigue, decrease in physical and mental performance, and gastrointestinal disorders are some of the early symptoms. However, the availability of food today makes it very unlikely that someone will become severely deficient in vitamins, especially if an effort is made to consume a daily dose of vegetables and fruits.

Do people with busy lifestyles, those who perform heavy physical work (construction workers, laborers, longshoremen, etc.), or extreme exercise (athletes) need to take megadoses of vitamins? There is no evidence that these healthy individuals need vitamin supplements as long as they maintain an adequate diet. There is also no scientific evidence to indicate that taking megadoses or a variety of vitamins will enhance athletic performance.[14,15] Such benefits claimed from the ingestion of large quantities of vitamins C and E are purely anecdotal. However, there is evidence that taking a daily multivitamin does no harm and makes good sense for most adults. But it is important to emphasize that vitamin supplements should never be a substitute for a healthy diet. It should only be a supplement.

The essential role of vitamins in human health is indisputable. What is less apparent is the amount of vitamins required for optimum health and whether vitamin supplements have a role in promoting health, physical and mental performance, or averting certain disease. This issue is often controversial and is not likely to be resolved in the near future. However, it is encouraging that in recent years significant research efforts are been made to better understand the potential health benefits of vitamins and vitamin supplements.

It is important to emphasize the following about vitamins:

- Vitamins are essential to the normal functioning of the body. Vitamin deficiency therefore can lead to poor health and even death. This in part has contributed to some people taking excessive amounts of vitamins.

- There is no evidence to support that megadoses of vitamins improve physical or mental performance. Conversely, there is evidence that vitamins E and A (beta carotene) may increase the risk of death, especially in some populations.

- Taking a multivitamin daily is likely to cause no harm and may even provide some nutritional benefits. However, multivitamin supplements should never be confused as being an alternative to healthy diet. Multivitamin supplements provide only a fraction of what a diet rich in fruits, vegetables, and whole grains provides. Furthermore, even the most wisely engineered vitamin supplement cannot come close to replacing healthy dietary habits.

Until more information is accumulated for scientists to have a better understanding of the complex role of vitamins in human health and performance, and thereby advise the public accordingly, it is prudent that the consumption of vitamin or herbal supplements be discussed with a physician.

■ MINERALS

While vitamins are organic, minerals are inorganic elements that have important roles in the metabolism and proper functioning of the body. We obtain them from the water and foods consumed. Seven minerals are classified as major and are 14 classified as trace. Like vitamins, it is important not to ingest more than the recommended daily amount of minerals. Several of the important minerals are discussed in the following sections.

Iron

Iron plays a key role in metabolism performance and overall health. It is important for the formation of hemoglobin and is involved in the transport of oxygen to the tissues as well as a number of biochemical reactions responsible for energy production.[16,17] Iron is absorbed by the body from iron found in the food consumed, such as meat and fish. In a healthy individual, the amount of iron absorbed by the body depends on two factors: (1) the amount of iron present in the food consumed, and (2) the body's need for iron. The total body iron is regulated by altering its rate of absorption.[16]

■ Requirements

The daily iron requirements for men are 10 mg; women require almost double that amount (18 mg) because of the iron losses of 5 to 45 mg that occur during the menstrual cycle. A typical diet contains about 6 mg of iron per 1,000 dietary calories. Men who consume about 2,000 calories per day can easily meet their daily iron requirements; however, women must consume 3,000 calories or more to meet their requirements. Because the average caloric intake of American women is about 1,660 calories per day, their average is about 10 mg of iron that results in a deficit of 8 mg. Indeed, nutritionists estimate that 30% to 50% of adult women have some degree of iron deficiency.

■ Health Consequences of Iron Deficiency

Iron deficiency causes a reduction in the size of red blood cells and the amount of hemoglobin they contain. Because hemoglobin is essential as it transports oxygen in the blood to all the tissues of the body, even in mild iron-deficiency states, having fewer hemoglobin molecules results in less oxygen delivered to the tissues. Oxygen is required for cells to produce energy. This is especially important during physical work when energy requirements increase. Those with extreme and prolonged conditions of iron deficiency—a condition referred to as *iron-deficient anemia*—will have a reduced physical working capacity and productivity. They will feel fatigued, sluggish, and lose their appetites.[16–19] The good news is that these conditions can be reversed when the body's iron requirements are restored.[17] It is prudent that women during their menstrual cycles ingest foods rich in iron to compensate for the problem of iron deficiency. These include meats, nuts, legumes, leafy green vegetables, egg yolks, oysters, and shellfish.

■ Prevention and Treatment

Inadequate nutrition is the major cause of iron deficiency. In our weight-conscious society, caloric intake is dramatically reduced, too often to health threatening levels, to acquire or maintain a desirable slenderness. The following steps can be taken to prevent iron deficiency:

1. Increase the consumption of foods that are iron-rich.

2. Increase physical activity. Doing so will achieve two things: (a) an increased caloric intake and therefore increased iron intake, and (b) help maintain a desirable body weight without severe dietary restrictions.
3. Take iron supplements when a large iron deficit exists. However, this should only be tried after consultation with a physician and an iron deficiency diagnosis is established.

■ Supplements and Health Concerns

It is important to emphasize that overconsumption of iron may be potentially harmful. There is some evidence that men with high levels of body iron stores are at an increased risk for coronary heart disease and heart failure.[18] In addition, a substantial number of individuals have a genetic abnormality (known as *hereditary hemochromatosis*) that leads to iron accumulation in the body's various tissues. Men with this abnormality experience abdominal pain and chronic fatigue; women can have menstrual dysfunction.

Some preliminary evidence supports that heavy physical activity such as sports training may increase the demand for iron and induce iron deficiency. Indeed, athletes (especially premenopausal women) may be at risk for iron deficiency.[19] If iron deficiency is present, performance usually decreases and this factor might be a strong incentive for young athletes to take iron supplements. It is essential, however, to keep in mind that: (1) iron deficiency observed in athletes is transient, occurring in the early stages of training and returning to pre-training levels within weeks; (2) iron supplements do not enhance performance in those with mild iron deficiency without anemia; and (3) iron supplements can cause excessive iron accumulation to toxic levels in the body and result in serious health problems.[2]

Sodium and Potassium

Sodium (salt) and potassium are referred to as *electrolytes*. They are dissolved in body fluids as electrically changed particles (ions). Electrolytes are involved in a number of bodily functions, including the electrical transmission of nerve signals (cell signaling), generation of the impulse in the cardiac cells that results in cardiac contraction and relaxation, muscle contraction, and fluid exchange within the body's fluid compartments.[2,28]

Potassium is found in higher concentrations within the cell (intracellular fluid), whereas sodium is concentrated outside the cell (extracellular fluid). These concentrations and the exchange of the electrolytes between the intra- and extracellular compartments are tightly controlled. Consequently, the controlled entry of sodium into the cell and the exit of potassium outside the cell have a crucial role in the generation of the heart impulse and the facilitation of the impulse throughout the heart and nerve fibers.

■ Consumption, Requirements, and Health Consequences

The daily requirement for salt is about 1.5 grams, but the typical diet in the United States and other Western countries contains about 10 times that amount. Our affinity for salt is not because of its importance, but because we acquired a taste for it. Before the invention of refrigeration, salt was a major means of preserving foods. The acquired taste for salt has been perpetuated by food manufacturing companies in their efforts to provide products to please the public's taste.

Excessive consumption of salt is implicated in the development or aggravation of hypertension (high blood pressure) in at least some people.[20] Societies from different parts of the world whose diet lacks sodium have no hypertension and no increases in blood pressure with age.[21] A progressive rise in blood pressure and hypertension is evident when people with low-salt diets and normal blood pressure adopt Western lifestyles and increase the sodium in their diet.[21] Experimental studies show that blood pressure decreases when dietary salt is restricted in hypertensive patients. The fall in blood pressure is associated with the degree of sodium restriction.[22] However, only some of the population in Western societies whose diet is high in sodium develop hypertension. This suggests that some may have a certain degree of sensitivity to sodium or that sodium excretion may be impaired.[23]

Inadequate potassium intake is also implicated in higher blood pressure.[24] These blood pressure effects appear to be more pronounced in patients consuming a high sodium diet.[24,25]

Although the association between high blood pressure and inadequate potassium intake is not as strong as with sodium,[24,25] it is recommended that an adequate dietary potassium be maintained to help regulate a normal blood pressure or lower it for those with an elevated blood pressure. Foods rich in potassium include bananas and all fruits, vegetables, beans, and unsalted nuts.

Potassium supplementation has been shown to be therapeutic in some hypertensive individuals. However, the risk of increased concentrations of potassium in blood (hyperkalemia) is a serious condition, so large dosage potassium supplements should be avoided.

■ Salt Intake and Physical Activity

Although excess salt intake is not advisable, the correct amount of salt is essential to maintain health and even sustain life. Exercising in hot environments can result in excessive loss of salt and water through sweat. Athletes can lose up to 10 pounds of water and about 8 grams of salt during strenuous activity. Consequently, muscle cramping and heat exhaustion may ensue. This is more common among "weekend exercisers" and not conditioned athletes.

The observation of cramping and heat exhaustion has prompted many coaches and athletes to consume excessive amounts of salt. However, this is not necessary. In addition to future health problems, doing so can also decrease performance. A slight increase in the demand for salt for the first two weeks of exercise in the heat may be necessary at times, especially if one sweats excessively. This can be remedied by drinking small amounts of fruit juices such as orange or tomato juice, or commercially available drinks (Gatorade, Powerade, etc.). Drinks with excessive sugars, preservatives, or other undesirable ingredients should be avoided.

Calcium

Calcium is essential in the formation and health of bones, muscle contraction, heart function, transmission of nerve impulses, regulation of blood pressure, blood clotting, and a number of other essential metabolic functions.

Calcium is readily available in the foods we eat. Foods rich in calcium include: milk and dairy products, fish, green vegetables, legumes, sesame seeds, almonds, dried figs, and some nuts. Requirements to facilitate peak bone mass are 1,300 mg/day for children (ages 9–18), 1,000 mg/day for adult men and women (ages 19–50), and 1,200 mg/day for those over the age of 50. Unfortunately, the daily calcium intake of many individuals, particularly women, is much less than the recommended values.

■ Calcium Deficiency and Osteoporosis

Osteoporosis is a condition where bones lose their mineral mass and density and progressively become porous. As the condition pro-

gresses, the bones become weaker and fractures occur easily. Healing of these fractures is very slow and, in a number of cases, incomplete. Most bone fractures occur in the spinal column, hip (neck of the femur), and wrist.

Approximately 25 million Americans are afflicted with osteoporosis. Of those, approximately 80% or more are women. Some reasons for women being more prone to osteoporosis than men are:

1. Women have smaller skeletal mass than men.
2. Rapid bone loss during and after menopause.
3. Traditionally, women are less physically active than men.

Bone loss starts at about the fourth decade in women and about the sixth in men. Women lose bone more rapidly than men, especially during 2 to 5 years immediately after menopause, with a continuous decline at a slower rate thereafter. Women can lose 3% to 5% of bone mass per year, which can lead to a total loss of between 30% and 50% during the course of their lifetime. When bone mass decreases by 30% or more below the average bone mass of healthy individuals who are in their 30s, the condition is classified as **osteoporosis**.

Osteoporosis is linked to genetic and lifestyle factors. Evidence suggests that a calcium deficiency in the diet or reduced calcium absorption by the body may be implicated in the disease.[26] Evidence also supports that decreased mechanical loading of the skeleton contributes to age-related bone loss. The bad news is that no pharmacological treatments are available to reverse the bone loss that has already taken place. The best strategy is to prevent osteoporosis.

Bone mass and bone strength increase rapidly during puberty, with a peak bone density achieved between the ages of 20 and 30. It remains constant between ages 30 and 45 and afterwards it begins to decline. The best approach to combat bone loss is to build strong bones early in life and reduce bone loss in later years. The period between ages 9 and 20 is critical in building up an optimal bone mass as a safeguard against losses later in life. Diets that are poor in calcium, alcohol consumption, smoking, and a sedentary lifestyle should be avoided in all ages but especially during puberty, when peak bone density occurs.

Table 4.2 outlines the dietary sources and functions of the major minerals.

■ WATER

Water is essential to our existence. It is vital for the formation of carbohydrates, proteins, and lipids; the digestive process; absorption and transport of nutrients and oxygen; the process of elimination of waste products out of the cells; and is the primary mechanism for heat removal.[27–29] It is found within every cell (intracellular) and between cells (extracellular), and accounts for about 50% to 70% of an individual's body weight.[27]

In normal environments, adults require about 2.5 liters of water daily. Approximately 1.2 liters of the water needs of the body are met through the intake of fluids, 1.0 liter is contained in the food we eat, and the remaining 300 ml are released when carbohydrates, proteins, and fats are metabolized.[17] Water is lost in the form of urine, feces, through the skin (mostly during sweating), and during respirations. However, in hot, humid environments the requirements for water can increase 2.4-fold, especially when work is performed in such environments. The water loss through sweating under these conditions is so severe that if water is not replenished, the body's ability to regulate temperature will be impaired and serious injury or death may occur.[17] A delicate balance in the volume of body fluids is maintained between water intake and loss.

Water is the most efficacious performance-enhancing aid.

■ Consequences of Water Loss

Water loss through sweat is a significant problem for the individual who exercises or works in a hot environment. This is especially true during the first 2 to 4 weeks of activity, before the body had a chance to acclimate.

Table 4.2 Dietary Sources and Functions of the Major Minerals

Mineral	Dietary Sources	Functions
Iron	Eggs, lean meats, green leafy vegetables, whole grains, legumes	Involved in energy metabolism
Sodium	Common salt	Nerve signal transmission, fluid balance, important electrolyte for heart function
Potassium	Bananas, leafy vegetables, potatoes, meats, milk	Nerve transmission, fluid balance, important electrolyte for heart function
Calcium	Milk and milk products, dark green vegetables	Bone formation, nerve signal transmission, heart function, blood clotting

Cooling of the body is accomplished to a major extent by the evaporation of sweat. In a hot environment, the sweat rate increases dramatically. If the environment is high in humidity, then the sweat rate is even higher. As an individual sweats, the volume of water in the body decreases. If this lost water is not replenished the consequences can be serious, ranging from a decline in physical and mental performance to electrolyte imbalance, cardiac arrhythmias, and even death. A loss of 2% to 3% of body weight in water significantly reduces the individual's aerobic capacity, especially in hot environments.[30-33] A loss of 5% of body weight or greater results in a progressive decrease in stroke volume, gradual elevation in heart rate, and a drop in blood pressure, a phenomenon known as the *cardiovascular drift*.[34] Further water losses can lead to heat stroke and possibly death.

■ Hydration During Exercise

When working or exercising in a hot environment, one must keep in mind that thirst is not a sufficient or reliable indicator of the need for water. In fact, by the time one feels thirsty, he or she is already in an early state of dehydration. Plenty of water must be taken before and during the activity to prevent dehydration. Although this is now common knowledge among athletes, too often the information is not applied correctly. Based on available evidence, the American College of Sports Medicine makes the following general recommendations on the amount and composition of fluid that should be ingested in preparation for, during, and after exercise or athletic competition[34]:

- Adequate fluid replacement helps maintain hydration and, therefore, promotes the health, safety, and optimal physical performance of individuals participating in regular physical activity.

- Individuals should consume a nutritionally balanced diet and drink adequate fluids during the 24-hour period before an event, especially during the period that includes the meal prior to exercise, to promote proper hydration before exercise or competition.

- Individuals should drink about 500 ml (about 17 ounces) of fluid about two hours before exercise to promote adequate hydration and allow time for excretion of excess ingested water.

- During exercise, athletes should start drinking early and again at regular intervals in an attempt to consume fluids at a rate sufficient to replace all of the water lost through sweating (i.e., body weight loss) or consume the maximal amount that can be tolerated.

- It is recommended that ingested fluids be cooler than ambient temperature (between 15° and 22°C [59° and 72°F]). It can be flavored to enhance palatability and promote fluid replacement. Fluids should be readily available and served in containers that allow adequate volumes to be ingested with ease and with minimal interruption of exercise.

- Addition of proper amounts of carbohydrates and/or electrolytes to a fluid replacement solution is recommended for exercise events of duration greater than 1 hour because it does not significantly impair water delivery to the body and may enhance performance. During exercise lasting less than 1 hour, there is little evidence of physiological or physical performance differences between consuming a carbohydrate-electrolyte drink and plain water.

- During intense exercise lasting longer than 1 hour, it is recommended that carbohydrates be ingested at a rate of 30 to 60 g/hour to maintain oxidation of carbohydrates and delay fatigue. This rate of carbohydrate intake can be achieved without compromising fluid delivery by drinking 600 to 1,200 ml per hour of solutions containing 4% to 8% carbohydrates. These carbohydrates can be in the form of sugars (glucose or sucrose) or starch (e.g., maltodextrin).

In addition, keep in mind the following:

- Gastric emptying increases progressively as the ingested water volume increases. To promote gastric emptying, it is advantageous to drink plenty of water prior to exercise.
- Avoid drinks that contain a lot of sugar, salt, or caffeine. If the solution of the drink consumed is more concentrated than that of the body's fluids, the drink will remain in the stomach longer and attract water. This will add to the dehydration of the individual. Researchers have shown that drinks containing over 2% sugar significantly retard water replacement that is lost during heavy exercise. Such drinks include all soft drinks. Drinks that contain caffeine (i.e., soft drinks) compound the problem because caffeine is a diuretic (it causes water loss from the body by frequent urination). The sugar content of the drink thus retards water emptying from the stomach and the caffeine contained in the drink causes water loss.
- Do not drink alcoholic beverages. Beer or any other beverage containing alcohol is not a good substitute for water replacement after exercise. Alcohol is a diuretic, so consumption of these beverages may cause greater water loss than water replacement. Keep in mind that the best drink to ingest is water. If you would rather drink a commercial product (e.g., Gatorade), mix half a glass of it with one glass of water. The sugar content in some of these drinks may be too high for optimum utilization by the body.
- The best approach is to drink plenty of water. You cannot go wrong with water.

■ Heat Illness

Excessive water loss occurs because of heavy sweating and or lack of adequate hydration when exercising in hot environments. It is common among those in poor physical condition or who are not acclimated to the hot environment. Regardless of the reason, excessive water loss will lead to the following symptoms or illnesses:

1. Muscle cramps resulting from excessive sodium (salt) loss.
2. Heat exhaustion due to large volumes of water loss.
3. Heat stroke where the body can no longer sweat. This is the most serious of the three.

Different people exhibit different symptoms, and often these symptoms appear rapidly. **Muscle cramps** are painful but not a serious condition. They are likely caused by excessive salt losses and can be easily remedied by ingesting a small amount of salt, drinking water, and cooling the body. **Heat exhaustion** is a common heat illness. Symptoms may include weakness, dizziness, heavy sweating, pale colored skin, muscle cramping, nausea, vomiting, and fainting. A decrease in blood volume consequent to profuse sweating is usually the cause. Water or commercially available drinks should be consumed immediately and the person should be taken to a shady area and cooled by wiping or spraying down the body with cool or cold water. **Heat stroke** is a serious illness. During heat stroke, the body's temperature rises to dangerous levels because of dehydration (not enough internal water for sweating to cool down the body) or an inability to dissipate heat. The symptoms are similar to heat exhaustion except that the individual does not sweat, has a hot skin temperature, hot red or dry flushed skin, rapid pulse, and difficulty breathing. The individual may act strangely, be disoriented and have hallucinations, be confused or agitated, and experience seizures and even coma. Immediate hospitalization is required. To prevent lasting organ damage, it is imperative to cool the body immediately.

■ SUMMARY

- Vitamins are essential for growth, vitality, health, general well-being, and for the prevention and cure of many health problems and diseases.
- Vitamin deficiency leads to poor health and even death. There is no evidence to support that megadoses of vitamins improve physical or mental performance.
- Multivitamin supplements provide only a fraction of what a diet rich in fruits, vegetables, and whole grains provides. Therefore, multivitamin supplements should never be confused as an alternative to healthy diet.
- Minerals are inorganic elements that have an important role in the metabolism and proper function of the body. Conversely, mineral deficiencies can be unhealthy.
- Some individuals may need mineral supplements, but it is important that they are consumed under the advice of a physician.
- Water is essential to our existence. It is vital for the formation of carbohydrates, proteins, and lipids; digestion, absorption, and transportation of nutrients and oxygen;

and elimination waste products out of the cells; and is the primary mechanism for regulating body temperature.

- Water loss through sweat is a significant problem for the individual who exercise or work in a hot environment. This is especially true during the first 2 to 4 weeks, before the body has a chance to acclimate.
- Excessive water loss has immediate deleterious effects on the body and, if not replaced, may cause death. Thus, adequate fluid replacement must be practiced to help maintain hydration, and thereby promote the health, safety, and optimal physical performance of individuals participating in regular physical activity.

■ REFERENCES

1. Vitamin preparations as dietary supplements and as therapeutic agents. Council on Scientific Affairs. *JAMA* 1987;257(14):1929–1936.
2. Wang TJ, Pencina MJ, Booth SL, et al. Vitamin D deficiency and risk of cardiovascular disease. *Circulation* 2008;117(4):503–511.
3. Molavi B, Mehta JL. Oxidative stress in cardiovascular disease: molecular basis of its deleterious effects, its detection, and therapeutic considerations. *Curr Opin Cardiol* 2004;19(5):488–493.
4. Griendling KK, FitzGerald GA. Oxidative stress and cardiovascular injury: Part I: basic mechanisms and in vivo monitoring of ROS. *Circulation* 2003;108(16):1912–1916.
5. Murray RK, Granner DK, Mayes PA. *Harpers' Biochemistry*. Stamford, CT: Simon & Schuster; 1996.
6. Greenberg ER, Baron JA, Tosteson TD, et al. A clinical trial of antioxidant vitamins to prevent colorectal adenoma. Polyp Prevention Study Group. *N Engl J Med* 1994;331(3): 141–147.

7. Greenberg ER, Baron JA, Karagas MR, et al. Mortality associated with low plasma concentration of beta carotene and the effect of oral supplementation. *JAMA* 1996;275(9): 699–703.

8. Rapola JM, Virtamo J, Ripatti S, et al. Effect of vitamin E and beta carotene on the incidence of angina pectoris. A randomized, double-blind, controlled trial. *JAMA* 1996;275(9): 693–698.

9. Hennekens CH, Buring JE, Peto R. Antioxidant vitamins—benefits not yet proved. *N Engl J Med* 1994;330(15):1080–1081.

10. Ballmer PE, Stahelin HB. Beta carotene, vitamin E, and lung cancer. *N Engl J Med* 1994;331(9):612–613.

11. Bjelakovic G, Nikolova D, Gluud LL, et al. Mortality in randomized trials of antioxidant supplements for primary and secondary prevention: systematic review and meta-analysis. *JAMA* 2007;297(8):842–857.

12. Gibbons RJ, Abrams J, Chatterjee K, et al. ACC/AHA 2002 guideline update for the management of patients with chronic stable angina—summary article: a report of the American College of Cardiology/American Heart Association Task Force on Practice Guidelines (Committee on the Management of Patients with Chronic Stable Angina). *Circulation* 2003;107(1):149–158.

13. Mosca L, Appel LJ, Benjamin EJ, et al. American Heart Association. Evidence-based guidelines for cardiovascular disease prevention in women. *Circulation*. 2004;109: 672–693.

14. Singh A, Papanicoulaou DA, Lawrence LL, et al. Neuroendocrine responses to running in women after zinc and vitamin E supplementation. *Med Sci Sports Exerc* 1999;31(4): 536–542.

15. Virk RS, Dunton NJ, Young JC, Leklem JE. Effect of vitamin B-6 supplementation on fuels, catecholamines, and amino acids during exercise in men. *Med Sci Sports Exerc* 1999;31(3):400–408.

16. Guyton AC. *Textbook of Medical Physiology*. Philadelphia: W.B. Saunders; 1991.

17. McArdle WD, Katch FI, Katch VL. *Exercise Physiology*, 5th ed. Baltimore: Lippincott Williams & Wilkins; 2001.

18. Herbert V, Shaw S, Jayatilleke E, Stopler-Kasdan T. Most free-radical injury is iron-related: It is promoted by iron, hemin, holoferritin and vitamin C, and inhibited by desferoxamine and apoferritin. *Stem Cells* 1994;12(3):289–303.

19. Frederickson LA, Puhl JL, Runyan WS. Effects of training on indices of iron status of young female cross-country runners. *Med Sci Sports Exerc* 1983;15(4):271–276.

20. Denton D. *The Hunger for Salt*. New York: Springer-Verlag; 1982.

21. Maddocks I. Blood pressures in Melanesians. *Med J Aust* 1967;1(22):1123–1126.

22. Cutler JA, Follmann D, Elliott L, Suh I. An overview of randomized trials of sodium reduction and blood pressure. *Hypertension* 1991;17(1 Suppl):I27–I33. (see comments)

23. Hamet P, Mongeau E, Lambert J, et al. Interactions among calcium, sodium, and alcohol intake as determinants of blood pressure. *Hypertension* 1991;17(1 Suppl):I150–I154.

24. Whelton PK, He J, Cutler JA, et al. Effects of oral potassium on blood pressure. Meta-analysis of randomized controlled clinical trials. *JAMA* 1997;277(20):1624–1632. (see comments)

25. Zoccali C, Cumming AM, Hutcheson MJ, et al. Effects of potassium on sodium balance, renin, noradrenaline and arterial pressure. *J Hypertens* 1985;3(1):67–72.

26. Heaney RP, Gallagher JC, Johnston CC, et al. Calcium nutrition and bone health in the elderly. *Am J Clin Nutr* 1982;36(5 Suppl):986–1013.

27. Antonio J, Jeffrey SR. *Sports Supplements*. Baltimore: Lippincott Williams & Wilkins; 2001.

28. Kleiner SM. Water: an essential but overlooked nutrient. *J Am Diet Assoc* 1999; 99(2):200–206.

29. Beetham WP Jr, Buskirk ER. Effects of dehydration, physical conditioning and heat acclimatization on the response to passive tilting. *J Appl Physiol* 1958;13(3):465–468.

30. Buskirk ER, Iampietro PF, Bass DE. Work performance after dehydration: effects of physical conditioning and heat acclimatization. *J Appl Physiol* 1958;12(2):189–194.

31. Kozlowski S, Saltin B. Effect of sweat loss on body fluids. *J Appl Physiol* 1964;19:1119–1124.

32. Saltin B. Aerobic and anaerobic work capacity after dehydration. *J Appl Physiol* 1964;19:1114–1118.

33. Ekelund LG. Circulatory and respiratory adaptation during prolonged exercise of moderate intensity in the sitting position. *Acta Physiol Scand* 1967;69(4):327–340.

34. Convertino VA, Armstrong LE, Coyle EF, et al. American College of Sports Medicine Position Stand. Exercise and fluid replacement. *Med Sci Sports Exerc* 1996;28(1):i–vii.

Muscular and Cardiovascular Systems and Exercise-Related Adaptations

Perhaps the most misunderstood system in the relationship between cardiovascular diseases and physical activity is the muscular system. However, the muscular system is the reason for all physiologic changes that lead to better health; it is the muscular system that makes it all possible. Changes in the body that lead to better health are the result of the increased muscular demands during physical work.

All organs adapt to support the muscles and meet this increased energy demand. The heart thus must get stronger in order to pump more blood to the working muscles, the vessels must get more efficient in delivering the blood and nutrients to the muscles, and the metabolic systems must form and utilize energy sources more efficiently to meet the increased metabolic demand of the working muscles. Indeed, without muscular work, there is no need for the heart to pump more blood and no need for more energy.

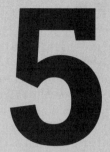

The Muscular System

We humans are able to move because of a sublime interaction of energy, chemical reaction, cell signaling, and the conscious and unconscious tensing or relaxing of the tissue fibers that comprise the muscular system. Movement becomes possible as certain muscles contract while reciprocal muscles relax. It is this well-coordinated effort of muscle relaxation and contraction that allows us to walk, jump, lift an object, or simply smile. Other functions such as digestion, heartbeat, and breathing also involve muscle contraction and relaxation, although we are less aware of this. This chapter explores the different types of muscles and their functions, especially as they relate to overall health.

■ MUSCLE TYPES AND FIBERS

It is obvious that physical activity is impossible without muscular action. Perhaps not as obvious is that muscles and muscular action play an integral role in the metabolism, structure, and function of the cardiovascular system and the overall health of the organism. It is the metabolic needs of the working skeletal muscles that demand the involvement of all other systems in the body. As a result of this challenge, all systems involved make specific adaptations to meet the particular demands imposed by the working muscles. Consequently, these systems—including the muscular system—become more efficient in performing their respective tasks and more resilient to injury and disease. Furthermore, these adaptations are dictated by the type of work performed by the muscles. For example, the types of muscular work (aerobic versus anaerobic) will dictate the specific adaptations in blood pressure, heart size, and metabolism. A general understanding of muscle structure and function is important to understand and appreciate the interaction between muscles, metabolism, and health.

Skeletal Muscles

The muscular system of the human body is comprised of over 650 skeletal muscles accounting for approximately 50% of body weight.[1,2] The main function of this system is to create movement. This is accomplished by an elaborate lever system created as muscles, which are attached to bones by tough connective tissue called **tendons**, move. This muscle-bone arrangement allows bones to move in a precise manner as dictated by the contracting muscles (**Figure 5.1**). Consequently, all movement becomes possible. For example, the extension of the lower arm is accomplished by the contraction of the triceps while an opposite movement is accomplished by the biceps.

In addition to making movement possible, muscles have other functions. For example, they stabilize the skeletal structure and provide postural support. They produce heat and help the body maintain a constant temperature. Muscles use energy even at rest. This increases the daily caloric expenditure and therefore fewer calories are left to be stored as fat. Muscles also help return the blood from the legs back to the heart. This is accomplished by the muscles of the legs that squeeze the veins with each contraction, thus pushing the blood towards the heart and then to be cycled back through the entire body.[1]

Muscle Fibers

Muscles are comprised of thousands of fibers bundled together to form a unit. Each muscle fiber contains even smaller units called **myofibrils**. It is these myofibrils that contain the actual mechanism of muscle contraction. This mechanism consists of four proteins: **actin**, **myosin**, **troponin**, and **tropomyosin**. As will

Figure 5.1   Structure of skeletal muscle.

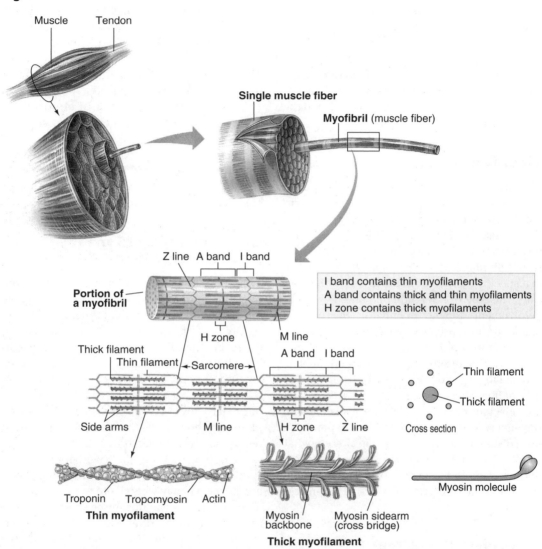

be discussed later, the interaction of these proteins regulates the myofibrils that makes muscular contraction possible (see Figure 5.1).

The mechanism and interaction of these four muscle proteins are the same for all muscle fibers. However, fibers possess unique properties that allow them to perform different types of work. Work that muscles perform can be generally categorized by the duration and intensity, the two factors that determine where and how much energy is necessary to perform the work (see Chapter 2). Accordingly, the muscles are equipped with two basic types of fibers. One is designed to perform low-intensity work over a long duration and the other is for high-intensity work over a relatively short duration. The two basic muscle fibers are the **slow-twitch** or **Type I fiber** and the **fast-twitch** or **Type II fiber**. Type II fibers are subdivided into *intermediate fibers*. As their name suggests, the characteristics of these fibers are somewhere in between the slow-twitch and the fast-twitch.

Fiber Recruitment

The different characteristics possessed by each type of fibers allow the muscle to perform within a wide range of work intensity and duration. Muscles accomplish this by selective recruitment of fibers for the task at hand. That is, not all fibers of a particular muscle engage in a specific task at the same time. On the contrary, the type of fiber, number, and percent of involvement depend mainly on the task at hand. Furthermore, fibers may engage and disengage at different times during work as dictated by the intensity of work and muscle (fiber) fatigue. In other words, the number and type of fibers best equipped for the task at hand are selected. Think of it as a car transmission. Engagement of the different gears depends on the speed of the automobile. In a somewhat similar but more elaborate fashion, muscle fibers engage and disengage based on the intensity, duration, and type of work. This makes good sense.

Characteristics of Type I (Slow-Twitch) Fibers

These fibers are mainly aerobic fibers. In other words, they are engaged by the muscle to contract predominately when oxygen is available. Thus, the required energy (adenosine triphosphate [ATP]) is produced via the aerobic pathways and are derived predominately from the metabolism of fats. Although they are

capable to perform anaerobically, Type I fibers' capacity for anaerobic metabolism is relatively limited. They are characterized by their ability to sustain work of low to moderate intensities over long durations. Type I fibers would be utilized in activities that include long distance running, swimming, biking, etc.

To accomplish this sustained effort, type I fibers contain certain properties that are conducive to aerobic metabolism. These properties include a higher activity of the enzymes that are responsible for aerobic metabolism (oxidative enzymes), more capillaries per fiber (higher blood supply), and more mitochondria.

Characteristics of Type II (Fast-Twitch) Fibers

Type II fibers are mainly anaerobic. Their contractions are explosive and generate more force but do not last a long time. Their blood supply is not as rich as that of the slow-twitch fibers and their fuel is predominately from carbohydrates, derived via a process that requires no oxygen (anaerobic) known as *glycolysis* (Greek for breakdown of glucose). They are thus rich in the anaerobic enzymes. These fibers are heavily used during activities that require explosive speeds or heavy work over a short period of time. Such activities include sprinting, shot-putting, discuss throwing, jumping, lifting a heavy weight, etc.

Type II fibers can further be subdivided into two intermediate fibers: *Type IIA* (or fast-oxidative-glycolytic [FOG]) and *Type IIB* (or fast-glycolytic [FG]) fibers. As the name implies, Type IIA fibers possess both oxidative and glycolytic properties. This makes them more versatile in the sense that they can perform relatively high-intensity activities and still derive a considerable portion of the required ATP via the aerobic pathways.

On the other hand, the Type IIB fibers have a very high capacity to perform anaerobically and a very low capacity for aerobic work. Those fibers are recruited heavily when the exercise intensity is near maximal. To further clarify the aerobic and anaerobic capacity of each fiber, the fiber with the most oxidative capacity is the Type I, followed by Type IIA and then Type IIB. Conversely, the fiber with the most anaerobic capacity is Type IIB, followed by Type IIA, and lastly Type I.[3] Some of the characteristics of the three types fibers are presented in **Table 5.1**.

Who Possesses What?

Do we all have these fibers? Do some people have more of one than the other? The answer is yes to both of these questions. We all have both types of fibers, but the percentage of each varies. For example, between 60% and 85% of the leg muscles of marathoners, long-distance runners, and cross country skiers are slow-twitch (Type I) fibers. On the other hand, 60% to 70% of the fibers for sprinters, discus, and javelin throwers, and shot-putters are Type II (fast-twitch) fibers (**Figure 5.2**).[3–9]

Can Fibers Be Altered?

Older studies support that changing from one fiber type to another through specific training is not possible, yet other studies advocate that fibers change if exposed to a certain type of training.[10,11] Which data are correct? It depends on the interpretation of the findings.

Changes are more likely to occur in Type IIA (intermediate) fibers. Let us take the example of an individual who possesses a relatively large percentage of Type IIA fibers (fast-oxidative-glycolytic) on the legs. If this individual engages in aerobic type of training, the activity of the aerobic enzymes along with all that fosters aerobic work capacity of these fibers will be

Table 5.1 Fibers and Their Characteristics

	Fiber Type			
Characteristic	**Type I**	**Type II**	**Type IIA**	**Type IIB**
Fiber diameter	Small	Large	Large	Large
Mitochondria density	High	Low	High	Low
Capillary density	High	Low	Medium	Low
Glycogen stores	Low	High	High	High
Triglycerides stores	High	Low	Medium	Low
Glycolytic enzyme activity	Low	High	High	High
Oxidative enzyme activity	High	Low	High	Low
Contraction time	Slow	Very Fast	Fast	Very Fast
Force production	Low	High	High	High
Resistance to fatigue	High	Low	Moderate	Low

Source: Essen B, Jensson E, Henriksson J, et al. Metabolic characteristics of fibre types in human skeletal muscle. *Acta Physiol Scand* 1975;95(2):153–165.

Figure 5.2 Distribution of Type II and Type I fibers in muscles of (A) men and (B) women athletes. Although there is some degree of variation, endurance athletes tend to have greater percentages of Type I fibers, whereas non-endurance athletes have greater percentages of Type II fibers.

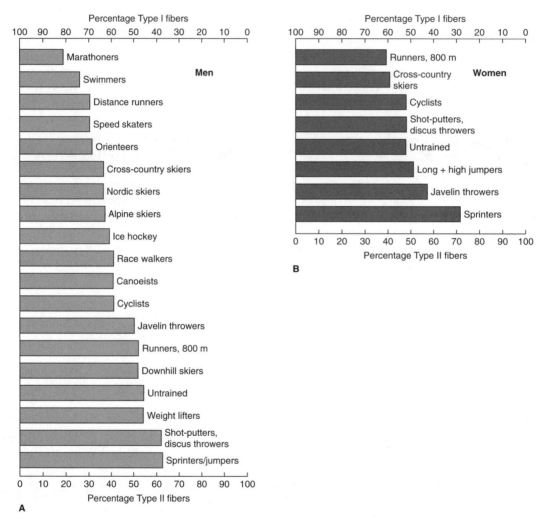

enhanced. Conversely, if the individual engages in anaerobic training, the glycolytic capacity of these fibers will be enhanced. Changes, however, require a great volume of work.

So, do fibers change with training? If change is defined as an increase in the ability of the fiber to perform a task not particularly designed for them, there is change. If change is defined as the fibers switching from predominantly Type I to Type II or vice versa, then the answer is a bit more complicated and not yet determined. Stating it in another way, change along the continuum within a fiber clearly occurs, but muscle fiber transformation from one fiber type to another is doubtful.

Type IIA muscle fibers possess aerobic or anaerobic properties. When these fibers are exposed to work (aerobic or anaerobic), they will adapt accordingly to accommodate the work imposed upon them. Type IIA fibers thus can behave more like aerobic or anaerobic fibers based on the work they endure.

Muscle Contraction: The Sliding Filament Model

Muscular contraction is the result of myofibril shortening. One way to visualize how muscles contract is to think of an expandable rod, like a curtain rod. Such a rod consists of two parts where each section has a specific length and one section slides into the other, allowing a change in the total length of the rod. Note that the actual length of each one remains the same, but the overall length of the rod can change according to the distance one piece moves inside the other.

This action is similar to what occurs with muscle contractions. As previously mentioned, myofibrils within the muscle fibers contain four different proteins. Two of these proteins (actin and myosin) are arranged in a way that resembles the two sliding parts of the rod. By design, they can bond with each another. The other two proteins (troponin and tropomyosin) are embedded between the actin and myosin to control the bond between them.

Each myosin filament consists of a tail and a head. Myosin heads, also known as **cross bridges**, are projected towards the actin filaments. In the resting state, troponin and tropomyosin block the sites and the bond between the head of the myosin protein cannot tightly bond to the actin site. When the muscle is activated to contract, troponin and tropomyosin interact, causing a position change in tropomyosin. This action leaves the actin sites exposed and the head of the myosin now bonds tightly with actin. The myosin heads then move in such a way that they pull on the actin, causing a sliding action similar to the action of two rods that slide past each other without changing length of each part. This action causes the length of the muscle to shorten (contract). As the bond is released, the two proteins slide back to their original position, resembling the two rods in an extended position. As thousands of these myofibrils go through the action of proteins sliding past one another, the muscles contract or relax. This is known as the **Sliding Filament Model** which was first proposed by Huxley in 1969[12] and later expanded upon by other researchers (**Figure 5.3**).[13,14]

Blood Supply

Muscles are designed to perform work that can vary in intensity, duration, and frequency. To meet these requirements, they need energy. Muscles have a rich blood supply to provide sufficient nutrients to accomplish these tasks. Muscle fibers are surrounded by **capillaries**, which are the smallest blood vessels that guarantee adequate oxygen and nutrients for that fiber. In sedentary individuals, each muscle fiber is surrounded by three to four capillaries; athletes have five to seven capillaries surrounding each muscle fiber.[1]

Muscle also has the capacity to control its own blood supply. During exercise, the arteries of the working muscles dilate and capillaries that are collapsed while the muscles are at rest now open to receive oxygenated blood. At maximum exercise, blood flow to the muscles can increase as much as 25 to 50 times compared to resting values.[1,15] Contractions of the muscles also serve another purpose. They

Figure 5.3   The sliding filament model.

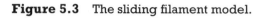

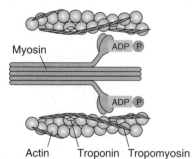

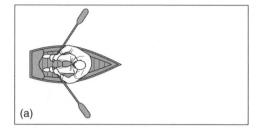

Myosin

ADP P

ADP P

Actin   Troponin   Tropomyosin

Resting

(a)

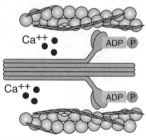

Ca^{++}

ADP P

Ca^{++}

ADP P

Step 1: Action potential

(b)

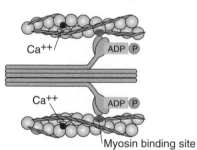

Ca^{++}

ADP P

Ca^{++}

ADP P

Myosin binding site

Step 2: Myosin-actin binding

(c) Catch

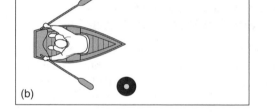

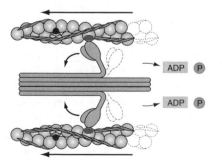

ADP P

ADP P

Step 3: Power stroke

(d) Drive

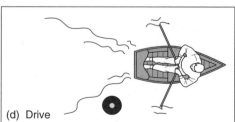

Figure 5.3 Continued

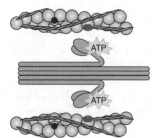

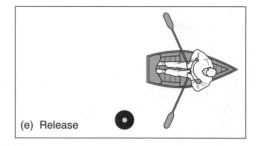

Step 4: ATP binding and actin-myosin release

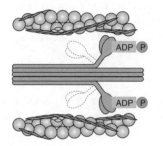

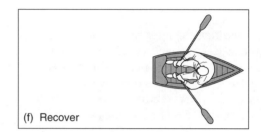

Step 5: ATP cleavage

squeeze the veins and return the blood back to the heart. This action allows for blood to quickly cycled through the heart and lungs, and then return to the muscles enriched with oxygen and nutrients.

Isometric muscular contractions that exceed 60% of the maximal force a muscle can generally cause a collapse of the blood vessels supplying blood to the contracting muscle. During such contractions, the energy to the muscle is provided by the anaerobic systems.

Muscle Soreness

Muscle soreness often follows after a day or two of intense exercise or work. It is more likely to occur in individuals engaging in new and usually intense activities, such as weight training or fast running. It also can occur in trained individuals following an interruption in their training or a change from one activity/sport to another.

Several myths surround the issue of muscle soreness. One misconception is that muscle soreness is due to lactic acid accumulation. It is known, however, that lactic acid is removed from the muscle within 40 to 60 minutes following an intense bout of exercise (muscle soreness usually occurs within a day or two.) Another misconception is muscle soreness signifies a "break-down" of the muscle. Furthermore, some believe that this is a "necessary evil" because a muscle has to be "broken-down" before it can be rebuilt to a stronger one. This myth feeds the "no pain, no gain" mentality of the past decades.

What are the reasons for muscle soreness? We do not know the precise causes; however,

Figure 5.4 An example of an eccentric contraction.

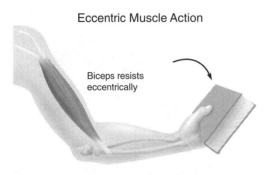

Eccentric Muscle Action

Biceps resists
eccentrically

we do know that the intensity of soreness and how long it lasts depend largely on the intensity and type of exercise performed. It is well established that exercises that involve **eccentric contractions** (activities that provide resistance against the elongation of the muscle; e.g., biceps muscle when lowering an object from the chest to the table [**Figure 5.4**]), are more likely to cause soreness than **concentric contractions** (activities where muscles shorten under tension; e.g., lifting the object from the table to your chest [**Figure 5.5**]).[16–18]

To some degree, muscle soreness is the result of small tears or damage to the muscle,[16–18] but

Figure 5.5 Concentric muscle contraction.

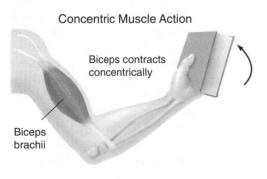

Concentric Muscle Action

Biceps contracts
concentrically

Biceps
brachii

certainly this damage is not necessary for the building of stronger muscle. Think about it. If that was the case, muscle would stop getting bigger and stronger as its soreness dissipated. Indeed, the opposite is true. Muscle soreness dissipates after about a week of engaging regularly in that activity, yet muscle strength, size, and performance continue to increase for weeks to come. In fact, it takes more than a week to see improvements. Muscle soreness also may be the result of some inflammation that occurs within the muscle fibers, muscle spasms, fluid retention causing pressure, and mild damage to the connective tissue from overstretching or a combination of the aforementioned factors.

■ Avoiding Muscle Soreness

There are several ways to avoid or at least reduce muscle soreness.

- Begin an exercise program gradually. Start with low intensity exercises and build gradually to a more intense regimen.
- If you are engaging in weight training, avoid working on eccentric exercises/contractions. Eccentric exercises or contractions are those that provide resistance against the relaxation of the muscle. It is the opposite of contraction. Such work is made possible by some machines and was hailed to be superior to the "normal" muscle contractions. Eccentric contractions cause more soreness and are not superior to the regular contractions.
- Low intensity work, hot baths, whirlpool spa, or anything that promotes blood flow to the affected muscle (such as massage) also helps to reduce the soreness and enhance recovery. The reason for this is that the heat increases blood flow to the muscles so recovery or perhaps "healing" occurs quicker.

Muscular Hypertrophy

It is well known that muscles respond to different work by adapting to accommodate the demand imposed upon them. These adaptations are specific to the type of work, muscular strength, or muscular endurance (see Chapter 2). Briefly, if a muscle or groups of muscles are exposed to exercises that require a great deal of strength (weight training with low repetitions and heavy resistance), accelerated protein synthesis is triggered and these muscles increase in size and strength to accommodate the excess weight. Conversely, if muscles are exposed to work that requires repetitive work with light resistance, they change accordingly to accommodate for the type of work.

Exposure of a muscle or group of muscles to adequate resistance training stimulates visible muscle growth in skeletal muscles, known as muscle **hypertrophy**. This adaptation is relatively similar for men and women, young and old.[19]

> Muscle hypertrophy is an adaptation to an increased work demand. It is independent of gender and age.

An interesting question is whether the increased muscle size and consequently muscular strength is the result of additional fibers created (known as *hyperplasia*) or the thickening of the existing fibers, or both? This has been the subject of research and great debate over the years, especially during the 1980s. Although possible hyperplasia may take place in some animal models, research supports that the formation of additional fibers in humans is unlikely. Therefore, increases in muscle strength and size in humans are the result of enlargement of existing muscle fibers.

> Muscle strength is the result of an increase in the diameter of the fibers and not their number.

Muscular Atrophy

Muscle atrophy means muscle degeneration or decline in strength and size from a lack of use or other causes. Muscle atrophy is an observable phenomenon that occurs within a relatively short time in muscles that are not used. The best example is the decline in the size of a broken limb as a result of a few weeks of immobilization imposed by plaster cast.

The reason for this decline or atrophy is based on a simple logic. That is, the body will respond to a demand (stimulus) imposed upon it and make the necessary changes to accommodate for this demand. In the absence of a stimulus, there is no response. In the case of a limb in the cast, the arm is not used and, therefore, there is no stimulus to trigger protein synthesis. The limb thus atrophies.

Age-Related Muscle Atrophy

Aging is associated with losses in muscle size and strength. It is estimated that we lose 10% of muscle mass from ages 25 to 50. After the age of 50, muscle mass loss is accelerated and by age 80 years, we lose another 40% of muscle mass.

The loss of muscle mass and strength observed with aging is not totally a function of aging, but can be the result of diminished use that accompanies aging.[20] Muscles respond to exercise training equally for young and old. Studies demonstrated that 10 weeks of weight training of nursing home residents (average age 87.1 years) resulted in significant improvements in muscle size and strength. The gains are similar to what have been observed in younger adults. Muscles thus respond to training regardless of age.[21–23]

Muscle atrophy and decline in strength are not entirely a function of aging but the result of diminished use.

■ TYPES OF MUSCULAR CONTRACTIONS

Muscles are capable of producing three types of contractions: isometric, isotonic, and isokinetic.

Isometric (Static) Muscle Contraction

Isometric is derived from the words *iso*, the Greek word for equal, and *metric*, Greek for measure or length. Indeed, during an **isometric** (or static) contraction, resistance is applied to the muscle or muscle group, but the muscle maintains a constant length and no joint movement occurs. Some even question the term muscular contraction applied to isometric state of the muscle, because the length of the muscle does not change. An example of an isometric contraction is pushing against an immovable object such as a wall (**Figure 5.6**).

Isometric contractions were popularized several decades ago and were hailed as the solution to building strength and fitness for busy executives. However, strength gains from isometric contractions are not practical because the increased strength observed is only at the joint angles where the contraction occurs.

Isotonic (Dynamic) Muscular Contraction

This contraction is characterized by movement of the joint as a result of muscles contracting. **Isotonic** (Greek for equal tension or resistance) suggests that the movement about the joint occurs under equal resistance. Indeed, resistance is constant throughout the range of

Figure 5.6 Isometric muscle contraction.

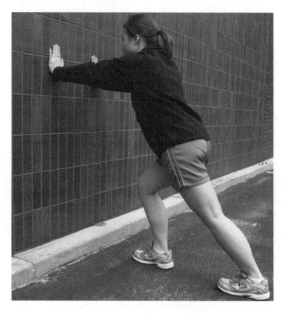

movement during dynamic isotonic contractions. For example, a 50-pound weight remains constant throughout the lift.

Isotonic contractions can further be classified as concentric or eccentric. As previously discussed, concentric contractions are those that occur when the length of the muscle involved in the contractions shortens (see Figure 5.5). Conversely, eccentric contractions are those where the muscle involved is lengthened (see Figure 5.4).

Isokinetic Contraction

Isokinetic (Greek for constant speed) **contractions** do not occur naturally. Rather they are artificially created contractions by the use of an apparatus. To put it in other terms, when a weight is lifted throughout the range of joint, the weight is constant but the resistance offered by the weight changes. This change in resistance is the result of changes in the mechanical advantage of

Figure 5.7 An isokinetic exercise apparatus.

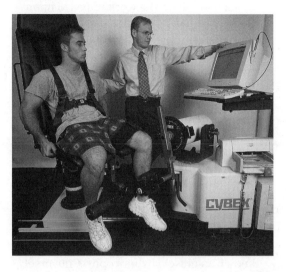

the joint as it moves. As the resistance decreases, the speed of contraction increases.

In isokinetic contractions, the apparatus maintains a constant speed of contraction by maintaining a constant resistance throughout the full range of motion. The theoretical advantage of isokinetic contractions is that it allows strength development throughout the range of motion by forcing the muscle to develop maximal tension throughout its full range of motion (**Figure 5.7**).

Excitation-Contraction Coupling

The mechanical and physiological events fundamental to the sliding filament are proposed in a model referred to as the **excitation-contraction coupling**. The events as we currently know them are presented here.[14,24]

■ Excitation

- A stimulus generated by a motor neuron (action potential) causes the release of the neurotransmitter acetylcholine into the synaptic clef of the **neuromuscular junction** (where neuron and muscle meet).
- Acetylcholine stimulates an impulse that reaches the muscle and spreads quickly throughout the muscle fiber by an elaborate channel system, which transverses throughout the fibers known as T-tubules. In turn, calcium is released.

■ Coupling

As you recall, in the resting state, the actin and myosin proteins are weakly connected. Actin sites where the myosin heads hook onto are blocked by the protein tropomyosin. After the impulse is generated and relatively large quantities of calcium are released, the following events take place.

- Calcium binds to troponin.
- This causes a shift in the position of the protein tropomyosin so that the actin sites are now exposed to the myosin heads.
- A strong bond is now formed between the actin and myosin proteins.
- Energy is released (ATP is used) and the two proteins are mutually attracted to each other. The myosin heads (cross bridges) now pull on the actin filaments, causing them to slide. Muscle contraction thereby occurs.
- Muscle relaxation occurs as ATP is used and ADP is formed (ATP to ADT). The process is repeated with a fresh amount of ATP released from the cross bridges.

Muscle Fatigue

Muscle fatigue is defined as a decline in the maximal force generated by a muscle. The causes of muscle fatigue vary with the type of work performed. For example, muscle fatigue from very intense work is the result of metabolite accumulation. Fatigue from low-intensity, long duration exercise such as running a marathon involves the failure of excitation-contraction coupling system.

■ SUMMARY

- All human movement is accomplished by an elaborate lever system created by approximately 650 skeletal muscles that are attached to bones by tough connective tissue called tendons. This muscle-bone arrangement allows bones to move in a precise manner as dictated by the contracting or relaxing muscles.
- Muscles are comprised of thousands of fibers bundled together to form a unit. Each muscle fiber contains even smaller units called myofibrils.
- Myofibrils contain the actual mechanism of muscle contraction. Muscular contraction is the result of an interaction of four proteins contained in the myofibrils: actin, myosin, troponin, and tropomyosin.
- Two basic muscle fibers have been identified: the slow-twitch or Type I fiber and the fast-twitch or Type II fiber. The slow-twitch type is designed for long duration–low intensity work (aerobic) and the fast-twitch fiber is designed for a high intensity–short duration activities (anaerobic work).
- There are also further subdivisions of the Type II fibers that are referred to as the intermediate. As the name suggests, the characteristics of these fibers are somewhere between the slow-twitch and the fast-twitch types.
- Type IIA muscle fibers possess both aerobic and anaerobic properties. When these fibers are exposed to work (aerobic or anaerobic), they will adapt accordingly to accommodate the work imposed upon them. Type IIA fibers thus can behave more like aerobic or anaerobic fibers based on the work to which they are exposed.
- Some researchers believe that a change from one fiber type to another through proper training is possible. Others, however, think that fibers do not change but only enhance their innate characteristics to better accommodate the work imposed upon them. Future studies are necessary to resolve this issue.
- Exposure of a muscle or group of muscles to adequate resistance training stimulates visible muscle growth in skeletal muscles, known as muscle hypertrophy. Conversely, cessation of such activity or total inactivity leads to muscle atrophy.
- Muscles are capable of producing three types of contractions: isometric, isotonic, and isokinetic.
- During an isometric contraction, resistance is applied to the muscle or muscle group, but the muscle maintains a constant length and no joint movement occurs.
- Isotonic contraction is characterized by movement of the joint as a result of muscles contracting. Isotonic contractions can be classified further as concentric or eccentric.
- Concentric contractions are those that occur when the length of the muscle involved in the contractions shortens. Eccentric contractions are those that the muscle involved is lengthened.
- Isokinetic contractions are artificially created by using an apparatus. The apparatus maintains a constant speed of contraction by changing the resistance.

■ REFERENCES

1. McArdle WD, Katch FI, Katch VL. *Exercise Physiology*, 5th ed. Baltimore: Lippincott Williams & Wilkins; 2001.
2. Johnson T, Klueber KM. Skeletal muscle following tonic overload: functional and structural analysis. *Med Sci Sports Exerc* 1991; 23(1):49–55.
3. Essen B, Jansson E, Henriksson J, et al. Metabolic characteristics of fibre types in human skeletal muscle. *Acta Physiol Scand* 1975; 95(2):153–165.
4. Thorstensson A, Larsson L, Tesch P, Karlsson J. Muscle strength and fiber composition in athletes and sedentary men. *Med Sci Sports* 1977;9(1):26–30.
5. Thorstensson A. Observations on strength training and detraining. *Acta Physiol Scand* 1977;100(4):491–493.
6. Komi PV, Rusko H, Vos J, Vinko V. Anaerobic performance capacity in athletes. *Acta Physiol Scand* 1977;100(1):107–114.
7. Gollnick PD, Armstrong RB. Enzyme activity and fiber composition in skeletal muscle of untrained and trained men. *J Appl Physiol* 1972;33(3):312–319.
8. Costill DL, Fink WJ, Pollock ML. Muscle fiber composition and enzyme activities of elite distance runners. *Med Sci Sports* 1976;8(2): 96–100.
9. Burke ER, Cerny F, Cestili D, Fink W. Characteristics of skeletal muscle in competitive cyclists. *Med Sci Sports* 1977;9(2):109–112.
10. Schantz P, Billeter R, Henriksson J, Jansson E. Training-induced increase in myofibrillar ATPase intermediate fibers in human skeletal muscle. *Muscle Nerve* 1982;5(8):628–636.
11. Demirel HA, Powers SK, Naito H, et al. Exercise-induced alterations in skeletal muscle myosin heavy chain phenotype: dose-response relationship. *J Appl Physiol* 1999;86(3):1002–1008.
12. Foss M, Kateyian S. *Fox's Physiological Basis for Exercise and Sport*, 6th ed. Boston: McGraw-Hill; 1998.
13. Huxley HE. The mechanism of muscular contraction. *Science* 1969;164(886):1356–1365.
14. Rayment I, Rypniewski W, Schmidt-Base K, et al. Three-dimensional structure of myosin subfragment-1: a molecular motor. *Science* 1993;261(5117):50–58.
15. Rayment I, Rypniewski W, Schmidt-Base K, et al. Structure of the actin-myosin complex and its implications for muscle contraction. *Science* 1993;261(5117):58–65.
16. Teague BN, Schwane JA. Effect of intermittent eccentric contractions on symptoms of muscle microinjury. *Med Sci Sports Exerc* 1995;27(10):1378–1384.
17. Sorichter S, Mair J, Koller A, et al. Skeletal troponin I as a marker of exercise-induced muscle damage. *J Appl Physiol* 1997;83(4): 1076–1082.
18. Lieber RL, Friden J. Muscle damage is not a function of muscle force but active muscle strain. *J Appl Physiol* 1993;74(2):520–526.
19. Charette SL, McEvoy L, Pyka G, et al. Muscle hypertrophy response to resistance training in older women. *J Appl Physiol* 1991;70(5): 1912–1916.
20. Larsson L. Physical training effects on muscle morphology in sedentary males at different ages. *Med Sci Sports Exerc* 1982;14(3): 203–206.
21. Sullivan VK, Powers DS, Criswell N, et al. Myosin heavy chain composition in young and old rat skeletal muscle: effects of endurance exercise. *J Appl Physiol* 1995;78(6): 2115–2120.
22. Powers SK, Lawler J, Criswell D, et al. Aging and respiratory muscle metabolic plasticity: effects of endurance training. *J Appl Physiol* 1992;72(3):1068–1073.
23. Powers SK, Lawler J, Criswell D, et al. Age-related changes in enzyme activity in the rat diaphragm. *Respir Physiol* 1991;83(1):1–9.
24. Vale RD. Getting a grip on myosin. *Cell* 1994; 78(5):733–737.

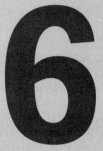

Metabolism and Physical Activity

nergy is required for all biological work. The energy for muscular work is derived mostly from the catabolism (breakdown) of carbohydrates or fats. The preference for one over the other depends largely on the type of exercise, its duration, and its intensity. Thus, interactions between physical activity or exercise and the derivation of the energy requirements for that activity are important, especially for those with certain chronic diseases such as diabetes mellitus. This chapter provides a basic understanding of how energy is derived and what determines the preference for a particular fuel source as well as the many factors that affect the derivation of energy and its use by the cells. All those who are involved in exercise programs and exercise-related research should become familiar with these interactions.

■ ATP: THE ENERGY FOR ALL LIVING CELLS

All living organisms require energy to sustain life and function. This energy is harnessed by plants through the process of photosynthesis from the sun (solar energy). Animals and humans obtain energy from the foods consumed, which are mostly carbohydrates and fats but also proteins. Then, through an elaborate process, our bodies extract the energy, mainly from carbohydrates (starches) and fats, and process it into an energy compound that the cells can use for each of their functions. This form of energy is known as **adenosine triphosphate (ATP)**.

ATP is an energy-packed compound. The energy is stored in the chemical bond that joins the phosphate with the rest of the compound (**Figure 6.1**). Considerable free energy is

Figure 6.1 Structure of adenosine triphosphate (ATP) showing the high energy phosphate bonds (A). Breakdown of ATP to adenosine diphosphate (ADP) and the release of energy (B).

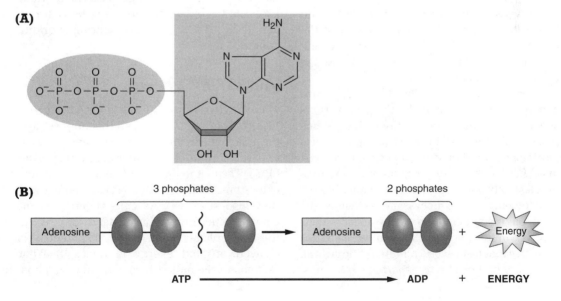

released when this bond is broken. When this occurs, the compound is left with only two phosphates and is now referred to as **adenosine diphosphate (ADP)**. ADP can pick up a phosphate and be transformed back to ATP if sufficient energy is available, for example, from the breakdown of carbohydrates and fats. It then releases energy again as one of its phosphates is cleaved off. This continues on for as long as energy is available.

ATP is present everywhere and in all cells. It provides energy for all biologic work. It even provides energy required for the metabolism of foods and its own formation. Think of it like the money we use for business transactions and in daily life. Indeed, ATP is often referred to as the **energy currency** of the body that can be generated and spent again and again.[1–3]

> ATP is the energy currency of the body that can be generated and spent again and again.

Formation

ATP is derived mainly from carbohydrates and fats. Proteins provide a small fraction of the energy requirements and only in special conditions. Each healthy cell of the body has the capacity to form its own ATP.

Because humans have the ability to perform a number of tasks and do them at various speeds, intensities, and durations, the systems responsible for the energy requirements of a particular type of task are also specific to that task. For example, for very intense activities that last only a few seconds but require a great deal of energy, the necessary ATP must be available instantaneously to the muscle cells involved in that activity. On the other hand, for activities that last several minutes to hours, the necessary fuel can be transported to the mus-

cle cells from either the liver, fat depots, or both; ATP can be formed continuously during the duration of the activity. It is easy to appreciate the logic that two different systems exist to meet the energy demands of entirely different types of activities.

Generally speaking, cells can form ATP from foods in two different ways: with and without the use of oxygen. Formation of ATP with the use of oxygen is referred to as **aerobic** (Greek word meaning *with air*). Conversely, the formation of ATP without oxygen is known as **anaerobic** (*without air*). It is important to keep in mind that the two systems (aerobic and anaerobic) are never turned off. Rather, they are working together in a harmonious way, sharing the responsibility for providing the energy for the entire body. However, at any time, one may be the predominant system providing most of the energy for the particular activity at hand.

Although the ATP is the same whether it is derived from fats or carbohydrates, the process by which the body extracts ATP from carbohydrates is different from that of fats. An understanding of these processes is important if one is to understand how the body forms and uses ATP at rest and during working conditions.

The ATP-PC System

There are two ways that ATP is formed anaerobically. The first way is also the simplest and the quickest. It involves the combination of two substances, ADP and **phosphocreatine (PC)**. The metabolic process begins as muscle cells store ATP to be used instantaneously and they also store PC. As cells require instant energy to perform upon demand, one of the three phosphates found on the ATP molecule is cleaved off and energy is released. What remains of the molecule is ADP. In turn, phosphate from PC is transferred to ADP to form a new ATP molecule. This process continues until all of the stored PC is depleted.

This process is known as the **ATP-PC system** (also the **phosphagen system**), shown in **Figure 6.2**. This system is essential in providing enough ATP for the muscles to function instantaneously for very intense activities (e.g., 50-yard dash, a heavy lift, high jump). After an all-out effort, the ATP-PC stores decline by approximately 80% within 8 to 10 seconds.[2]

ATP from Carbohydrates

As previously mentioned, the primary function of carbohydrates is to supply energy for all cellular work. The formation of ATP from carbohydrates is a relatively quick process designed to provide quick energy to meet the body's needs when the activity lasts more than 5 seconds. Indeed, when the body requires the necessary energy to sustain an activity at a maximum effort, the anaerobic process that generates ATP is referred to as **glycolysis** (Greek for *glucose degradation*). It begins immediately and peaks within 30 seconds. However, glycolysis starts to subside after about 60 seconds and approaches baseline levels within 3 minutes.

Glycolysis is a purely anaerobic process. It is a series of 10 chemical reactions controlled by different enzymes (**Figure 6.3**). It takes place in the **cytoplasm** (also known as **cytosol**), the watery environment of the cell (**Figure 6.4**). Glycolysis generates four molecules of ATP for every one unit of glucose. Two of the generated ATP are required to power glycolysis, leaving a net gain of two ATP. The generation of ATP through glycolysis thus is not an economical process. However, the maximal rate of ATP formation for a given period of time through glycolysis is three times faster than ATP formation via the aerobic pathways.[3] This is essential during maximal or near maximal exercise lasting approximately 7 to 60 seconds. During such tasks, most of the required ATP is supplied by glycolysis.[2,3]

> Formation of ATP via glycolysis is not an economical process. Rather, it takes place rapidly. The maximal rate of ATP formation for a given period of time through glycolysis is three times faster than ATP formation via the aerobic pathways.

Figure 6.2 The ATP-PC system. When ATP is degraded to ADP, the phosphate from the stored phosphocreatine (PC) binds to ADP to form ATP.

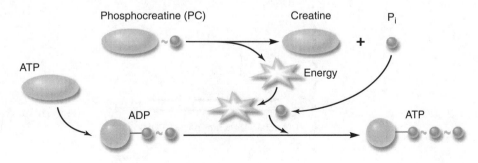

Figure 6.3 Glycolysis.

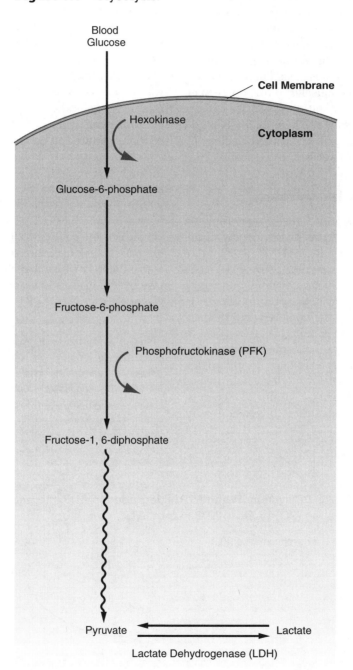

Figure 6.4 Cell depicting cytoplasm (where glycolysis occurs) and mitochondrion (aerobic metabolism).

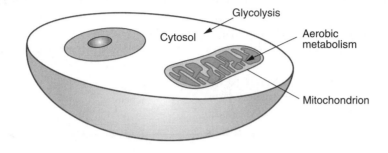

Regulation of Glycolysis

Glycolysis is regulated precisely by: (1) concentrations of key enzymes; (2) concentrations of fructose 1,6-bisphosphate; (3) oxygen availability; and (4) glucose availability. The key enzymes that control the rate of glycolysis are hexokinase, phosphofructokinase (PFK), and lactate dehydrogenase (LDH) (see Figure 6.3).

Hexokinase controls the entry of glucose into the cell. As blood glucose enters the cell, it is immediately *phosphorylated* (that is, a phosphate is attached to the end of the molecule) by hexokinase to form glucose 6-phosphate (G-6-P). *This form of glucose cannot exit the muscle cell and must be used in that cell.* Entry of glucose into the cell and the formation of G-6-P are regulated by the concentrations of G-6-P within the cell. As the concentration increases, it inhibits the activity of hexokinase and consequently the entry of glucose into the cell and formation of G-6-P. This provides the first step in the regulation of glycolysis.

The key regulatory step in glycolysis occurs during the conversion of fructose 6-phosphate (F-6-P) to fructose 1,6-bisphosphate. PFK is the enzyme that controls this step and the entire glycolytic process. PFK can be viewed as the "gatekeeper" of glycolysis. The activity of PFK is limited by several factors including a rise in lactate concentrations, ATP formation, increased levels of citrate, and free fatty acids.

Finally, LDH is involved the conversion of pyruvate to lactate. The formation of lactate allows glycolysis to proceed for awhile longer as well as the formation of ATP under anaerobic conditions. Lactate, therefore, is the "unsung hero" and not the "villain" of muscular soreness as it has been perceived in the past.

The harmonious interaction of these factors results in the precise regulation of glycolysis and ultimately ATP formation. This process can be summarized as follows:

As intense (anaerobic) work begins, ATP concentrations are reduced within seconds. This enhances the activity of PFK and formation of ATP is increased. As work becomes more intense, the point is reached where glycolysis is overwhelmed and lactate concentrations increase. This inhibits PFK, ATP formation decreases, and work intensity is reduced (i.e., the individual slows down).

This slowing down allows the aerobic pathways to take over and the formation of citrate and ATP is increased. The increased concentrations of citrate and ATP further inhibit PFK and glycolysis gears down.

■ LACTATE

Lactate is the end product of carbohydrate metabolism via the anaerobic pathways (glycolysis). At rest, most of the product of glycolysis is pyruvate with a small accumulation of lactate in the blood. This small concentration of blood lactate at rest is a reminder to the reader that glycolysis is never turned completely off. Blood lactate concentrations remain relatively low and close to resting levels during low-intensity physical activities.

However, as the activity increases in intensity, lactate production by the working muscles also increases and lactate concentrations in blood rise. The concentration of lactate in the blood during exercise is influenced by a number of factors including heredity, the fitness status of the individual, age, and most important, the intensity of the activity performed.[3]

Lactate is the end product of carbohydrate metabolism via the anaerobic pathways (glycolysis).

Routes of Lactate

There are four possible routes of the lactate produced by the working muscles (**Figure 6.5**):

1. It is used as energy by the same muscles that produce it.
2. It is used as energy by other muscles not participating in exercise.
3. It is used for energy by the heart.
4. It is converted back to glucose by the liver.

Most of the lactate produced by the working muscles is used by the same muscle for energy. Muscles are comprised of different types of fibers. Some are designed to do high-intensity

Figure 6.5 Routes of lactate. About 70% of the lactate is used by the same muscle that produces it. The rest is carried by the blood to the heart and other muscles to be used for energy, and to the liver where it is converted to glucose and released into the bloodstream.

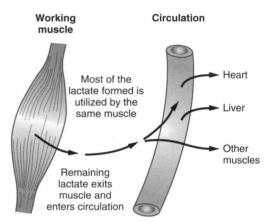

work (anaerobic) and others are designed to do low-intensity (aerobic) work. During high-intensity work, the muscle recruits (engages) the anaerobic fibers to perform. These fibers produce most of the lactate. This lactate is carried by the blood to the fibers that are not engaged (aerobic fibers). The aerobic fibers are not deprived of oxygen and have a great ability to use lactate as fuel. They shuttle lactate to their aerobic pathways where lactate is converted to ATP and used by these fibers for their energy needs.[2–4] Muscle thus is not only the major site of lactate production but also is a primary tissue of lactate removal.[4]

Almost all of the remaining lactate is removed and carried mainly to the liver, heart, and other muscles by the circulating blood. The heart and the muscles use lactate for fuel while the liver converts lactate back to glucose and releases it into the bloodstream. Eventually, this glucose finds its way back to the working muscle and the muscle again is using to meet its energy needs.[2,3] Nothing is wasted. The muscle that produces lactate either uses it or releases it to be used by other organs. Lactate should not be viewed as waste product of glucose metabolism. It is only a source of energy that has been chemically altered to temporarily allow certain functions to continue.

By approximately 25 minutes of recovery following exhaustive exercise, about half of the accumulated lactate is removed from the blood and muscle.[5] The removal is nearly complete within 60 minutes.[6] If following the intense activity one engages in light exercise that involves the same muscles (such as walking after a fast run), the removal is faster. There are two reasons for this fact. First, because the intensity of the activity is light (aerobic), no lactic acid is generated. Second, blood flow to the muscle increases and, therefore, the shuttling of lactate within the muscle or its removal outside of the muscle (in the liver and heart) is enhanced.

To some extent, lactate may even acts as a "protector" for the muscle. The higher the lactate accumulation, the slower and more sluggish muscle contractions become. Eventually, when a certain level of lactate is reached, muscular contractions become painful enough that the individual is forced to either terminate the activity or reduce its intensity considerably.

Threshold

As mentioned earlier, low concentrations of lactate exist even at rest. During low-intensity exercise, blood lactate levels remain close to resting levels. As the exercise intensity increases progressively, a progressive increase in the contribution of ATP by the anaerobic pathways (glycolysis) occurs. Consequently, lactate production also increases. At some point, the capacity of the muscle to deal with

the lactate internally is surpassed. Excess lactate is removed from the muscle by the circulating blood and lactate levels rise suddenly in the blood. The level of exercise intensity or oxygen consumption that coincides with a lactate level of about 2.5 times that of resting levels (or 2.5 mM/l) is known as the **lactate threshold.** Another common term used to describe this level is the **anaerobic threshold**. To avoid confusion, the sudden rise in blood lactate levels during incremental exercise here will be referred to as the *lactate threshold*.

■ Significance

Our capacity to work continuously below the lactate threshold is great. We can work for many hours with little rest. Examples of work under the lactate threshold include retail clerking, most routine daily activities, office work, and most factory assembly line work.

However, we only have a limited capacity to work above the lactate threshold. Working conditions above the lactate threshold include occupations that require moderate to heavy lifting, speed, or near maximum effort. Under such working conditions, frequent rest periods are necessary.

■ How Is It Determined?

The lactate threshold is determined in the laboratory under controlled exercise conditions. During such conditions, blood is drawn for measuring blood lactate levels and/or the oxygen and breathing rates are monitored closely. The lactate threshold for healthy, untrained individuals occurs at about 55% to 60% of the individual's maximal oxygen capacity.[7,8] This is the maximum amount of oxygen that one can utilize to do work. This is termed **maximal oxygen capacity** or **maximal oxygen consumption** and abbreviated as $\dot{V}O_2max$.

■ Can the Lactate Threshold Be Altered?

Yes, it can, but remember that the lactate threshold is determined by two primary factors: genetics and the level of physical fitness.

Because there is little we can do about our genetic make-up, the lactate threshold can only be changed by physical activity. There are two important facts to consider. First, it is well established that individuals engaging in aerobic activities regularly develop a greater capacity to utilize oxygen. In other words, they have higher $\dot{V}O_2$max. Second, the lactate threshold for trained and highly trained individuals occurs at about 75% and not at 50% as is the case with sedentary individuals.[7,8] Let us now take three individuals with same body weight of about 175 lbs. One is sedentary, the other is an average exerciser (defined as one who exercises regularly 3–4 times per week, for several months), and the third is a marathoner runner. The $\dot{V}O_2$max of these three individuals is presented in **Table 6.1**.

Let us now see how the lactate threshold is affected. Let us assume that the onset of the lactate threshold for all three individuals is at approximately 50% of their $\dot{V}O_2$max. One can easily see in Table 6.1 that the lactate threshold for the sedentary individuals is reached at 1.5 liters of oxygen consumption, for the moderately fit individuals at 2 liters, and for the marathon runner (high fit) at 3 liters (**Figure 6.6**).

The differences become even greater when we consider the fact that the lactate threshold

Figure 6.6 Theoretical representation of the anaerobic threshold. Note that the sedentary individual reaches the anaerobic threshold at 1.5 liters of O_2, whereas the high-fit individual reaches it at 3 liters of O_2.

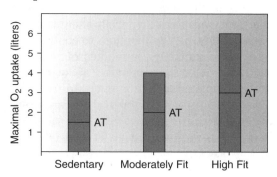

of highly trained (high-fit) individuals occurs at about 75% to 80% of $\dot{V}O_2$max and between 50% and 75% for moderately trained individuals. We can then assume that the marathon runner will reach lactate threshold at 4.5 liters of oxygen (6/0.75 = 4.5).

This is all illustrated in **Figure 6.7**. As you can see, the four units of lactate (y axis) that represents lactate threshold are reached at 50% of maximum oxygen consumption for the sedentary (low-fit) individuals, whereas the same lactate level is reached at 75% of maximal oxygen consumption for the high-fit individual. This means that when the sedentary individual reaches his or her maximum capacity to utilize

Table 6.1 Differences in $\dot{V}O_2$max According to Intensity and Duration of Exercise

Type of Exercise	$\dot{V}O_2$max
Sedentary	3 liters O_2
Average Exerciser (moderately fit)	4 liters O_2
Marathon Runner (high fit)	6 liters O_2

Figure 6.7 Anaerobic threshold for sedentary and fit individuals.

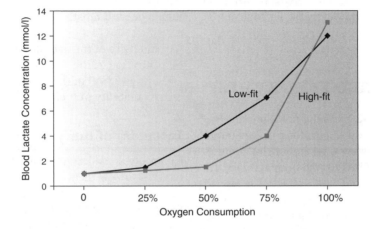

Source: Adapted from *ACSM's Resource Manual for Guidelines for Exercise Testing and Prescription*, 5th ed.

oxygen (3 liters/minute), the highly trained athlete will not even be breathing hard.

As you may recall, without oxygen, only carbohydrates can be used to form ATP. However, when oxygen is available, carbohydrates, fats, and proteins can be used to form ATP. Formation of ATP via the aerobic pathways takes place within the mitochondria of the cells (Figure 6.4).[3,9,10] Mitochondria can be thought of as the "power plants" of the cell.

Aerobic formation of ATP consists of two phases and involves the interaction of two metabolic processes: the **Krebs cycle** and the **electron transport chain**. As shown in **Figure 6.8**, in Phase 1 (the Krebs cycle), acetyl CoA is formed from the catabolism of pyruvate (a product of glucose metabolism when adequate oxygen is available), fats, and proteins. Acetyl CoA enters the Krebs cycle and as it goes through a complex series of steps, hydrogen atoms and ATP are released. The loose hydrogen atoms then enter into Phase 2—the electron transport chain—where significant quantities of ATP are generated. The complete oxidation of one molecule of glucose (glycolysis, Krebs cycle, and electron transport chain)

Figure 6.8 Aerobic metabolism.

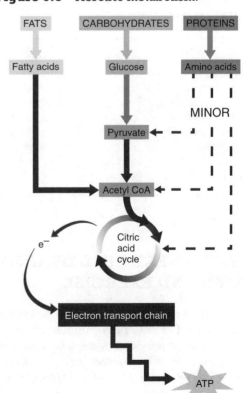

yields a net gain of 30 ATP molecules.[3] However, some authors estimate the ATP formation from glucose oxidation to be as high as 38 molecules.[2]

PREFERRED FUEL AT REST

Generally speaking, fat is the predominant fuel source at rest and during prolonged, low-intensity exercise. However, an important point is that the preferred fuel for the body is a mixture of carbohydrates and fats. Indeed, the use of pure fat for energy is detrimental for the body and, in some cases, may be fatal. Under normal conditions, the body uses both fats and carbohydrates to meet its energy demand.

Normally, 60% to 70% of the required ATP at rest is derived from fat and the remaining 30% to 40% from carbohydrates.

The preferred fuel for the body is a mixture of carbohydrates and fats. Using pure fat for energy is detrimental for the body and, in some cases, may be fatal. Under normal conditions, the body uses both fats and carbohydrates to meet its energy demand. The percent contribution of each depends on a number of factors, but the most important factors are the duration, intensity, and frequency of the activity.

PREFERRED FUEL DURING WORK AND EXERCISE

Another important point to emphasize is that the energy required to perform most types of physical tasks is provided by the interaction of aerobic and anaerobic sources, not by one system exclusively. The percent contribution of either system (aerobic or anaerobic) and the type of fuel (carbohydrates or fat) that will be used predominantly to meet the ATP requirements depend mostly on four factors:

1. Intensity of the activity or exercise
2. Duration of the exercise session
3. Fitness level of the individual
4. Availability of fuel

Intensity of Activity

Generally speaking, the lower the intensity of exercise or physical activity, the higher is the contribution of fats to meet the energy requirements of the activity. The greatest amount of fat utilization occurs at an exercise intensity of about 40% to 60% of maximum oxygen uptake.[11-16] Low-intensity activities include a fast walk, biking or jogging at low speeds, swimming, dancing, gardening, long distance, etc. Theoretically, such activities can last forever. For example, one can walk at a gentle pace over fairly level terrain for many hours without ever running out of breath.

The contribution of anaerobic sources (PC and glycolysis) to meet the energy of an activity is directly related to the intensity of the activity. As the intensity increases, carbohydrate utilization also increases progressively with a concomitant decrease in the utilization of fats. For activities that require maximum or near maximum effort, nearly all of the ATP is derived form carbohydrates.[11,12,14] Such activities include running, biking or rowing at high speeds, weight lifting, or lifting and carrying heavy weight, etc. The duration of such activities depends greatly on the intensity. At maximum or near maximum intensities, the activity can only be sustained for about 1 to 3 minutes. Bouts of the same activity can be performed following a few minutes of recovery between bouts.

Two scenarios better describe the metabolic events that unfold during physical work or dif-

Figure 6.9   From rest to maximal effort, contributions and interactions of three energy systems relative to different intensities and duration (from maximum effort lasting only a few seconds to lower intensities of 2 and 10 minutes).

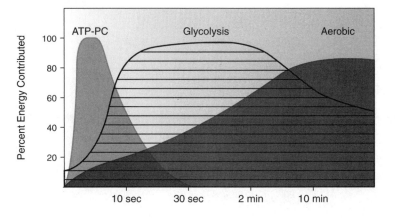

ferent intensities (energy systems involved and fuel preference). The first is an individual going from rest to running at maximal speed, an effort lasting only a few seconds to minutes (**Figure 6.9**). The second is a long distance run lasting 2 or more hours (**Figures 6.10 and 6.11**).

■ From Rest to an All-Out Effort and Beyond

The transition from resting conditions to an all-out effort requires significant amounts of ATP. This energy is supplied predominately

Figure 6.10   Energy contribution of fats progressively increases as exercise duration increases.

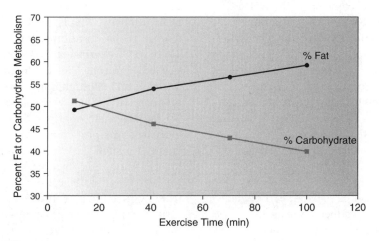

Source: Courtsey of Powers.

Figure 6.11 Exercise intensity as a determinant of the source of fuel. Note the progressive shift to carbohydrates as exercise intensity increases and concomitant decline in fat utilization.

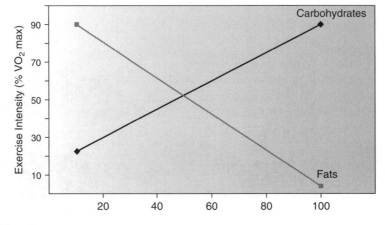

Source: Adapted from Powers.

anaerobically in a well-coordinated interaction of the ATP-PC and glycolytic systems.

- During the initial 7 to 10 seconds of the activity, the ATP requirements are met almost exclusively by the ATP-PC system. This allows time for the glycolytic pathway to progressively increase its capacity to maximum levels.
- By the time the capacity of the ATP-PC system is almost exhausted (about 10 seconds into the activity), the glycolytic system is operating at maximum capacity. Glycolysis now can meet all of the energy requirements of the system operating at maximum intensity for approximately 1 minute.
- At the end of that first minute, the glycolytic pathway is greatly "exhausted" and the intensity of the activity is progressively reduced. The intensity of the activity (individual's speed) is reduced.
- As the speed is reduced, the aerobic pathways begin to progressively share more of the burden to meet the energy

demand. As the intensity of activity falls below a certain level, the energy demands are almost exclusively met by the aerobic system.

Fuel Preference as Dictated by the Duration and Intensity of the Activity

The duration of exercise is influenced inversely by its intensity. That is, the higher the intensity, the lower the duration will be and visa versa. The fuel for exercise also depends on its intensity and duration. This is illustrated in Figures 6.10 and 6.11. Note that low intensity activities that last longer than 30 minutes depend mostly on fat for their energy.[11–17] As the duration increases, the percentage of fat providing the energy for such activity becomes progressively higher. About 80% or more of the ATP needed for activities that last 2 or more hours comes from fat (see Figure 6.10).

In contrast, as exercise intensity increases, the contribution of fat for energy decreases and carbohydrate contribution increases (see

Figure 6.11). At a maximal effort, approximately all energy is derived from carbohydrates.

■ DETERMINANTS OF EXERCISE DURATION

The duration of an anaerobic activity is largely determined by its intensity. The higher the intensity, the shorter the duration will be. The duration of a predominantly aerobic activity is determined by the availability of glucose.

As previously stated, the necessary fuel for aerobic activities is provided by the interaction of both aerobic and anaerobic sources and not by one system exclusively. The onset of exercise stimulates a rapid increase in glucose transport to the working muscles to meet the increased energy demands. As blood glucose is transported to the muscles, the liver releases glucose into the bloodstream. This action ensures that blood glucose concentrations remain constant throughout the exercise. This normal blood glucose level is maintained until

glycogen stores in the liver are depleted. The duration of exercise for an individual at a given intensity depends largely on the liver glycogen stores prior to the initiation of exercise. When liver glycogen stores are depleted, hypoglycemia ensues and the individual no longer can sustain the exercise. This phenomenon is commonly known as "hitting the wall." For most people, hypoglycemia occurs after approximately 2 hours of continuous exercise. The onset of hypoglycemia can be prevented or more accurately, delayed if sufficient carbohydrates are ingested during the activity or glycogen stores are increased days prior to the activity, a practice known as *carbohydrate loading* or *super-compensation*.

The rate of depletion of the liver glycogen stores depends on the intensity of the activity. The higher the intensity of the activity the quicker glycogen stores are depleted. High-intensity activities deplete glycogen stores within 30 minutes. Similar glycogen depletion is achieved at lower exercise intensities but longer durations (**Figure 6.12**).

Figure 6.12 Exercise intensity and muscle glycogen depletion.

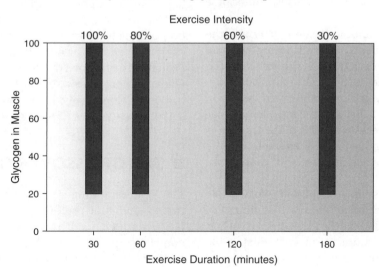

> The duration of exercise for an individual at a given intensity depends largely on the liver glycogen stores prior to the initiation of exercise.

Fitness Level of the Individual

The higher aerobic fitness levels of the individual, the higher the portion of ATP is derived from fats at any intensity.[13] This is one more reason that high-fit individuals can exercise longer at any given exercise intensity. The significance of fitness and fuel preference is presented in more detail in the section about the lactate threshold.

Availability of Fuel

The availability of fuel is an issue only with the smaller of our energy sources, that is, phosphocreatine and carbohydrates, and not with fat, which theoretically is inexhaustible. Phosphocreatine availability could increase with creatine supplementation and carbohydrate availability can increase with a carbohydrate-rich diet, carbohydrate loading, and carbohydrate supplementation during endurance exercise.

There is also another issue concerning the availability of fuel to the cell during physical activity or exercise. That is the cell's preference when different substrates of fuel are available. Naturally, the availability of fuel will determine what substance the muscles will use to derive the necessary ATP if the muscle is capable of using this fuel. For example, if there is no glucose available, the cells cannot use glucose.

This of course is a simplified explanation. What is emphasized is the role that fitness of the individual plays in the utilization of fuel. In this regard, the more fit an individual is the higher the percentage of energy will be derived

from fat oxidation at any exercise/work intensity. That is, if the amount of available fat between identical twins is the same, but one twin is highly fit, that individual will use more of the available fat than the less-fit twin. This is another reason why fit people can do more exercise than those who are sedentary.

> The intensity of the activity is directly related to the contribution of ATP derived from anaerobic metabolism. That is to say, the higher the intensity of the work, the greater the percent of anaerobically derived ATP.
>
> The duration of the activity is directly related to the contribution of ATP derived from aerobic metabolism. This means that the longer the duration, the greater the percent of aerobically derived ATP.

Availability of Free Fatty Acid for Energy

As mentioned earlier, the availability of free fatty acid (FFA) concentration is one of the factors that will determine the fuel preference of the working muscle. When all else is equal, the higher the FFA concentration, the greater the FFA utilization. An individual's FFA concentration is largely determined by the duration of exercise [17] and his or her nutritional status.[15–18] Prolonged fasting or a diet low in carbohydrates results in a progressive increase in FFA concentrations.[19] Conversely, high carbohydrate consumption decreases FFA concentrations.

■ THE CROSSOVER CONCEPT

The understanding of interaction between fitness and fuel preference during exercise has been advanced by the concept that the contribution of carbohydrates and fat to the total energy requirements for any activity is determined by the relative exercise intensity.[20-22]

As stated, fat oxidation predominates during rest and at low exercise intensities. A progressive increase in the exercise intensity is reflected by a progressive decrease in fat oxidation, which is mirrored by a concomitant increase in carbohydrate oxidation. At some point, the predominant fuel for the total energy requirements shifts from fat to carbohydrates. Brooks refers to this as *the crossover point*.[18-20] The crossover point usually occurs at approximately 50% of $\dot{V}O_2$max. Indeed, several contemporary studies have shown that during hard-intensity exercise (at approximately 75% $\dot{V}O_2$max), carbohydrates provide the predominant substrate.

The significance of the crossover point is that it represents a theoretical means by which one can understand the effects of exercise intensity and endurance training adaptations on the balance of carbohydrate and lipid metabolism during sustained exercise. For this reason, it is important to realize that the crossover point is not absolute. Rather, it can be altered by proper exercise training. According to this concept, endurance training results in muscular biochemical adaptations that enhance greater fat utilization for fuel at the same (and even higher) rate of submaximal exercise workloads in comparison to the amount of fat utilization when undergoing the same work prior to training. Another way of stating this phenomenon is that the workload that will require 50% of the energy contribution from carbohydrates and 50% from fats will shift to a higher percentage of fat usage for fuel after exercise training. This is illustrated in **Figure 6.13**.

The pattern of substrate utilization in an individual at any point in time therefore depends on the interaction between exercise intensity-induced responses (which increases carbohydrate utilization) and endurance training-induced responses (which promote lipid oxidation).

> The utilization pattern of glucose or fats during work depends largely on the interaction between the type of work (aerobic or anaerobic) performed and the type of training of the individual.

Figure 6.13 Theoretical energy contribution of fats and carbohydrates before and after training.

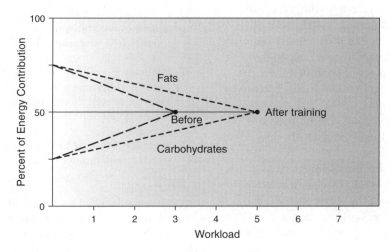

■ SUMMARY

- ATP is the form of energy present in all cells. It provides energy for all biologic work. It is replenished mainly through the oxidation of carbohydrates and fats. It even provides energy required for the metabolism of foods and its own formation. ATP is the energy currency of the body.
- ATP is formed either with the use of oxygen (aerobic) or without (anaerobic).
- The ATP-PC (or the phosphagen system) is an anaerobic system that provides ATP for the muscle cells instantaneously for very intense activities (e.g., 50-yard dash, a heavy lift, high jump) or short durations.
- Glycolysis is an anaerobic process for the formation of ATP. It is characterized by a rather quick generation of ATP necessary for the energy demands of intense physical activities.
- Lactate is the end product of carbohydrate metabolism via the anaerobic pathways (glycolysis). Most of the lactate produced by the working muscles is used by the same muscle for energy. The remaining is used by the heart for energy or converted to glucose by the liver.
- The lactate threshold is the level of lactate in the blood that marks the shift from aerobic to anaerobic metabolism. In general, the higher the intensity required to reach this lactate level, the higher the aerobic capacity of the individual. The lactate threshold thus can be changed by aerobic training.
- Generally speaking, the intensity and duration of the activity determines the fuel source required.
- The predominant fuel source at rest and during prolonged exercise of relatively low-intensity is fat. Conversely, during high-intensity short-duration activities, the predominant fuel source is carbohydrates.

■ REFERENCES

1. Guyton AC, Hall J. *Human Physiology and Mechanisms of Disease.* Philadelphia: W.B. Saunders; 1997.
2. McArdle WD, Katch FI, Katch VL. *Exercise Physiology*, 5th ed. Baltimore: Lippincott Williams & Wilkins; 2001.
3. Mougios V. *Exercise Biochemistry*. Champaign, IL: Human Kinetics; 2006.
4. Brooks GA. Intra- and extra-cellular lactate shuttles. *Med Sci Sports Exerc* 2000;32(4): 790–799.
5. Karlsson J, Saltin B. Oxygen deficit and muscle metabolites in intermittent exercise. *Acta Physiol Scand* 1971;82(1):115–122.
6. Hermansen L, Stensvold I. Production and removal of lactate during exercise in man. *Acta Physiol Scand* 1972;86(2):191–201.
7. Davis JA, Frank MH, Whipp BJ, Wasserman K. Anaerobic threshold alterations caused by endurance training in middle-aged men. *J Appl Physiol* 1979;46(6):1039–1046.
8. Gollnick PD, Bayly WM, Hodgson DR. Exercise intensity, training, diet, and lactate concentration in muscle and blood. *Med Sci Sports Exerc* 1986;18(3):334–340.
9. Guyton AC. *Textbook of Medical Physiology*. Philadelphia: W.B. Saunders; 1991.
10. Murray RK, Granner DK, Mayes PA. *Harpers' Biochemistry*, 24th ed. Stamford, CT: Simon & Schuster; 1996.
11. Gollnick PD. Metabolism of substrates: energy substrate metabolism during exercise and as modified by training. *Fed Proc* 1985;44(2): 353–357.
12. Gollnick PD, Reidy M, Quintinskie JJ, Bertocci A. Differences in metabolic potential of skeletal muscle fibres and their significance for metabolic control. *J Exp Biol* 1985;115: 191–199.
13. Holloszy JO, Coyle EF. Adaptations of skeletal muscle to endurance exercise and their metabolic consequences. *J Appl Physiol* 1984;56(4): 831–838.
14. Newsholme EA. The control of fuel utilization by muscle during exercise and starvation. *Diabetes* 1979;28(Suppl 1):1–7.

15. Romijn JA, Coyle EF, Sidossis LS, et al. Regulation of endogenous fat and carbohydrate metabolism in relation to exercise intensity and duration. *Am J Physiol* 1993;265(3 Pt 1): E380–E391.

16. Sidossis LS, Gastaldi A, Klein S, et al. Regulation of plasma fatty acid oxidation during low- and high-intensity exercise. *Am J Physiol* 1997;272(6 Pt 1):E1065–E1070.

17. Holloszy JO, Kohrt WM, Hansen PA. The regulation of carbohydrate and fat metabolism during and after exercise. *Front Biosci* 1998;3: D1011–D1027.

18. Coyle EF, Jeukendrup AE, Wagenmakers AJM, Saris WHM. Fatty acid oxidation is directly regulated by carbohydrate metabolism during exercise. *Am J Physiol* 1997;273(2 Pt 1): E268–E275.

19. Galbo H, Holst JJ, Christensen NJ. The effect of different diets and of insulin on the hormonal response to prolonged exercise. *Acta Physiol Scand* 1979;107(1):19–32.

20. Brooks GA. Importance of the "crossover" concept in exercise metabolism. *Clin Exp Pharmacol Physiol* 1997;24(11):889–895.

21. Brooks GA. Maximal metabolic rate and the balance of substrate utilization in aging. *Am J Physiol* 1997;273(3 Pt 1):E655–E656.

22. Brooks GA, Mercier J. Balance of carbohydrate and lipid utilization during exercise: the "crossover" concept. *J Appl Physiol* 1994; 76(6):2253–2261.

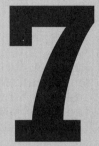
The Cardiovascular System

■ STRUCTURES AND FUNCTIONS OF THE CARDIOVASCULAR SYSTEM

The cardiovascular (CV) system consists of the heart and a network of approximately 100,000 miles of blood vessels. Its primary function is to rapidly transport oxygen and nutrients to the tissues upon demand. An equally important function is the removal of all metabolic waste products such as carbon dioxide, creatine, and urea.

In addition, the CV system plays an essential role in body temperature regulation. Vasodilation and vasoconstriction of the blood vessels control the distribution of blood so the body core temperature is maintained at a consistent level despite environmental changes. Heat produced by organs, deep tissues, and working muscles is carried via the blood to the skin surface where it dissipates.

Finally, the CV system distributes hormones and secretes certain agents involved in the control of blood volume, which determines blood pressure values that affect the overall function of the CV system.

Heart: The Incredible Pump

The size of the human heart in an average sized adult is about 12 cm long (about 5 inches), 9 cm wide (3.5 inches) at its broadest point, and

6 cm thick (2 inches). It is approximately the size of a clenched fist and weighs about 10 to 12 ounces in men and 8 to 10 ounces in women.[1,2] Its main function is to pump the necessary blood throughout the body. It does so persistently beat by beat, minute after minute, hour after hour for life. At rest, the heart pumps about 5 liters of blood per minute. During hard work, the heart of the average fit individual can pump 20 liters of blood per minute. An athlete's heart can pump over 30 liters. Even with the most conservative estimates, the heart beats about 45 million times and pumps over 3.0 million liters of blood in one year. It does this year after year for a lifetime. This enormous amount of work performed by the heart and the simplicity of its design is astonishing. To fully appreciate how the heart accomplishes this task, it is important to understand its structure and function of its components.

■ Structure of the Heart

The heart is partitioned into four distinct areas: the **apex**, **base** or **posterior**, **anterior**, and **inferior**. The *apex* of the heart is formed by the tip of the left ventricle, which points to the left. The atria (mainly the left) form the *base* or *posterior* wall of the heart. The *anterior* part is comprised of the right atrium and ventricle, and the *inferior* surface of the heart is formed by both ventricles (primarily the left) and lies along the diaphragm (**Figure 7.1**).

The interior surface of the heart (the one in contact with the blood) and the valves are lined with a single layer of endothelial cells known as the **endocardium** (*endo*, Greek word for inside). The outer layer of the heart is the **pericardium** (*peri*, Greek for around). Between these surfaces is the thickest muscular layer of the heart wall, known as the **myocardium** (**Figure 7.2**).

Figure 7.1   External anatomy of the heart.

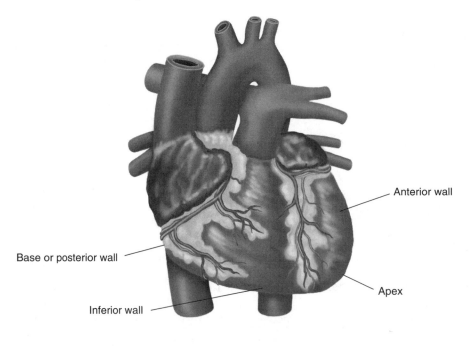

Anterior wall

Base or posterior wall

Apex

Inferior wall

Figure 7.2   Internal anatomy of the heart.

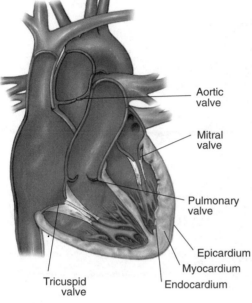

Aortic valve

Mitral valve

Pulmonary valve

Epicardium
Myocardium
Endocardium

Tricuspid valve

The cardiac muscle (myocardium) is similar to the skeletal muscles in a number of ways. The cardiac muscle is striated. It is comprised of myofibrils that contain actin and myosin filaments that are almost identical to those found in skeletal muscles. Contraction of the myocardial cells is thought to occur according to the sliding filament theory that governs the contraction of skeletal muscles (see Chapter 6).

Several differences exist between the two muscle types, however. For example, the myocardial fibers are arranged in series (i.e., end-to-end) and are connected by structures known as **intercalated disks**, which are not found in skeletal muscle. These intercalated discs have a very low electrical resistance and are designed to propagate the nerve impulse from one fiber to the next. The electrical impulse thus can travel from fiber to fiber virtually unimpeded. This allows all cardiac muscle fibers to contract nearly simultaneously when stimulated.[1,2]

The entire cardiac muscle follows an **all-or-none law**. That is, when stimulated, either all or none of the cardiac muscle fibers will contract. Consequently, the heart functions as a unit. This action is known as **functional syncytium**. Cardiac muscle differs from skeletal muscle in that only the individual units that are stimulated follow the all-or-none law. This allows the upper and lower heart chambers to contract independently

The myocardium is also a predominately aerobic muscle, more so than skeletal muscles. It has an abundance of mitochondria and blood supply and is capable of using lactate, free fatty acids, and glucose as fuel sources. Finally, the myocardial cells have the innate ability to initiate an impulse. That is, if all of the nerves regulating the heart are severed, the cardiac cells will continue to initiate an impulse that will cause the heart to contract in a rhythmic fashion. The cardiac cells also have the ability to transmit the impulse from cell to cell throughout the heart and respond to an impulse with a pumping action.

Physiologic properties of cardiac muscle cells are:

- Automaticity—Ability to initiate an impulse
- Excitability—Ability to respond to an impulse
- Conductivity—Ability to transmit an impulse
- Contractility—Ability to respond with pumping action

■ Cardiac Chambers

The heart is comprised of four chambers (**Figure 7.3**). The two top chambers are the right and left atria and the lower chambers are the right and left ventricles. The ventricles are comprised mainly of cardiac muscle. These are the

Figure 7.3 Chambers of the heart.

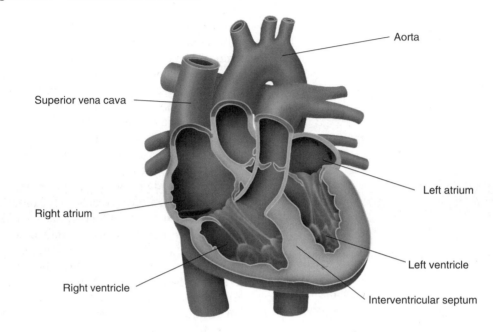

"muscular pumps" that generate the necessary force to push the blood out of the heart. The thick wall shared by the two ventricles is the **interventricular septum**. The atria are less muscular and serve as blood reservoirs for the respective ventricles.

The right ventricle pumps non-oxygenated blood through the pulmonary artery to the lungs. The left ventricle pumps oxygenated blood through the aorta to the body. The pressure generated by the left ventricle is four to five times higher than that generated by the right ventricle. For this reason, the left ventricle is considerably thicker than the right ventricle.

■ Cardiac Valves

Blood flow from the atria to the ventricles is controlled by the opening and closing of one-way valves. These valves have movable inner edges that open passively. When the pressure

in the atria exceeds the pressure in the ventricles during diastole, they open. This allows blood to flow freely into the respective ventricles. The **mitral** or **bicuspid valve** is situated between the left atria and left ventricle. It allows blood to flow from the atria to the ventricle. The **tricuspid valve** is situated between the right atria and ventricle. It allows blood to flow from the right atria to the ventricle. As the blood empties from the atria and fills the ventricles, a progressive rise in ventricular pressure occurs with a concomitant fall in atria pressure. As the pressure gradient rises, the valves are forced shut, thus preventing the backflow of blood to the respective atria during systole that is about to take place.

Two other valves control the blood flow from the ventricles to the regions outside of the heart, namely lungs and periphery. These valves are composed of three leaflets (also called *cusps* or *semilunar*, for their half-moon shape), which are flexible tissue that control the direction of blood flow through the valve. The **aortic valve** allows blood to flow from the left ventricle out to the body. The **pulmonary valve** allows the flow of blood from the right ventricle to the lungs (see Figure 7.2).

■ Coronary Arteries

The heart is an aerobic organ. In other words, the heart generates the necessary adenosine triphosphate (ATP) mainly through the aerobic pathways. However, it has only limited capacity to generate ATP through the anaerobic pathways. For this, the heart requires a constant and abundant supply of oxygenated blood. After just minutes without it, the heart suffers irreversible damage.

Blood is carried to the heart by two main arteries, the left and right coronary arteries. These two arteries rise from the root of the aorta, the main artery that provides the exit for all blood pumped out of the left ventricle, which is located just above the aortic valve. Both the right and left coronary arteries branch off to smaller and smaller vessels so that the entire heart is assured of adequate blood supply (**Figure 7.4**).

The **left main coronary artery** travels down the front of the heart. About one third of the way down, it divides into two other vessels, the **left anterior descending (LAD) coronary artery** and the **circumflex**. The LAD coronary artery continues downwards towards the apex of the heart. Along the way, it branches into smaller vessels that supply the anterior surface of the entire left ventricle and part of the interventricular septum. The circumflex wraps around the lateral portion of the left ventricle and branches off marginal vessels that reach the posterior wall of the heart.

Figure 7.4 The coronary arteries.

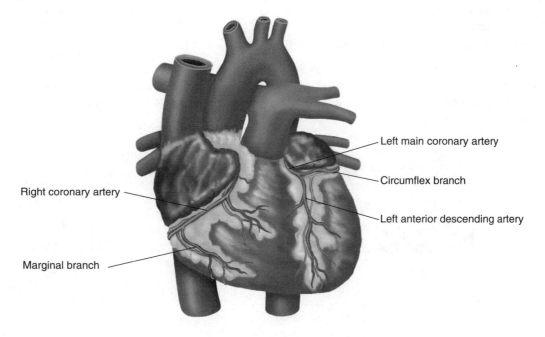

Left main coronary artery

Circumflex branch

Right coronary artery

Left anterior descending artery

Marginal branch

The **right coronary artery (RCA)** extends from the aorta to the right side of the heart and wraps around it, supplying blood to the right-side inferior and posterior walls of the ventricles, and part of the intraventricular septum.

■ Cardiac Cycle

The *cardiac cycle* is the time period between the beginning of one heartbeat to the beginning of the next. During this time, the heart undergoes a contraction and relaxation phase. The contraction phase is known as **systole**. During this phase, blood is pumped out of the heart chambers and into the lungs and all other tissues of the body.

During the cardiac cycle, the heart goes through contraction, known as *systole*, and relaxation, known as *diastole*.

The relaxation phase of the heart begins at the end of systole and is known as **diastole**. Three important events occur during diastole. *First*, the heart rests. In fact, the heart spends more time in diastole (resting) than systole

(working). In fact, at a resting heart rate of 60 beats per minute (one contraction per second; bpm), the heart rests 60% and works 40% of that time. As the heart rate increases, (e.g., with exercise), the situation is reversed. This action is illustrated in **Figure 7.5**.

Second, the relatively long resting interval gives time for the chambers of the heart to fill with blood. Generally, speaking, the longer the diastolic phase, the more blood can enter the ventricles. As explained later, this is an important factor in cardiac performance.

Third, the heart receives its blood supply and nutrients necessary to perform its work. During systole, the forceful contractions of the myocardium squeeze the coronary arteries and increase the pressure within them. Consequently, blood flow to these arteries ceases. As relaxation begins, the pressure in the coronary arteries drops. During this period, blood that is present in the aorta flows into the coronary vessels. It is only during diastole that blood can flow to the coronary arteries and perfuse the myocardium.

Blood flow to the myocardium occurs only during diastole.

Figure 7.5 Heart rate and time spent in systole and diastole. Note that the heart at rest spends 60% of the time in diastole and 40% in systole. The reverse occurs during peak exercise.

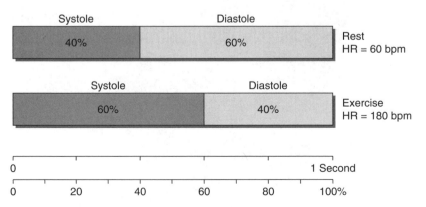

Figure 7.6 Pulmonary circulation.

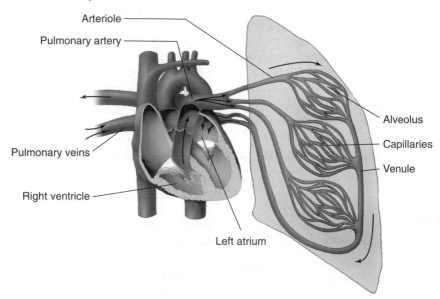

Arteriole

Pulmonary artery

Alveolus

Capillaries

Venule

Pulmonary veins

Right ventricle

Left atrium

■ Circulation

The cycle of blood entering and exiting the heart is illustrated in **Figures 7.6** and **7.7**, which describe the **pulmonary circulation** and **systemic circulation**. The systemic circulation provides blood to all tissues of the body except the lungs. For this reason, it is frequently called the *greater circulation* or *peripheral circulation*.

When the ventricles are filled with blood, a contraction occurs and blood is forced out. With each contraction, the right ventricle forces its non-oxygenated blood out through the pulmonary artery and to the lungs. There, the blood is enriched with oxygen. The now oxygen-rich blood returns from the lungs via the pulmonary veins and then enters the left atrium and eventually the left ventricle via the mitral valve. This completes the **pulmonary circulation** (see Figure 7.6). Note that during pulmonary circulation, the oxygenated blood is carried by the veins and non-oxygenated blood is carried by the arteries.

Figure 7.7 Systemic circulation.

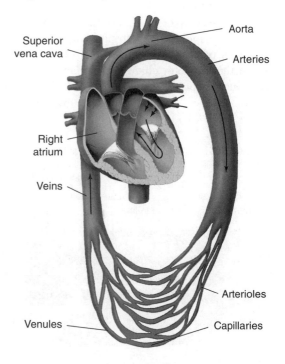

Superior vena cava

Aorta

Arteries

Right atrium

Veins

Arterioles

Venules

Capillaries

The left ventricle contracts and forces the oxygenated blood out via the aorta and throughout the body via the network of arteries. As the oxygenated blood reaches the various tissues, oxygen and nutrients are released to the tissues while carbon dioxide and other metabolic waste products are picked up and carried back to the lungs. Blood returns to the right atrium via two great veins, the **superior vena cava** and **inferior vena cava**. This blood enters the right ventricle and the cycle is repeated. This completes the systemic circulation (see Figure 7.7).

Blood Vessels: Structure and Function

The walls of all blood vessels except capillaries consist of three layers: the adventitia, media, and intima (**Figure 7.8**).

The **adventitia** layer is a connective tissue sheath that surrounds the vessel and binds it to surrounding tissue.

The **media** layer is a smooth muscle that provides the mechanical strength and contractile power of the vessel. This layer is responsible for the diameter change (vasodilation and vasoconstriction) of the vessel.

Figure 7.8 The structure of the arteries.

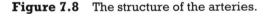
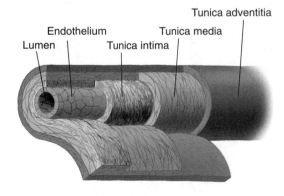

The **intima** (innermost layer) is composed of a sheet of endothelial cells that rests on a thin layer of connective tissue. The endothelial layer is in direct contact with the blood. In atherosclerosis, the deposition of cholesterol and plaque formation occurs within the tissues of this layer. Because of the importance of this endothelial layer, a more detailed discussion follows.

■ Endothelium

The endothelium is comprised of a single layer of endothelial cells that line the inner wall of the blood vessels (see Figure 7.8). The vascular endothelium of an average size individual contains approximately 10,000,000,000,000 endothelial cells that weigh 1.5 kg and cover almost 700 m^2, an area equivalent to six tennis courts. This makes the endothelium the largest endocrine organ in the body.[3]

Prior to 1970, the endothelium was thought to be a passive, semipermeable layer of cells between the smooth muscle of the vessel wall and blood. In the next three decades, the work of several scientists revealed that the endothelium is an organ that manages vital activities and plays a major role in homeostasis, vasoactivity (dilation and constriction of the vessel), immunologic and inflammatory events, and cellular proliferation.[4] In 1998, Dr. Luis Ignarro and Dr. Robert Furchgott were awarded the Nobel Prize of Medicine for their work that led to our understanding of the many functions of the endothelium.

Primary Functions of the Endothelium Understanding endothelium function is one of the most important achievements in medicine within the last 50 years. For those interested in exercise-related research, understanding endothelial function opens new horizons for research that will revolutionize our understanding of cardiovascular function during exercise as well as its protective effects against cardiovascular disease.

Blood vessels are the conduits for blood flow. Their function is to maintain adequate blood flow to the muscles and organs upon demand. The main mechanism for blood flow regulation for each organ is vasodilation or vasoconstriction of the blood vessels that bring blood to that organ. Naturally, for blood to flow unimpeded and upon demand to the organs, blood vessels must dilate and constrict upon demand as well as maintain a smooth surface for minimum resistance to the flow of blood. All of these requirements are accomplished by the endothelium. More specifically, a healthy endothelium synthesizes and releases various substances that control and maintain a balance between:

- **Relaxation and constriction (vasoactivity).** This ensures that the vessels respond to the demand of blood flow to a specific organ by the appropriate degree of dilation or constriction. It also controls blood pressure.
- **Antithrombotic and prothrombotic activities.** This prevents the formation of thrombus (antithrombotic) and internal bleeding (prothrombotic). The balance of these two activities prevents a heart attack and stroke.
- **Anti-inflammatory and pro-inflammatory actions.** This prevents endothelial damage.
- **Growth stimulation and growth inhibition.** This regulates vascular growth

and adhesion of leukocytes, thus maintaining healthy blood vessels.

> The endothelium is comprised of a single layer of endothelial cells that line the inner wall of the blood vessels. Its main function is to manage the behavior of the vessel (dilation and constriction) and protect it against damage.

Endothelial Dysfunction Endothelial cells can be damaged by several factors such as smoking, obesity, high blood cholesterol, and aging.[5–7] When the endothelium is damaged, synthesis and release of these substances is inhibited, and vasodilation is impaired. This condition, known as *endothelial dysfunction*, plays a critical role in the pathogenesis of chronic diseases such as hypertension, diabetes, and atherosclerosis.[4,8–10]

■ Nitric Oxide

In 1980, Furchgott and Zawadzki demonstrated that healthy endothelium releases a factor that induces relaxation and the consequent vasodilation of the blood vessel.[11] They coined this factor as *endothelium-derived relaxing factor (EDRF)*. In 1987, Palmer and colleagues[12] showed that EDRF was actually nitric oxide (NO).

NO is a gas molecule synthesized from the amino acid L-arginine. The reaction involves the enzyme nitric oxide synthase (NOS; **Figure 7.9**).

Figure 7.9 Nitric oxide (NO) synthesis.

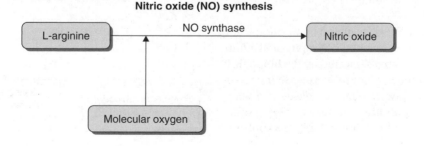

Nitric oxide (NO) synthesis

L-arginine → NO synthase → Nitric oxide

Molecular oxygen

Three types of NOS have been identified: type I, neural (nNOS); type II, inducible (iNOS); and type III, endothelial (eNOS). Both eNOS and nNOS are involved in cardiovascular physiology.

In 1992, *Science* voted NO the "molecule of the year" and described it as follows:

It [NO] helps maintain blood pressure by dilating blood vessels, helps kill foreign invaders in the immune response, is a major mediator of penile erections, and is probably a major biochemical component of long-term memory...these are a few of its benefits.[13]

Others described NO as "a startlingly simple molecule that unites neuroscience, physiology, and immunology, and revises scientists' understanding of how cells communicate and defend themselves."[14]

Indeed, it is hard to find a major physiologic effect that does not involve NO. Once NO is released from the endothelial cells, its half life is only about 5 seconds. This is perhaps the reason it has escaped detection for so long. The released NO diffuses into the lumen and into the smooth muscle cells of the vessel. There, NO that diffuses into the lumen inhibits platelet aggregation and that into the smooth muscle cells causes the vessel wall to relax. Conversely, NO inhibition results in vasoconstriction within the cardiovascular system and the consequential increase in blood pressure. Simply stated, NO constitutes the basis of endothelial-related vasoactivity of the coronary, systemic, cerebral, and pulmonary arteries.

Release of NO is regulated by hormonal and physical (exercise) stimuli. The physical stimulus is the shear stress exerted by the blood flow within the blood vessel.[15] NO release increases when blood flow velocity increases and when blood flow is pulsatile. During exercise or other physical work, blood flow velocity and pulsatil-

ity are increased. This leads to an increase in NO release by the vessel and the consequent vasodilation and increase in blood flow to the working muscles (**Figure 7.10**).

In addition to the increase in blood flow, the NO release during exercise lowers peripheral resistance. The lower resistance is essential to maintain blood pressure values within physiologic limits despite the increase in blood flow.

■ **Arteries**

The aorta is the main trunk of a series of vessels (**Figure 7.11**). It rises from the left ventricle and divides into the ascending aorta, the curved portion known as the arch and the descending aorta. The latter is subdivided into the *thoracic* (the part of the descending aorta in the chest area) and *abdominal aorta* (the part in the stomach area). Smaller branches expand to the arms, chest, and organs. The main arteries of the lower extremities are the *iliac arteries* that branch into smaller arteries to supply blood to the legs.

Figure 7.10   Nitric oxide release with exercise.

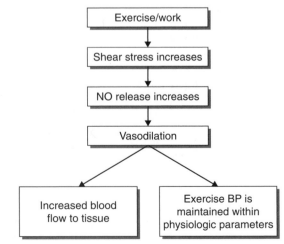

Figure 7.11 Heart, aorta, and other main arteries and veins.

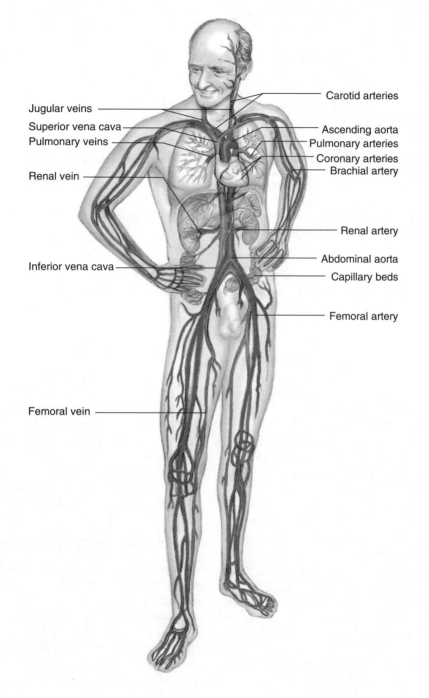

Jugular veins

Superior vena cava

Pulmonary veins

Renal vein

Inferior vena cava

Femoral vein

Carotid arteries

Ascending aorta

Pulmonary arteries

Coronary arteries

Brachial artery

Renal artery

Abdominal aorta

Capillary beds

Femoral artery

The main function of the arteries is to transport blood under high pressure to the tissues. For this reason, arteries have strong vascular walls.[2] In addition to conducting blood, each aforementioned vessel is constructed to play a specific role in circulation. The largest arteries such as the aorta and the arteries of the legs have thick, muscular walls with large quantities of **elastin**, a protein that is six times more extensible than rubber. This allows the arteries to expand by approximately 10% as blood is pushed through in systole and recoils during diastole. The expansion accommodates the force generated by the contracting left ventricle and the ejected blood. The recoil maintains a constant flow of blood through arterial system.[16]

> The main function of the arteries is to transport blood under high pressure to the tissues. For this reason, arteries have strong vascular walls.

Arterioles The conduit arteries branch progressively to form smaller and smaller vessels, known as **arterioles**. Their function is to control blood flow to the capillaries.

Arterioles are medium to small sized vessels. They have strong muscular walls that make these vessels capable of expanding up to sevenfold in diameter or closing the arteriole completely. They thus have the capability to regulate blood flow to the capillaries in response to the needs of the tissues.[2,16] Arterioles also can contract to reduce blood loss in case of a serious injury.

> The main function of the arterioles is to control blood flow to the capillaries.

Capillaries Arterioles branch into very fine, thin-walled vessels called **capillaries**. The main role of the capillaries is to exchange nutrients, fluid, oxygen, and carbon dioxide between the blood and surrounding tissues. The capillaries then converge to small venules and in turn, venules converge to veins. Thus, the systemic circulation is formed.[16]

Capillaries are numerous tiny vessels with thin walls permeable to small molecular substances. Their function is to exchange fluids, nutrients, gases, and other substances between the blood and the interstitial fluid. For this reason, the large cross-sectional area of the capillary bed provides low resistance to blood flow and slow blood velocity. This allows the red blood cell sufficient time for gas exchange.

> The main function of capillaries is to exchange fluids, nutrients, gases, and other substances between the blood and the interstitial fluid.

■ Venules and Veins

The **venules** collect blood from the capillaries. They gradually join together and progressively form larger vessels, called the **veins**, which in turn transport blood back to the heart via the superior and inferior vena cava. The pressure in the venous system is low. For this reason, vein walls are thin. Even so, the wall is muscular and allows the veins to expand or contract and thereby act as a blood reservoir.

Conduction System of the Heart

Arrhythmias (irregular heart beats) range from benign to fatal. Increased physical activity has been shown to foster arrhythmias and also to suppress them.[17–19] The intensity of exercise appears to play a role in the generation or suppression of arrhythmias.[19] However, the association between physical activity and arrhythmias has not been investigated extensively. This is an exciting area for exercise-related research. A basic understanding of the conduction system of the heart is necessary for all those interested in the relationship between cardiovascular disease and physical activity.

■ Overview

Rhythmic contractions of the heart are possible because of the generation of electrical impulses and their well-coordinated propagation throughout the heart. These impulses are synchronized by the conduction system of the heart. This system is comprised of specialized cells that initiate and electrically coordinate the contraction of the heart chambers.

The impulse is initiated by a specialized area of cardiac cells referred to as the **sinoatrial node (SA node)**. The SA node is located on the superior wall of the right atrium and at the entrance of the superior vena cava (**Figure 7.12**). The intrinsic rate of impulse generation by the SA node is approximately 60 to 100 impulses per minute. Naturally, this rate fluctuates according to the demands of the system and other factors. The generated impulse spreads rapidly throughout both atria by special fibers known as the **internodal tracks**, resulting in a contraction by the atria.

The impulse then reaches another specialized area of cardiac tissue, also located in the right atrium near the base of the interatrial

Figure 7.12 Main components of the cardiac conduction system.

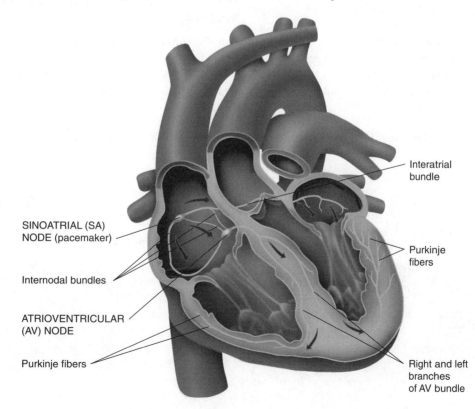

septum (Figure 7.12): the **atrioventricular node (AV node)**. Next, the impulse travels to the **bundle of His**, located distally to the AV node. The bundle of His then divides into the **right** and **left bundle branches**, which innervate (i.e., to supply with nerves) and conduct the impulse to the right and left ventricles, respectively. In turn, these two branches extend into smaller branches and eventually terminate in tiny fibers known as the **Purkinje fibers**. These fibers transmit the impulse first to the muscles that control the heart valves and then throughout the entire ventricular tissue. This allows the valves to close before a ventricular contraction and thus prevent any regurgitation of blood flow to the atria.[20]

■ Cardiac Action Potentials

Action potential describes the state of a nerve fiber or a cardiac cell. When nerve fibers remain undisturbed (resting state), the membrane of the fiber is at a state referred to as **resting potential**. However, when the permeability of the membrane to sodium is changed by any factor or factors, a sequence of events is likely to occur that changes the resting state of the cells and subsequently, the resting potential. The sequence of potential changes is known as the **action potential**.[2]

There are two types of action potential. The first type is the **fast response**. It occurs in the cardiac muscle cells and the conducting fibers (Purkinje fibers). The second type is the **slow response**. This is found in the SA and AV nodes.

■ Basic Electrophysiology

Generation of an impulse becomes possible mainly by the well-coordinated and tightly controlled exchange of sodium and potassium (known as *electrolytes*) inside and outside of the cardiac cells. This becomes possible by an elaborate system that will be discussed briefly in the following sections.

Ion Channels The exchange of sodium and potassium is made possible through specialized ion channels found in the cell membrane (**Figure 7.13**). These ion channels are highly

Figure 7.13 Channel activity during the different phases of the action potential.

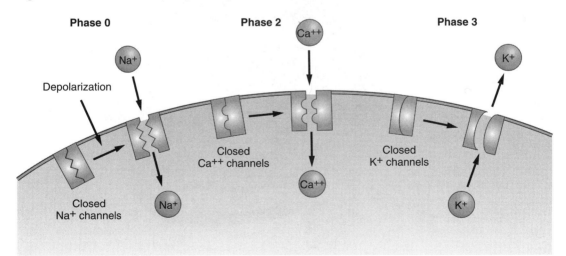

selective. That is, they are designed to only allow a specific ion through the membrane. For example, sodium ions can only pass through certain channels and, thus, these channels are referred to as **sodium channels**. Likewise, potassium ions can only pass through **potassium channels** and calcium ions through the **calcium channels**.

In addition, these channels allow the specific ions to pass through only at certain times. That is, the channels are **gated**. This means that at any given moment the channel is in either in an open or closed state. The opening and closing of the cardiac channels is precisely coordinated and depends upon the voltage across the membrane. Thus, these channels are known as **voltage-sensitive**.[20]

Resting State of the Myocardial Cells   If a fine microelectrode is placed in the cell when the cell is at rest (quiet), it will record approximately –90 mV. In other words, the intracellular potential of cardiac muscle cells is –90 mV below the extracellular level. As stated previously, this is referred to as the *resting potential.*

This resting potential is generated and maintained by tightly controlled differences in ion concentrations inside and outside of the cell membrane. Briefly, this process is as follows:

- Sodium (Na^+) and calcium (Ca^{++}) concentrations are substantially higher outside of the cell compared to the inside. Conversely, potassium concentrations within the cell greatly exceed concentrations outside the cell (**Figure 7.14**).
- The environment inside the cell is *negatively charged* with respect to the outside. This is because the negatively charged proteins within the cell are unable to exit.

Figure 7.14   Ion concentrations inside and outside the cell.

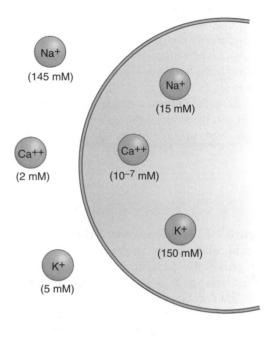

- Despite the tight control of sodium and potassium ion movement inside and outside of the cell, there is a slow but steady leak of sodium and potassium through the cell membrane. Because the cell membrane is much more permeable to potassium ions and far less to sodium and calcium ions, relatively more potassium leaks out than sodium leaks in.

This creates an environment with two opposing forces at work.

1. The first force is created by the concentration gradient. The low concentrations of potassium outside of the cell along with the high membrane permeability of potassium favor a net diffusion of potassium from inside to outside of the cell.

2. The counterforce is electrostatic. As the positively charged potassium exits the cell, the environment inside becomes progressively more negative due to the negatively charged proteins that remain inside the cell. Consequently, potassium is attracted back into the cell.

The balance between these two opposing forces determines the resting membrane potential, which is approximately –90 mV in the cardiac muscle cells (**Figure 7.15**).

Figure 7.15 Resting potential of cardiac muscle cells. The resting membrane potential of the cardiac cell is determined by the balance between the concentration gradient that favors outward movement of potassium and the electrical force that favors the entry of the positively charged potassium into the cell.

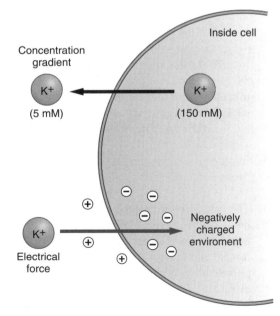

Sodium-Potassium Pump As mentioned earlier, some sodium and potassium leak through the cell membrane. If left unchecked, the concentrations of both sodium and potassium will reach equilibrium across the cell membrane and therefore the resting and action potential of the cell will be disrupted. To maintain the proper concentrations and balance between these two electrolytes (sodium and potassium), the cell membrane is equipped with a mechanism known as the **sodium-potassium pump**. This pump captures the sodium ions that leak into the cell and the potassium ions that leak outside of the cell, and returns them to their respective environments. In this process, three sodium ions are moved out of the cell for every two potassium ions returned inside the cell. This allows a more precise control of the resting membrane potential.

Action Potential of Cardiac Muscle Cells We already know that the resting potential of the cardiac muscle cells is about –90 mV. When this voltage is altered, the cell membrane permeability to ions is also altered. The change of the resting potential occurs when the cell is "provoked" by an impulse generated by the SA node or neighboring cells. Generation of the impulse will be discussed later. For now, the discussion is focused on the development of the action potential in the cardiac muscle cells.[16,20]

The cell's resting potential of –90 mV is known as *phase 4*. At this state, sodium and potassium channels are closed and the sodium potassium membrane is maintaining the proper electrolyte concentrations outside and inside the cell environment (**Figure 7.16**). The four phases of the action potential are:

Phase 0: When an impulse reaches the cardiac muscle cell, it progressively changes the membrane potential to

Figure 7.16 Action potential of cardiac muscle cells.

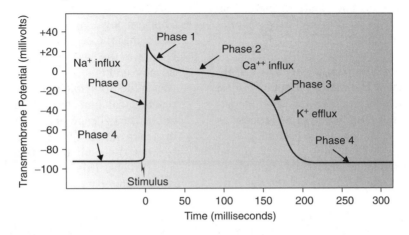

positive. As the membrane becomes progressively less negative and then a threshold of about −70 mV is reached (*action potential threshold*), sodium channels swing wide open and sodium ions rush into the cell. The sodium channels stay open for a very short time and then close again. During that time, sodium entry into the cell drives the transmembrane potential into a positive range of about +10 mV to −20 mV. This is the *depolarization phase* of the cell.

Phase 1: Following depolarization (within milliseconds), repolarization begins and the membrane potential drifts towards zero.

Phase 2: As the membrane potential returns to zero (phase 1), calcium channels, which begin to open during phase 0 and after sodium channels close, are now fully open and calcium enters the cell. The balance between calcium entering the cell and the persistent outward flow of potassium mediates the membrane at a voltage of about 0 mV for a relatively long period (about 200–400 ms). This

is known as the *plateau*. The plateau is significant because it allows the cardiac cells to sustain the contraction necessary to achieve the pumping action.

Phase 3: This final phase begins as the calcium channels close and potassium exits the cell, returning the membrane to a progressively more negative state and finally back to −90 mV (phase 4). Phase 3 is the final period of repolarization.

Significance of Phase 3 Phase 3 of the cardiac muscle cells is much longer than that of skeletal muscle cells. The longer period is necessary to allow the ventricles sufficient time to pump the blood out and refill prior to the next cardiac cycle.

Phase 3 is also subdivided into the **absolute refractory period** and **relative refractory period**. During the absolute refractory period, the cardiac muscle cells are absolutely unexcitable. That is, if another stimulus comes along, they will not depolarize regardless of the strength of that stimulus.

Conversely, during the relative refractory period, the cells can depolarize prematurely (before phase 4 is achieved) if they are provoked by a stimulus of adequate strength. This situation can lead to *cardiac arrhythmias* (abnormal heart beats).

Generation of an Impulse: The Slow Response Action Potential Depolarization of the SA node cells and the subsequent generation of an impulse follow the same process as other cardiac cells (as just explained) with some variations. Specifically, the cells of the SA node do not require any provocation to initiate an action potential. They are endowed by the property of automaticity and depolarize spontaneously in a rhythmic fashion. These are known as **pacemaker cells**. The action potential of these cells is depicted in **Figure 7.17**.

The following differences exist between the action potential of the cardiac muscle cells and pacemaker cells:

- The resting membrane potential of the pacemaker cells is –60 mV, which is substantially less negative that that of the cardiac muscle cells (–90 mV).
- This less negative current favors sodium influx into the cell and the progressive change of the membrane potential to less negative value.
- When the threshold potential of –40 mV is reached, calcium channels open, calcium enters the cell, and phase 0 begins. The upstroke of phase 0 is less rapid and reaches lower amplitude than cardiac muscle cells. This is true because the fast sodium channels are inactivated and phase 0 relies solely on the relatively slower calcium channels.
- Repolarization of the pacemaker cells is similar to that described for cardiac muscle cells.

As the SA node cells depolarize, the generated impulse reaches cardiac muscle cells and provokes the events that lead to the depolarization of cardiac cells as described.

Figure 7.17 Action potential of the pacemaker cells (SA node). Note that the resting membrane potential of these cells is –60 mV, substantially less negative that that of the cardiac muscle cells (–90 mV).

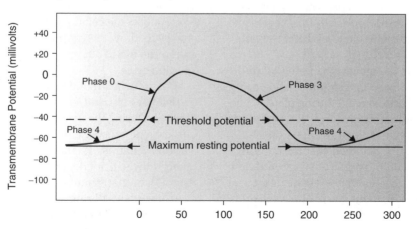

Cardiac Parameters and Function

■ Heart Rate

The importance of providing adequate blood supply to various organs is obvious. In addition to the SA node, with its intrinsic rate of heart contractions at between 60 and 100 times per minute for adults, the heart has a back-up system. If the SA node fails to initiate an impulse within a certain time, the next potential pacemaker site is the AV node, which has a firing rate of 40 to 60 times per minute. Finally, when both sites fail to discharge, the ventricles take over with a rate of 15 to 40 times per minute. Blood flow and life thus can be sustained. (**Figure 7.18**)

The normal heart rate at rest in healthy adults ranges between 60 to 100 bpm. A heart rate of less than 60 bpm is referred to as **bradycardia** (slow heart rate) and above 100 bpm as **tachycardia** (fast heart rate).

> Bradycardia is a resting heart rate of less than 60 bpm and tachycardia is above 100 bpm.

A low heart rate (below 60 bpm) does not always mean that something is wrong. In fact, in some cases it is quite the opposite. For example, athletes generally have a low heart rate, generally around 40 bpm. Certain medications

Figure 7.18 Pacemaker sites and intrinsic rates.

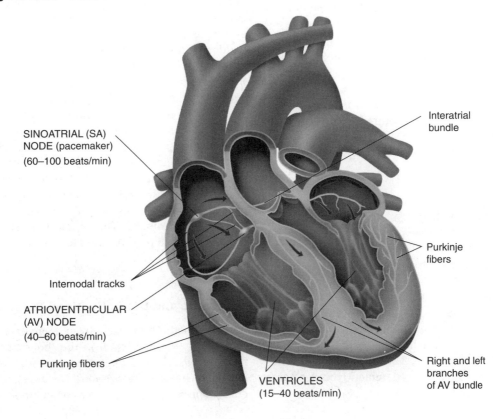

SINOATRIAL (SA)
NODE (pacemaker)
(60–100 beats/min)

Interatrial
bundle

Internodal tracks

Purkinje
fibers

ATRIOVENTRICULAR
(AV) NODE
(40–60 beats/min)

Purkinje fibers

VENTRICLES
(15–40 beats/min)

Right and left
branches
of AV bundle

also lower the heart rate. These medications are called *beta-blockers* and are discussed in greater detail in Chapter 12.

The heart rate is precisely regulated by the balance between the **sympathetic** and **parasympathetic nervous systems**.[21,22] As part of the "fight or flight" response, when the body reacts to a fear-based stimulus, the sympathetic nervous system responds immediately. Blood pressure increases, the heart beats faster, and the digestive system slows down. The sympathetic fibers release the neurotransmitter **norepinephrine** (also known as **noradrenaline**) onto the pacemaker of the heart and acts to cause immediate changes. In addition, and for longer effects, the hormone **epinephrine** (also known as **adrenaline**) is released into the bloodstream by the medulla of the adrenal gland, a hat-shaped organ located on the top of each kidney. The hormones epinephrine and norepinephrine are known as **catecholamines**.

Release of catecholamines (sympathetic stimulation of the heart) has the following effects:

- Increased heart rate (*chronotropic effect*)
- Increased force of contraction (*inotropic effect*)
- Increased rate of relaxation (*lusitropic effect*)

Acetylcholine is the chemical mediator for the parasympathetic system. Parasympathetic stimulation decreases the heart rate and the force of its contractions. It also slows down the digestive system and blood pressure so the body can rest.

If both the sympathetic and parasympathetic systems are blocked, the intrinsic heart rate will be about 105 bpm. The average resting heart rate of most healthy adults is approximately 70 to 80 bpm. This is evidence that the heart rate at rest is predominantly under parasympathetic control.

■ Heart Rate Variability

In healthy individuals, the heart rate at rest exhibits a certain degree of variability in the time interval between beats. The normal variability in heart rate is known as *heart rate variability (HRV)*.

The natural rhythmic phenomenon known as *respiratory sinus arrhythmia (RSA)* fluctuates the heart beat with the phase of respiration. More specifically, the heart rate at rest accelerates during inspiration and decelerates during expiration. Biofeedback techniques use the strategy of slow and controlled expiration to help slow down the heart rate. RSA is predominantly mediated by parasympathetic efferent activity to the heart. A reduced HRV thus is used as a marker of reduced vagal activity.

The clinical relevance of HRV became apparent with the recognition of a significant relationship between the autonomic nervous system and cardiovascular mortality, including sudden cardiac death.[23,24] In the late 1980s, studies confirmed that HRV was a strong and independent predictor of mortality after an acute myocardial infarction (heart attack).[25–27]

Evidence for an association between propensity for lethal arrhythmias and signs of either increased sympathetic or reduced vagal activity spurred efforts to develop quantitative markers of autonomic activity. Depressed HRV is a predictor of mortality and arrhythmic complications that is independent of other recognized risk factors.[28,29] This is another area of exercise-related research that has not yet been fully explored.

■ Systolic and Diastolic Blood Pressure

As discussed previously, from heartbeat to heartbeat (cardiac cycle), the heart goes through *systole* (Greek for contraction) and *diastole* (Greek for relaxation). During systole, enough pressure is mounted to push blood out of the left ventricle of the heart, through the large aorta, and onwards to the blood vessels throughout the body. During this phase, the arteries expand to accommodate the increased amount of blood. The pressure generated by the heart during this phase (systole) is known as the **systolic blood pressure**.

Under normal conditions, systolic blood pressure must be (and is) greater than diastolic to overcome the diastolic pressure, open the aortic valve, and send the blood throughout the body.

At the end of this phase, the heart begins to relax (diastole). The heart chambers expand to receive the new supply of blood that will be ejected in the following beat. The large arteries that had expanded to accommodate the large quantities of blood they received during systole are now recoiling. This recoiling action helps to maintain the necessary pressure for the blood to continue traveling throughout the body during diastole. The pressure that the blood exerts on the blood vessels during the relaxing phase of the heart (diastole) is known to as the **diastolic blood pressure**.

Systolic blood pressure is the pressure generated by the myocardium during systole. Diastolic blood pressure is the pressure the blood exerts on the blood vessels during diastole.

■ Rate-Pressure Product

Myocardial oxygen consumption (the metabolic demand of the heart) can be estimated by the **rate-pressure product**, which is calculated by multiplying the heart rate times the systolic blood pressure.

Rate-Pressure Product =
Heart Rate × Systolic Blood Pressure

A higher rate-pressure product indicates a higher workload for the heart and therefore a greater demand for oxygen. Although the myocardial oxygen demand at rest is almost always met, the rate-pressure product becomes important during physical work for sedentary individuals, especially for patients with heart disease.

■ Left Ventricular End-Diastolic Volume and End-Systolic Volume

Following each contraction (systole), the relaxation (diastolic) phase of the heart begins. It is during diastole that the ventricles fill with blood. The volume of blood present in the left ventricle during diastole is about 100 ml. This is known as the **end-diastolic volume (EDV)** or **left ventricular (LV-EDV)**. Similarly, the blood left in the ventricle at the end of systole is referred to the **end-systolic volume (ESV)** or **left ventricular (LV-ESV)**.

■ Ejection Fraction

The percentage of the EDV that is forced out by the left ventricle with every contraction is known as **ejection fraction (EF)**.

A healthy heart pumps out about 60% to 70% of the blood that is present in the left ventricle at the end of the relaxation period (diastole). Because at the end of the relaxation period, the left ventricle fills with about 100 ml of blood (about 4 oz), 60 to 70 ml of it (just over 2 oz) are pumped out.

In heart failure or when the heart is injured (as in the case of a myocardial infarction [heart attack]), the ejection fraction may be reduced. The reduction varies from individual to individual. Tests are available to determine the severity of the myocardial infarction and the heart's capacity to do work. Generally speaking, the greater the injury (the severity of the myocardial infarction), the lower the ejection fraction. An ejection fraction below 50% is usually considered the threshold for heart failure. It follows that the lower the ejection fraction, the more serious the condition. Commonly, a patient who has suffered a heart attack might have an ejection fraction of 40% or even 20% and yet do relatively well. The decline in the ejection fraction can continue over the years, especially if proper medical therapy is not provided.

Ejection fraction is the percentage of the end of diastolic volume that is pumped out by the left ventricle with each contraction.

■ Preload and Afterload

At the end of diastole, the blood within the ventricle (LV-EDV) exerts certain tension on the walls of the ventricle. This tension is known as the **preload**. In clinical terms, preload is the stress on the left ventricular wall at the end of the diastolic phase, approximated by the LV-EDV.

For the left ventricle to empty its content (the blood within the ventricle at the diastole) and deliver the blood throughout the body, it must generate enough force to overcome the resistance offered by the closed aortic valve and—most importantly—the pressure exerted by the blood within the aorta (above the aortic valve), otherwise known as the diastolic pressure. The ventricular wall tension generated by the left ventricle during systole is known as the **afterload**. It is approximately equal to the systolic blood pressure.

Preload is the stress on the left ventricular wall at the end of the diastole. Afterload is the ventricular wall tension generated by the left ventricle during systole.

■ Stroke Volume

Stroke volume is the amount of blood the heart pumps out per contraction. Expressing it in another way, stroke volume is the difference between the EDV and ESV.

$$\text{Stroke Volume} = \text{LV-EDV} - \text{LV-ESV}$$

In many ways, it is similar to the ejection fraction. The difference is that the ejection fraction expresses the percentage of blood that is pumped, while the stroke volume expresses the actual amount of blood in milliliters that the left ventricle pumps out. At rest, the stroke volume of a healthy heart is about 60 to 70 ml.

Stroke volume is the amount of blood the left ventricle pumps out with each contraction.

■ Cardiac Output

The volume of blood pumped out by the left ventricle in one minute is known as **cardiac output**. It is calculated by the heart rate and stroke volume:

$$\text{Cardiac Output} = \text{Heart Rate} \times \text{Stroke Volume}$$

The cardiac output of a healthy adult heart at rest is approximately 5,000 ml (5 liters or about 1.3 gallons).

Cardiac output is the volume of blood pumped out by the left ventricle in 1 minute. It is a by-product of heart rate and stroke volume.

■ Frank-Starling Mechanism of the Heart

One of the intrinsic mechanisms that regulate stroke volume and cardiac output is the ability of the heart to adjust to the changing volume of blood entering the heart and the ventricles. The mechanism is referred to as the **Frank-Starling mechanism of the heart**, named in honor of Otto Frank and Ernest Starling, the two physiologists who described heart muscle behavior in separate studies.

The Frank-Starling mechanism states that the force of the contractions by the heart (left ventricle) will increase (within physiologic limits) proportionally to the amount of blood entering the left ventricle. An analogy is that the heart acts similarly to a slingshot. The more the slingshot band is pulled back, the greater the force generated and the pebble is flung further. In a similar fashion, the more blood flowing into the ventricle during diastole, the more the ventricle stretches. Consequently, the force generated by the ventricle increases and the amount of blood pumped out with each contraction (stroke volume) increases.

The Frank-Starling mechanism of the heart states that tension applied to the cardiac muscle results in muscular contraction. The strength of the contraction (up to a point) is directly proportional to the degree of the applied tension.

■ CARDIOVASCULAR ADAPTATIONS TO EXERCISE

Physical activity or exercise is defined as work. According to the laws of physics, for work to be performed, equivalent energy must be spent. When the body is subjected to this extra work, it makes the necessary adjustments to meet the energy demand. For example, as exercise begins, the rate and depth of breathing increase to provide the extra oxygen needed for the increased workload. The heart rate increases to provide the extra blood to the muscles involved in the task. Fuel from the liver and fat deposits is released to meet the increased demand for energy. These are the immediate (acute) changes the body makes to accommodate the extra workload. When exercise ceases, all systems return back to resting levels.

In addition to the acute changes occurring in the body during physical exertion, other changes take place. These changes occur at a slower pace and over a period of time (weeks or months), and only if proper exercise or physical activity is performed on a regular basis. When this is the case, the activity itself becomes the stimulus for chronic changes to the systems involved in performing the specific physical activity. There are three reasons for these changes:

1. To make the systems involved in the task more efficient in performing the given task.
2. To make the system capable in performing more work.
3. To make the systems more resilient to injury.

These changes provide the basis for the beneficial effects of exercise on the human body.

One example of these chronic changes can be experienced when engaging in jogging. At first the task is difficult. However, after continuing to jog for a few weeks, the task gradually becomes easier. As improvements continue over time, it is conceivable that someone who could jog for only a few kilometers gradually can increase his or her fitness to be able to complete running a marathon.

Acute Adaptations

A change from rest to work/exercise increases the energy demand proportionally to the work at hand. To meet this increased demand, the body responds with an array of changes in all of the systems involved. The response is immediate and specific to the type and intensity of work. The acute cardiovascular responses to the increased demand (work) are summarized in **Table 7.1**.

■ Exercise Heart Rate

As one begins to exercise or perform physical work, the heart rate increases. The reason for this increase is to adequately supply the muscles with the nutrients needed to perform the work. The increase is gradual and directly related to the intensity of the activity. Naturally, the heart rate does not increase indefinitely. A maximum heart level is reached for every individual during maximum efforts. This maximum heart rate is determined by the age of the individual. This rate can be estimated with surprising great accuracy by subtracting the individual's age from 220.

■ Left Ventricular End-Diastolic Volume

Following each systolic phase of the cardiac cycle, the diastolic phase begins and ventricular filling occurs. Four factors influence ventricular filling.

1. Size of the ventricle.
2. Compliance of the ventricle; that is, the ability of the ventricle to relax during the diastolic phase of the cardiac cycle.
3. LV filling pressure, which is the pressure by which blood enters the ventricle.
4. Duration of the diastolic phase.

During exercise and especially at higher heart rates, the diastolic phase is shortened progressively. Despite this decrease, the EDV remains optimal even at peak exercise heart rates. Primarily this is due to the improved relaxation and ventricular filling that occur during exercise. Only at heart rates beyond maximal levels will EDV begin to decline.[30]

Table 7.1 Summary of Acute Responses with Exercise

Heart Rate	Increases
Systolic Blood Pressure	Increases
Diastolic Blood Pressure	No change or decreases slightly
Rate-Pressure Product	Increases
End-Diastolic Volume	Increases
End-Systolic Volume	Decreases
Stroke Volume	Increases
Cardiac Output	Increases
Peripheral Resistance	Decreases

End-diastolic volume remains optimal even at peak exercise heart rates primarily because of the improved relaxation and ventricular filling that occur during exercise.

■ Exercise and Left Ventricular End-Systolic Volume

Myocardial contractions are more vigorous during exercise. This forces more blood out of the ventricle, thus reducing end-systolic volume.

■ Exercise and Stroke Volume

Stroke volume increases as the intensity of exercise increases. It levels off at approximately 60% of the maximum heart rate. The maximal stroke volume for a moderately active individual is about 100 to 120 ml. For an elite endurance athlete, stroke volume can reach up to 200 ml.

The increase in stroke volume for both moderately active individuals and athletes is the outcome two factors: (1) increased LV-EDV due to quicker filling of the ventricle with more blood, and (2) more vigorous contraction of the left ventricle resulting in lower LV-ESV. Adequate stroke volume can be maintained until maximal heart rates are reached. However, as the heart rate exceeds maximal levels, the diastolic phase is reduced substantially and with it the filling time, resulting in a reduction in end-diastolic volume and in turn stroke volume.[30]

Stroke volume increases during exercise. The primary reason for this increase is the increase in LV-EDV and more vigorous contraction of the left ventricle that results in lower LV-ESV.

■ Exercise and Cardiac Output

Cardiac output is defined as the volume of blood that the left ventricle pumps out in 1 minute. It is the product of stroke volume and heart rate.

Cardiac Output = Stroke Volume × Heart Rate

Cardiac output increases progressively with the increase in the intensity of exercise and levels-off at some point. This point is determined by a number of factors, including age, fitness level, and genetics.

During light work, such as a brisk walk, cardiac output can easily increase to about 10 to 12 liters per minute. During heavy work, for example, when running to catch the bus or playing a game of tennis, the cardiac output of a healthy adult of average fitness can increase to five times the resting level (25 L/min). Even more amazing is that maximal cardiac output of an elite endurance training athlete (marathon running, cross-country skiing, etc.) can be as high as 40 liters per minute. This large cardiac output is the result of the large stroke volume observed in such elite athletes. This is one of the reasons why trained athletes can do so much more work.

Cardiac output increases up to five times the resting in healthy adults of average fitness and up to eight times in elite athletes. This large increase observed in athletes is primarily the result of the large stroke volume.

■ Cardiovascular Drift

During submaximal prolonged exercise (over 30 to 60 min), a progressive fall in stroke volume occurs and is a concomitant rise in heart rate (**Figure 7.19**). Because these changes are

Figure 7.19 Cardiovascular drift. Note that a decrease in stroke volume is compensated by a concomitant increase in heart rate. Consequently, cardiac output is maintained constant.

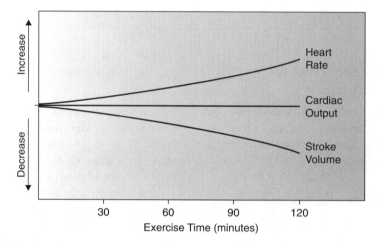

equal in magnitude, cardiac output is maintained throughout the exercise period. The increase in heart rate and decline in stroke volume is referred to a *cardiovascular drift*.[31,32] These actions are the result of the reduction in venous return to the heart perpetuated by an increase in blood flow to the skin, which dissipates heat, and a reduced plasma volume due to dehydration.[33] If prolonged exercise is performed under hot and humid conditions, therefore, the decrease in stroke volume and the concomitant increase in heart rate are exaggerated.[34]

■ Exercise and Blood Pressure

As the cardiac output increases during exercise, the systolic blood pressure also increases. Blood pressure during peak exercise can rise from approximately 120 mm Hg at rest to 180 or 200 mm Hg in healthy adults. The increase is directly related to exercise intensity. Generally speaking, the more intense the exercise, the higher the systolic blood pressure will rise.

Eventually, systolic blood pressure plateaus at approximately 200 mm Hg or less. Similar to the exercise heart rate, there is a plateau of blood pressure. However, the blood pressure plateau is not determined by age.

In some individuals, exercise blood pressure can rise above 200 mm Hg. Some studies suggest that this increase in exercise blood pressure is associated with future development of hypertension,[35,36] heart disease, and cardiovascular mortality.[37–39] However, other studies found no relationship.[40,41] More details about blood pressure during exercise are presented in Chapter 12.

Failure of systolic blood pressure to rise adequately during exercise is a sign of poor cardiac function. More importantly, a drop in blood pressure of more than 10 mm Hg below resting levels with increase in exercise intensity in most cases is an ominous sign of severe heart disease.[42,43]

The diastolic blood pressure in healthy individuals remains very close to resting levels or is slightly decreased. In fact, a decrease in diastolic blood pressure of about 5 to 10 mm Hg is normal. On the other hand, a rise in diastolic blood pressure of 10 mm Hg or higher may be observed in older individuals who have high blood pressure.

Large increases in both systolic and diastolic blood pressure are observed with exercises that involve resistance, such as weight training, weight lifting, and isometric contractions.[44–48] This increase is attributed to the cardiovascular system's attempt to overcome the pressure exerted by the contracting muscles on the blood vessels and maintain blood supply to the working muscles.[47,49] Blood pressure also increases by 15% more during work involving arm muscle versus legs. This is probably occurs because the relatively smaller arm muscles offer greater resistance to blood flow than the large muscles in the leg.[49]

> In healthy individuals, systolic blood pressure during exercise increases progressively and proportionally to the increase in the workload. Failure of systolic blood pressure to rise or a substantial drop (usually below resting levels) in pressure may indicate the presence of heart disease.

■ Rate-Pressure Product

As mentioned earlier, the increased demand for blood from the working muscles during work or exercise increases the workload to the heart. In turn, the metabolic demand of the heart (oxygen and nutrients) also increases. The metabolic demand of the heart can be estimated by the **rate-pressure product (RPP)**, which is calculated by multiplying the heart rate times the systolic blood pressure:

> RPP = Heart Rate × Systolic Blood Pressure

A higher rate-pressure product indicates a higher workload for the heart. Naturally, an increase in either the heart rate or systolic blood pressure will result in a greater workload for the heart. Because both the heart rate and systolic blood pressure increase with exercise, the RPP also increases. It is desirable and (healthy) that the workload of the heart at any absolute workload is low.

■ Peripheral Resistance

Peripheral resistance is defined as the impediment of the blood flow within blood vessels. Resistance is affected by a number of factors including the diameter of the blood vessels. During exercise, blood vessels of the exercising muscles dilate. This results in a decrease in the total peripheral resistance and consequently, blood pressure is maintained at physiologic levels (approximately 200/80 mm Hg at peak exercise for most healthy individuals). It is estimated that if peripheral resistance did not decrease, blood pressure would reach over 1,000/400 mm Hg at peak exercise.

> Total peripheral resistance decreases during exercise, and consequently blood pressure is maintained at physiologic levels.

Chronic Adaptations

Chronic adaptations are the result of long participation in a specific form of exercise on a regular basis that consists of adequate intensity, duration, and frequency. When the body is subjected to such exercise (physical stress), the demand for oxygen and nutrients for the muscles involved in the activity (i.e., leg muscles) increases. The body makes changes to accommodate this demand. These changes made are on the heart, blood vessels, and muscles involved in the activity. Ultimately, all changes lead to a more efficient system that not only can handle more work but also is more resilient to injury. A summary of the exercise-related chronic adaptations is presented in **Table 7.2.**

■ Resting Heart Rate

One of the easily observable changes following long-term exercise is a decrease in the resting heart rate. The average resting heart rate considered as normal in healthy adults is approximately 75 to 80 bpm. The resting heart rate can decrease substantially by 10 to 20 bpm within only a few weeks of regular exercise training of proper duration and intensity. It is common for athletes to have a resting heart rate of about 50 bpm and some exceptional athletes even as low as 35 to 45 bpm.

Significance   A lot of valuable information is packed in that heartbeat. Rhythm, sound, and rate all tell us something about the health of the person. Some have even advanced the theory that we are born with so many beats. When they finish, we finish. Animals with a low heart rate live longer than those with higher heart rates. For example, the resting heart rate of the mouse is about 600 bpm and it lives only a few years, the dog lives about 15 years and its heart rate is about 100 bpm, the horse and the elephant have heart rates of about 50 bpm and both live about 20 years, and the whale lives for about 35 years with a heart rate of less than 20 bpm.

There is no direct proof that this theory applies to humans. However, those with low resting heart rate tend to live longer than those with high heart rate.[50–52] In humans, sedentary individuals have a higher risk of developing and dying from heart disease as well as other causes. They also have a higher resting heart rate than people who are regularly physically active.

The heart rate of sedentary individuals is 80 to 90 bpm. Those who engage in mild exercise such as daily walk, have a resting heart rate of 60 to 70 bpm. Elite athletes such long distance runners, soccer players, and bikers have a resting heart rate between 30 and 40 bpm. Physically active individuals live longer than those who are sedentary.

To appreciate the importance of low resting heart rate and maximum heart rate, let us now present a hypothetical but very likely situation. Two individuals, both 40 years old, with a very similar genetic make-up but different fitness levels are presented in Table 7.2. Let us also assume that the one individual is physically active and has a resting heart rate of 60 bpm. The other individual is sedentary with a resting heart rate of 85 bpm. Although this situation is hypothetical, these heart rate values are within the limits of the average sedentary and physically active individuals.

The maximum heart rate of these individuals is 180 bpm (220 − 40 = 180). Both individuals

Table 7.2 Hypothetical Model of Heart Rate Response for Active and Sedentary Individuals During a Physical Challenge

	Age	HR at Rest	2*Resting HR	3*Resting HR	Max HR
Active	40	60 bpm	120 bpm	180 bpm	180
Sedentary	40	85 bpm	170 bpm	225 bpm*	180

*not physiologically possible

are now asked to engage in physical activity that would double their resting heart rate. This means that the heart rate of the physically active individual will now increase to 120 bpm (60 × 2 = 120) and that of the sedentary individual to 170 bpm (85 × 2 = 170).

As indicated in Table 7.2, at twice the resting HR, the physically active individual will be working at 66% of his or her maximum heart rate: (120/180) × 100 = 66%. At this intensity, exercise can be maintained for hours. On the other hand, doubling the heart rate for the sedentary individual will require that he or she works at 94% of the maximum heart rate: (170/180) × 100 = 94%. At this intensity, exercise can be sustained only for a few minutes. Furthermore, exercising at three times the resting heart rate is impossible for the sedentary individual, but attainable by the active individual.

> Resting HR decreases with exercise training. This allows the heart to perform more efficiently. Therefore, athletes can perform at substantially higher workloads than sedentary individuals.

■ Exercise and Heart Rate Variability

Findings from experimental studies support that regular exercise training has a positive effect on the autonomic system and promotes autonomic balance in normal subjects.[53,54] Other studies also have demonstrated that regularly performed exercise had a positive effect on the modulation of the parasympathetic and sympathetic systems in heart failure patients before and after cardiac transplant.

In an experimental study, the investigators induced an acute myocardial ischemia in seven conscious dogs and recorded the likely occurrence of ventricular fibrillation during myocardial ischemia (a lethal arrhythmia if not corrected). The dogs were then randomly assigned to 6 weeks of either daily exercise training or cage rest followed by exercise training. After 6 weeks of daily treadmill training, the same dogs were subjected to another episode of experimentally induced myocardial ischemia. This time, the investigators noted that exercise resulted in a marked improvement of vagal tone, as indicated by a 74% increase in heart rate variability. In addition, they noted a 44% improvement in the ventricular electrical stability. This resulted in 100% reduction in the incidence of ventricular fibrillation measured during acute myocardial ischemia, and all animals survived the new ischemic test.

Hull et al. reported that the most likely mechanism to explain the striking change in the risk for ventricular fibrillation was the shift in autonomic balance characterized by increased cardiac vagal activity. These results suggest that exercise training in healthy individuals may decrease their likelihood of developing lethal arrhythmias during acute myocardial ischemia.[55]

■ Exercise Heart Rate

As fitness improves, the heart rate at a specific workload decreases. For example, let us assume that one begins to run at the speed of a 15-minute mile. The heart rate during this endeavor is 130 bpm. As fitness improves (and within only 3–4 weeks), the heart rate during the same run (assuming the same weather conditions) will be lower. It is conceivable that the heart rate can decrease as much as 10 to 15 beats during the same run (workload) within 4 to 6 months of regular exercise.

■ Resting Blood Pressure

In general, blood pressure is lowered with exercise training. This is more evident in pre-hypertensive and hypertensive individuals. Study findings show that moderate intensity aerobic exercise training can lower blood pressure by about 10.5 mm Hg for systolic and 7.6 mm Hg for diastolic pressure.[56]

■ Exercise Blood Pressure

Similar to the reduction in heart rate, blood pressure also will be lower during the same exercise workload as the individual's fitness level improves. Again, it is conceivable that blood pressure can be lower by about 10 to 20 mm Hg within 3 to 4 months of regular exercise.

The mechanisms for the reduction in blood pressure are not well understood. Ultimately, lower catecholamine levels and reduction in peripheral resistance, cardiac output, or both all play a role. A detailed discussion of blood pressure response during exercise and the possible mechanisms governing this response is presented in Chapter 13.

■ Significance of Lower Heart Rate and Blood Pressure

As mentioned earlier, the metabolic demand of the heart can be estimated by the rate-pressure product (RPP), calculated by multiplying the heart rate times the systolic blood pressure. A higher RPP indicates a higher workload for the heart. Naturally, a relatively lower workload for the heart at any absolute workload is desirable and healthy. To illustrate this further, let us return to the example of an individual walking at the speed (exercise intensity) of 15 minutes per mile. The individual's heart rate during this exercise is 130 bpm and the systolic blood pressure 160 mm Hg (which are likely heart rate and blood pressure values). Based on this information, the individual's rate-pressure product is:

$$RPP = \text{Heart Rate} \times \text{Systolic BP}$$
$$130 \times 160 = 20{,}800$$

If this individual continues training for 4 to 6 months, a conservative estimate is that the heart rate during the same exercise (workload) is likely to decrease to 120 bpm and the systolic blood pressure to 150 mm Hg. The rate-pressure product is now

$$120 \times 150 = 18{,}000$$

As you can observe, the RPP is lower by 2,800. This indicates that the work the heart has to do to provide the muscles with the blood necessary to perform the same amount of work is now substantially lower. This is achieved because the heart has now become a more efficient pump. In general, a more efficient heart is a healthier heart and less likely to suffer an injury.

This is particularly important for patients who are at high risk for cardiovascular diseases. In our study of middle-aged and older Stage II hypertensive patients (resting systolic blood pressure [SBP] ≥ 160 mm Hg or diastolic BP [DBP] ≥ 100 mm Hg without treatment), we observed that the rate-pressure product was significantly reduced at all submaximal workloads after 16 weeks of low-intensity aerobic training (**Table 7.3**). This reduction was the result of lower blood pressure at these workloads.

It is also worth noting that after 16 weeks of training, their peak exercise capacity increased. Yet, despite the greater workload, their peak SBP value was lower by 20 mm Hg. Consequently, the RPP was lower.[57]

■ Left Ventricular End-Diastolic Volume

End-diastolic volume at any absolute workload will be higher following an improvement in exercise capacity (i.e., after exercise training). This is the result of the following changes:

Table 7.3 Exercise Heart Rate, Systolic Blood Pressure and Rate-Pressure Product Before and After 16 Weeks of Aerobic Exercise Training

	Heart Rate		Systolic Blood Pressure		Rate-Pressure Product	
	Baseline	Post Training	Baseline	Post Training	Baseline	Post Training
Rest	77 ± 11	68 ± 9	138 ± 12	131 ± 15	10,533	8798
3 METs	137 ± 16	134 ± 15	198 ± 34	171 ± 24	27,335	22,779
4 METs	146 ± 16	139 ± 12	213 ± 31	188 ± 25	31,172	26,039
5 METs	153 ± 15	146 ± 14	219 ± 24	187 ± 30	33,476	27,179
Peak Exercise	153 ± 15	153 ± 11	219 ± 24	199 ± 34	33,476	30,407

Source: Kokkinos, P.F., et al., Effects of aerobic training on exaggerated blood pressure response to exercise in African-Americans with severe systemic hypertension treated with indapamide +/– verapamil +/– enalapril. *Am J Cardiol* 1997;79(10):1424–1426.

First, the heart rate at any absolute, submaximal workloads will be lower following training. For example, an individual jogging at the speed of 10 minutes per mile before and after 4 months of exercise training, assuming that all conditions are similar (weather, health state of the individual, etc.), will have an exercise heart rate that is significantly lower following training. This is also evident in the aforementioned study of hypertensive patients (Table 7.3). Second, the size (cavity) of the left ventricle increases following training. Third, filling pressure increases. Fourth, the ventricle becomes more compliant (more relaxed) during the diastolic phase, thus allowing greater filling with oxygenated, nutrient-rich blood. The lower heart rate at an absolute workload allows for a longer filling time. This along with the increased cavity size and greater distensibility of the ventricle results in increased end-diastolic volume at absolute workloads, the aforementioned adaptations ensure that

end-diastolic volume is maintained even at maximum heart rates despite the progressive decrease in the diastolic phase and the higher peak workload achieved following exercise training.[58]

■ Left Ventricular End-Systolic Volume and Stroke Volume

The increase blood volume at the end of the diastolic phase (end-diastolic volume) results in greater distention of the left ventricle. According to the Frank-Starling law of the heart, the contractility of the ventricle will increase. As a result, the end-systolic volume at an absolute workload will be lowered following exercise training.

Consequently, the stroke volume will increase significantly at absolute workloads. In addition, stroke volume at maximal exercise also increases. In fact, the peak exercise stroke volume of elite athletes is almost double compared to normal subjects.[33] This increase is almost exclusively the result of the increases in LV-EDV.[58-60] The increase in LV-EDV leads to greater stretch of the left ventricle and a more forceful contraction (Frank-Starling's law) even at peak exercise.

The increase in stroke volume is evident at rest and during exercise. The increase is necessary to compensate for the decrease in heart rate and maintain a normal cardiac output. As you recall, cardiac output is the product of stroke volume and heart rate.

Cardiac Output = Heart Rate × Stroke Volume

As heart rate decreases, a proportional increase in the stroke volume must occur in order to maintain the same cardiac output. Although this may not sound as a rational or beneficial response at first, as you will see later, it is not only rational but highly beneficial for the body.

The exercise-related increase in stroke volume is almost exclusively the outcome of the increased left ventricular EDV that occurs with training.

■ Cardiac Output

Cardiac output at rest does not change as a result of exercise training. If you think about it, there is no reason for it to change. At rest, one needs the same amount of blood to carry out all bodily functions and sustain life regardless of the level of fitness. The profound changes in cardiac output following exercise training are seen during exercise. The cardiac output can reach 30 liters in moderately trained individuals and 40 liters in elite athletes. Because maximal heart rate does not change considerably with training, the main factor responsible for the increase in cardiac output thus is the increased stroke volume observed following exercise training.

■ Peripheral Resistance

The increase in cardiac output is compensated for by a concomitant decrease in peripheral resistance during exercise. This results in lower blood pressure at any workload and even at peak exercise. This is suggested by our findings in the study with hypertensive patients.[57] Although we did not assess peripheral resistance, the lower peak blood pressure following exercise training (219 vs. 199 mm Hg) at the same peak heart rate (153 bpm) strongly suggests that the peripheral resistance was lower in these patients (see Table 7.3).

■ IMPORTANCE OF THESE CHANGES: PUTTING IT ALL TOGETHER

To appreciate the changes that occur with exercise training in the heart and its function, one needs to consider all three factors: heart rate, stroke volume, and cardiac output. To illustrate this further, let us use the example of two identical twins. One twin exercises regularly (fit) and the other is sedentary. As mentioned before, the amount of blood required to sustain all body functions at rest (cardiac output) is similar for all individuals. The cardiac output of these two individuals at rest thus will be about 5,000 ml. The difference in the heart function of the twins can be seen in how the heart manages to pump 5,000 ml of blood per minute.

The resting heart rate of the fit twin is 50 bpm. Because cardiac output is a function of heart rate and stroke volume, the stroke volume of the active twin will be 100 ml/min. Thus, the required 5,000 ml of blood per minute (50 beats/minute × 100 ml) to sustain body functions at rest is provided.

The resting heart rate of the sedentary twin is 80 bpm. Because he also needs 5,000 ml of blood per minute to sustain body functions at

Table 7.4 Select Cardiac Parameters for Physically Active and Sedentary Individuals

	Resting HR	**Resting Stroke Volume**	**Resting Cardiac Output**
Active	50 bpm	100 ml	5,000 ml
Sedentary	80 bpm	63 ml	5,040 ml

rest, his stroke volume must be approximately 63 ml (80 bpm × 63 ml = 5,040 ml; **Table 7.4**).

The differences become even more evident during work or exercise. Let us assume that both individuals are 20 years of age and are both engaging in bicycling. The maximum heart rate of both is 200 bpm (220 − 20 = 200). Let us next assume that both individuals are biking at a certain speed that requires double the amount of blood required per minute at rest (resting cardiac output) or 10,000 ml of blood. Let us also assume that the stroke volume remains the same (in reality it does not). This means that both individuals will have to double their

heart rates to meet this demand. Thus, the heart of the physically fit (trained) individual will now be 100 bpm and the heart of the sedentary individual 160 bpm. Let us now assume that the workload increases and it now requires for the heart to increase the cardiac output three times the resting cardiac output or 15,000 ml per minute. This again will require the heart rate to triple. So the heart rate of the fit individual will increase to 150 bpm and the heart of the sedentary individual will have to increase to 240 bpm (**Table 7.5**). However, there is a problem. The maximum heart rate for these two individuals is 200 bpm. This means that the

Table 7.5 Heart Rate at Rest and During Exercise for Physically Fit and Unfit Individuals

	Heart Rate	**Stroke Volume**	**Cardiac Output**
Rest			
Individual (fit)	50 bpm	100 ml	5,000 ml
Individual (unfit)	80 bpm	63 ml	5,000 ml (about)
Exercise—Fit Individual			
2 x Resting HR	100 bpm	100 ml	10,000 ml
3 x Resting HR	150 bpm	100 ml	15,000 ml
Exercise—Unfit Individual			
2 x Resting HR	160 bpm	63 ml	15,000 ml
3 x Resting HR	240 bpm	63 ml	(physiologically impossible)

sedentary individual will not be able to continue at this rate. He or she will have to stop or slow down. On the other hand, the fit individual can continue at this pace for quite awhile because the exercise heart rate of 150 bpm is only 75% of his or her maximum heart rate.

To make matters worse, the stroke volume (as mentioned) also increases with exercise training. More accurately, both stroke volume and cardiac output increase during exercise. However, the maximum values achieved are greater in the trained than non-trained individuals. Let us then assume that both individuals will eventually reach a maximum heart rate (a valid assumption). At that point, the true values are likely to be similar to those presented in **Table 7.6**.

Thus, it becomes obvious why the trained individual can perform more work for a longer period of time.

■ Oxygen Extraction

Another important adaptation that occurs with exercise training is the ability of the exercising muscles to extract more oxygen from the blood delivered to them. This is known as the **arteriovenous-oxygen difference (a-$\bar{v}$ O$_2$ difference; Figure 7.20**). More specifically, if oxygen in the arterial blood is measured prior to entering the working muscle environment, and then measured again as it is leaving the muscle (venous blood), the difference repre-

Figure 7.20 Oxygen content in arterial and venous blood. The difference (referred as a-$\bar{v}$ O$_2$ difference) is the amount of oxygen utilized by the muscle.

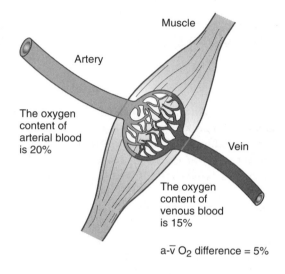

Muscle

Artery

The oxygen content of arterial blood is 20%

Vein

The oxygen content of venous blood is 15%

a-$\bar{v}$ O$_2$ difference = 5%

sents the amount of oxygen extracted from the blood by the muscle. This difference widens after training, as a result of the muscle extracting more oxygen from the blood.[61]

■ Maximum Oxygen Consumption: The Whole Picture

The exercise-induced adaptations just discussed work synergistically so that a rise in the

Table 7.6 Hypothetical Model of Maximal Values Achieved During Peak Exercise in Fit and Unfit Individuals

	Maximum Heart Rate	Maximum Stroke Volume	Maximum Cardiac Output
Fit	200 bpm	200 ml	40,000 ml
Unfit	200 bpm	120 ml	24,000 ml

maximum oxygen ($\dot{V}O_2$max) utilized by the body during maximal work. This represents the hallmark of cardiorespiratory fitness. Oxygen uptake is the product of cardiac output (HR × SV) and oxygen extraction (**a-$\bar{v}$ O_2 difference**).

$$\dot{V}O_2\text{max} = \text{Cardiac Output} \times \text{a-}\bar{v}\,O_2\text{ Difference}$$

Changes in $\dot{V}O_2$ max thus are the result of changes in either cardiac output, a-$\bar{v}$ O_2 difference, or both.

Note that $\dot{V}O_2$max can increase as much as 14 times from rest to peak exercise for sedentary individuals (oxygen consumption at rest is about 250 ml/min) and over 20 times for elite athletes (**Table 7.7**).[33] The $\dot{V}O_2$max increases linearly with the increase in cardiac output. Because the maximal heart rate does not change with exercise training, the increase in $\dot{V}O_2$max can only be attributed to increases observed in cardiac output and the ability of the muscle to extract more oxygen, known as an increase in a-$\bar{v}$ O_2 difference. Studies have shown that approximately 50% of the increase in $\dot{V}O_2$max can be attributed to the increase in maximal stroke volume and the remaining 50% to the increase in a-$\bar{v}$ O_2 difference.[59,60]

■ Frank-Starling Mechanism During Exercise

As stated previously, the Frank-Starling mechanism of the heart states that the force of the contractions by the left ventricle will increase (within physiologic limits) proportionally to the amount of blood entering the left ventricle. Consequently, the stoke volume and cardiac output increase.

The Frank-Starling mechanism at work is evident in the example of the two individuals (fit and sedentary) just presented. We know that the resting cardiac output is about 5,000 ml regardless of the fitness state of the individual. However, the resting heart rate of the fit individual is lower than that of the sedentary (50 bpm vs. 80 bpm). This allows longer time between heart beats and therefore the diastolic phase of the cardiac cycle is prolonged. In turn, the amount of blood entering into the ventricles increases. A greater stretching of the ventricle thus takes place and a greater force is generated to push the excess blood out of the heart. Consequently, stroke volume is increased and cardiac output is maintained constant at approximately 5,000 ml.

Similarly, during exercise at any absolute workload, the heart rate of fit individuals will be lower than the unfit. Once again the diastolic phase is longer, allowing for greater end

Table 7.7 Maximal Values for Oxygen Consumption, Heart Rate, Stroke Volume, and Cardiac Output for Sedentary Individuals and Athletes

	$\dot{V}O_2$max (ml/min)	Heart Rate (bpm)	Stroke Volume (ml/beat)	Cardiac Output (ml/min)
Athletes	6,250	190	205	38,950
Sedentary	3,500	195	112	21,840

Source: Used with permission from Rowell LB. *Human Circulation Regulation During Physical Stress.* New York: Oxford University Press; 1986.

diastolic volume and more time for the heart to rest. Consequently, a greater stroke volume is achieved by athletes at absolute workloads.

■ Exercise and Left Ventricular Hypertrophy: The Athlete's Heart

In 1892, Sir William Osler wrote, "In the process of training, the getting of wind as it is called, is largely a gradual increase in the capability of the heart . . . the large heart of athletes may be due to the prolonged use of their muscles, but no man becomes a great runner or oarsman who has not naturally a capable if not a large heart."[62] In the years to follow, this observation was ignored and physicians until the early twentieth centuries held the view that vigorous athletic activities were detrimental to the heart.[63] This myth was dispelled by the

work of two Austrian physicians who examined athletes involved in 16 different sports and documented that the heart size was substantially larger than the heart of the average population. However, upon reexamination at 6-month intervals, they found no serious problems as a result of the increased heart size.[64]

By the early 1990s, advances in echocardiography allowed cardiologists to study the athletic heart in great detail. It is now common knowledge that structural and functional changes occur with exercise as an adaptation to the increased physical workload.[65,66] The exercise-related changes in the structure and function of the heart are now commonly referred to as the *athletic heart syndrome* or *athlete's heart*.

Exercise-related heart adaptations are highly specific to the type of exercise (**Table 7.8**). For

Table 7.8 Differences in LVDD and Wall Thickness in 947 Athletes Versus Controls

Sport	Left Ventricular Diastolic Dimension (cm)	Walls (cm)
Cross Country Skiing	5.41	0.98
Pentathlon	4.35	0.98
Soccer	3.11	0.76
Cycling	5.91	2.02
Swimming	4.9	1.71
Canoeing	4.23	1.71
Rowing	3.87	2.13
Weight Training	1.32	1.23
Long-Distance Track	3.47	1.49
Tennis	2.69	1.0
Boxing	2.25	0.94
Taekwondo (Karate)	2.07	0.23
Water Polo	2.02	1.38
Volleyball	1.43	0.39
Wrestling/Judo	1.25	1.21

Source: Adapted from Spirito P, Pellicia A, Proschan MA, et al. Morphology of the "athlete's heart" assessed by echocardiography in 947 elite athletes representing 27 sports. *Am J Cardiol* 1994;74:804.

example, purely aerobic exercises such as jogging result in predominately left ventricular cavity enlargement, with some increase in left ventricular wall thickness.[67] This type of hypertrophy (increase in size in a particular tissue or organ) is known as *eccentric hypertrophy*. In contrast, working against high resistance in exercises such as weight training leads to a substantial hypertrophy of the left ventricular wall, known as *concentric hypertrophy*. Exercises that incorporate both aerobic and resistance training, such as rowing and to some degree cycling, can lead to both concentric and eccentric hypertrophy.[66] However, it is important to emphasize that most sports associated with left ventricular end-diastolic enlargement also are associated with increases in wall thickness. The increase in either alone (wall thickness or LV end-diastolic dimension [LV-EDD]) will not be physiologically desirable. LV dilation without a comparable increase in wall thickness will lead to an inappropriate increase in wall tension that is detrimental to the heart.[68]

In general, the changes are considered to be a normal physiologic adaptation to the particularly rigorous training of athletes. They are not associated with the diastolic dysfunction, arrhythmias, or adverse prognosis that are observed in hypertension-induced LV hypertrophy [69,70] and regresses quickly when training is discontinued.[71] However, a distinction must be made between the purely athletic heart syndrome and the changes that occur in **hypertrophic cardiomyopathy** that can also occur in athletes. This is a pathologic condition seen in patients (and athletes) with primary myocardial disease or significant valvular disease. The structural cardiac changes in these individuals are usually much greater than those induced by exercise only. The distinction between these two conditions (true athlete's heart or structural changes resulting from heart disease) is crucial because the risk for sudden deaths in young athletes increases when structural heart changes are the result of myocardial or valvular diseases.[72,73] This distinction can be made only by a cardiologist.

Exercise-related heart changes are highly specific to the type of exercise. Generally such changes are considered to be a normal physiologic adaptation to the particularly rigorous training of athletes.

■ Endothelial Function

Endothelial function is impaired with advancing age and a sedentary lifestyle. Evidence supports that the age-related decline in endothelial function can be attenuated—and even reversed—by adequate exercise training. In a cleverly designed study, endothelial function was assessed in 68 healthy men 22 to 35 or 50 to 76 years of age who were either sedentary or endurance exercise trained. Among the middle aged and older sedentary men, endothelial function was impaired by about 25% compared to young men. In contrast, there was no age-related difference in the endothelial function among the endurance-trained men.

Following the baseline assessments, 13 of the previously sedentary middle-aged and older men completed a 3-month, home-based aerobic exercise intervention (primarily walking). After the exercise intervention, endothelial function improved by approximately 30% and to levels similar to those in young adults and middle-aged and older endurance-trained men. These findings demonstrate that regular aerobic exercise can prevent the age-associated loss in endothelium function and restore levels in previously sedentary middle-aged and older healthy men.[74] **Table 7.9** summarizes data from several studies that have examined the before

Table 7.9 Summary of Exercise-Related Chronic Adaptation as Compared to Before Exercise Training

Resting Heart Rate	Lower
Exercise Heart Rate at Absolute Workloads	Lower
Exercise Blood Pressure at Absolute Workloads	Lower
Rate-Pressure Product at Absolute Workloads	Lower
Rate-Pressure Product at Peak Exercise	Lower
End-Diastolic Volume at Absolute Workloads	Lower
End-Diastolic Volume at Peak Exercise	Lower
End-Systolic Volume at Absolute Workloads	Lower
End-Systolic Volume at Peak Exercise	Lower
Stroke Volume at Absolute Workloads	Higher
Stroke Volume at Peak Exercise	Higher
Peak Cardiac Output	Higher
Peripheral Resistance	Lower
Oxygen Extraction (a-$\bar{v}$ O_2 Difference)	Higher
Maximum Oxygen Uptake ($\dot{V}O_2$max)	Higher

Sources: Kokkinos PF, Narayan P, Fletcher RD, et al. Effects of aerobic training on exaggerated blood pressure response to exercise in African-Americans with severe systemic hypertension treated with indapamide +/– verapamil +/– enalapril. *Am J Cardiol* 1997;79(10):1424–1426.

Bersohn MM, Scheuer J. Effects of physical training on end-diastolic volume and myocardial performance of isolated rat hearts. *Circ Res* 1977;40(5):510–516.

Saltin B, Blomqvist G, Mitchell JH, et al. Response to exercise after bed rest and after training. *Circulation* 1968;38(5 Suppl):VII1–78.

Scheuer J, Tipton CM. Cardiovascular adaptations to physical training. *Annu Rev Physiol* 1977;39:221–251.

Rowell LB. *Human Cardiovascular Control.* Gary, NC: Oxford University Press; 1994.

and after effects of exercise on the circulatory system.

Another interesting point about that study is that the exercise intensity necessary to improve endothelial function was relatively low (primarily walking). This is clinically important because low exercise intensities can easily be tolerated by most middle-aged and older individuals.

■ C-Reactive Protein and Physical Activity

Although the mechanisms of atherosclerosis are still not completely understood, it is now accepted that atherosclerosis is a chronic inflammatory disease of the arterial wall known as the **"response-to-injury"** theory.[75–77] This theory states that the atherosclerosis develops as a result of repetitive injury and ongoing inflammatory process of the inner arterial wall (endothelial layer) of large and medium-sized arteries. C-reactive protein (CRP) is released during systemic inflammation and CRP levels in blood rise. A more sensitive CRP test, called a *highly sensitive C-reactive protein* (hs-CRP) assay, is available for clinical use. A dose-response relationship between hs-CRP and coronary heart disease exists that is independent of other risk factors.[78]

Because increased physical activity is associated with a reduced incidence of coronary disease, it has been hypothesized that one of the mechanisms by which physical activity protects against cardiovascular disease is by reducing the inflammatory process within the arterial wall. This is another exciting area of exercise-related research. However, available data are currently limited.

■ SUMMARY

- The cardiovascular system consists of the heart and a network of approximately 100,000 miles of blood vessels. Its primary function is to rapidly transport oxygen and nutrients to the tissues upon demand.
- The primary function of the heart is to pump the necessary blood throughout the body. At rest, the heart pumps about 5 liters of blood per minute. During hard work, the heart of the average fit individual can pump 20 liters of blood per minute. The athlete's heart can reach over 30 liters.
- The cardiac cycle is the time period between the beginning of one heartbeat to the beginning of the next. During this time, the heart undergoes a contraction and relaxation phase.
- The contraction phase is known as systole. During this phase, the blood is pumped out

of the heart chambers and into the lungs and all other tissues of the body.
- The relaxation phase of the heart begins at the end of systole and is known as diastole. Blood returns to the heart and fills the heart chambers during diastole. The cycle is then repeated.
- The endothelium is comprised of a single layer of endothelial cells that line the inner wall of the blood vessels. A healthy endothelium synthesizes and releases various substances that control and maintain a balance between dilation and constriction of blood vessels and the unimpeded blood flow to the organs.
- When the endothelium is damaged, synthesis and release of these substances is inhibited and with vasodilation is impaired. This condition known as endothelial dysfunction plays a critical role in the pathogenesis of chronic disease such as hypertension, diabetes and atherosclerosis.
- The rhythmic contractions of the heart are possible because of the generation of electrical impulses and their well-coordinated propagation throughout the heart.
- The impulse is initiated by a specialized area of cardiac cells referred to as the sinoatrial node (SA node) and propagated by the conduction system of the heart.
- The generation of an impulse becomes possible mainly by the well-coordinated and tightly controlled exchange of sodium and potassium (known as electrolytes) inside and outside the cardiac cells.
- The heart rate is precisely regulated by the balance between the sympathetic and parasympathetic nervous system. The sympathetic fibers release the neurotransmitter norepinephrine on to the pacemaker of the heart.

- For longer effects, the hormone epinephrine or adrenaline is released into the blood stream by the medulla of the adrenal gland. Acetylcholine is the mediator for the parasympathetic system.
- An increase in heart rate and force of contractions is the result of adrenaline increase. Conversely, acetylcholine release by the parasympathetic system results in a decreased heart rate and force of contractions.
- The pressure generated by the left ventricle during systole is known as the systolic blood pressure. The pressure that the blood exerts on the blood vessels during the relaxing phase of the heart (diastole) is known to as the diastolic blood pressure.
- Myocardial oxygen consumption (metabolic demand of the heart) can be estimated by the rate-pressure product, which is calculated by multiplying the heart rate times the systolic blood pressure.
- Ejection fraction (EF) refers to the percentage of blood that is pumped out by the left ventricle with every contraction. The EF of a healthy heart is about 60% to 70%.
- Stroke volume is the amount of blood the heart pumps out per contraction.
- Cardiac output is the amount of blood pumped by the left ventricle in 1 minute. It is the product of the heart rate and the stroke volume. The resting cardiac output is approximately 5,000 ml.
- The Frank-Starling mechanism states that the force of the contractions by the left ventricle will increase (within physiologic limits) proportionally to the amount of blood entering the left ventricle.
- Work or exercise imposes an increased demand on the organism. Consequently,

acute and chronic adaptations occur to compensate for the imposed demand.
- Acute adaptations during exercise include an increase in heart rate, systolic blood pressure, stroke volume, end diastolic volume and cardiac output. In addition, end systolic volume and peripheral resistance decrease.
- Exercise-induced chronic adaptations include a decrease in resting heart rate and blood pressure and an increase in stroke volume.
- During exercise at absolute and peak workloads, favorable changes occur in heart rate, blood pressure, left ventricular filling and emptying, and peripheral resistance. Collectively, these changes result in a more efficient cardiac function.
- These changes are consistent with the Frank-Starling mechanism of the heart. Consequently, the stoke volume and with it cardiac output increase.
- Ultimately, the exercise-induced adaptations work synergistically to increase the maximum oxygen utilized by the body during maximal work. This represents the hallmark of cardiorespiratory fitness.
- Approximately 50% of the increase in maximal oxygen uptake following exercise training is attributed to the increase in maximal stroke volume and the remaining 50% to the increase in a-$\bar{v}$ O$_2$ difference.
- Structural and functional cardiac changes occur with exercise as an adaptation to the increased physical workload. These changes are highly specific to the type of exercise and commonly are referred to as the athletic heart syndrome or athlete's heart.
- Generally, the changes are considered to be a normal physiologic adaptation to the particularly rigorous training of athletes. They are not associated with the

abnormalities observed in the hypertensive heart and regresses quickly when training is discontinued.

- The heart changes observed in athletes as a result of the vigorous training are healthy. However, changes in the heart can occur as result of heart disease or genetic abnormalities. Such changes, referred to as hypertrophic cardiomyopathy, are considered pathological and are associated with increased risk of sudden death in young athletes.
- The decline in endothelial function as a result of aging and physical inactivity can be attenuated and perhaps reversed by adequate exercise training.

■ REFERENCES

1. Berne RM, Levy MN. *Physiology*, 2nd ed. St. Louis, MO: C.V. Mosby Company; 1988.
2. Guyton AC, Hall J. *Human Physiology and Mechanisms of Disease*. Philadelphia: W.B. Saunders Company; 1997.
3. Gimbone M. Vascular endothelium: nature's blood container. In J. Gimbrone, ed. *Vascular Endothelium in Homeostasis and Thrombosis*. Edinburgh, UK: Churchill Livingston; 1986:1–13.
4. Petty RG, Pearson JD. Endothelium—the axis of vascular health and disease. *J R Coll Physicians Lond* 1989;23(2):92–102.
5. Egashira K, Inou T, Hrrooka Y, et al. Effects of age on endothelium-dependent vasodilation of resistance coronary artery by acetylcholine in humans. *Circulation* 1993;88:77–81.
6. Celermajer DS, Sorensen KE, Georgakoupoulos D, et al. Cigarette smoking is associated with dose-related and potentially reversible impairment of endothelium-dependent dilation in healthy young adults. *Circulation* 1993;88(5 Pt 1):2149–2155.
7. Casino PR, Kilcoyne CM, Quyyumi AA, et al. The role of nitric oxide in endothelium-

dependent vasodilation of hypercholesterolemic patients. *Circulation* 1993;88(6): 2541–2547.
8. Johnstone MT, Creager SJ, Scales KM, et al. Impaired endothelium-dependent vasodilation in patients with insulin-dependent diabetes mellitus. *Circulation* 1993;88(6):2510–2516. (see comments)
9. Panza JA, Casino PR, Badar DM Quyyami AA. Effect of increased availability of endothelium-derived nitric oxide precursor on endothelium-dependent vascular relaxation in normal subjects and in patients with essential hypertension. *Circulation* 1993;87(5): 1475–1481.
10. Panza JA, Casino PR, Badar DM, Quyyami AA. Role of endothelium-derived nitric oxide in the abnormal endothelium-dependent vascular relaxation of patients with essential hypertension. *Circulation* 1993;87(5):1468–1474.
11. Furchgott RF, Zawadzki JV. The obligatory role of endothelial cells in the relaxation of arterial smooth muscle by acetylcholine. *Nature* 1980;288(5789):373–376.
12. Palmer RM, Ferrige AG, Moncada S. Nitric oxide release accounts for the biological activity of endothelium-derived relaxing factor. *Nature* 1987;327(6122): 524–526.
13. Koshland DE Jr. The molecule of the year. *Science* 1992;258(5090):1861.
14. Culotta E, Koshland DE Jr. NO news is good news. *Science* 1992;258(5090):1862–1865.
15. Ohno M, Gibbons GH, Dzau VJ, Cooke JP. Shear stress elevates endothelial cGMP. Role of a potassium channel and G protein coupling. *Circulation* 1993;88(1):193–197.
16. Levick J. *An Introduction to Cardiovascular Physiology*, 4th ed. London, UK: Arnold; 2003.
17. Furlanello F, Bertoldi A, Dallago M, et al. Atrial fibrillation in elite athletes. *J Cardiovasc Electrophysiol* 1998;9(8 Suppl):S63–S68.
18. Karjalainen J, Kujala UM, Kaprio J, et al. Lone atrial fibrillation in vigorously exercising middle aged men: case-control study. *BMJ* 1998;316(7147):1784–1785.
19. Mozaffarian D, Furberg CD, Psaty BM, Siscovick D. Physical activity and incidence of

atrial fibrillation in older adults. The Cardio-vascular Health Study. *Circulation* 2008;118: 800–807.

20. Lilly LS. *Pathophysiology of Heart Disease*, 2nd ed. Baltimore: Williams and Wilkins; 1998.

21. Saul J. Beat-to-beat variations of heart rate reflect modulation of cardiac autonomic out-flow. *News Physiol Sci* 1990;5:32–37.

22. Spyer K. Central nervous mechanisms con-tributing to cardiovascular control. *J Physiol* 1994;474:1–19.

23. Levy M, Schwartz PJ. *Vagal Control of the Heart: Experimental Basis and Clinical Implications*. Armonk, NY: Futura; 1994.

24. Lown B, Verrier RL. Neural activity and ventricular fibrillation. *N Engl J Med* 1976; 294(21):1165–1170.

25. Bigger JT Jr, Fleiss J, Steinman RC, et al. Fre-quency domain measures of heart period variability and mortality after myocardial infarction. *Circulation* 1992;85(1):164–171.

26. Kleiger RE, Miller JP, Bigger JT Jr, Moss AJ. Decreased heart rate variability and its asso-ciation with increased mortality after acute myocardial infarction. *Am J Cardiol* 1987;59 (4):256–262.

27. Malik M, Farrell T, Cripps T, Camm AJ. Heart rate variability in relation to prognosis after myocardial infarction: selection of optimal processing techniques. *Eur Heart J* 1989; 10(12):1060–1074.

28. Heart rate variability: standards of measure-ment, physiological interpretation and clini-cal use. Task Force of the European Society of Cardiology and the North American Soci-ety of Pacing and Electrophysiology. *Circula-tion* 1996;93(5):1043–1065.

29. Huikuri HV, Seppänen T, Koistinen MJ, et al. Abnormalities in beat-to-beat dynamics of heart rate before the spontaneous onset of life-threatening ventricular tachyarrhythmias in patients with prior myocardial infarction. *Circulation* 1996;93(10):1836–1844.

30. More RL. *ACSM's Advanced Exercise Physi-ology. The Cardiovascular System: Cardiac Function*. Baltimore: Lippincott Williams & Wilkins; 2006:326–342.

31. Åstrand PO, Cuddy CE, Salton B, Steinberg J. Cardiac output during submaximal and maxi-mal work. *J Appl Physiol* 1964;19:268–274.

32. Saltin B. Circulatory response to submaximal and maximal exercise after thermal dehydra-tion. *J Appl Physiol* 1964;19:1125–1132.

33. Rowell BL. *Human Circulation Regulation During Physical Stress*. New York: Oxford University Press; 1986.

34. Powers SK, Howley ET, Cox R. A differential catecholamine response during prolonged exercise and passive heating. *Med Sci Sports Exerc* 1982;14(6):435–439.

35. Miyai N, Arita M, Miyashita K, et al. Blood pressure response to heart rate during exer-cise test and risk of future hypertension. *Hypertension* 2002;39(3):761–766.

36. Singh JP, Larson MG, Manolio TA, et al. Blood pressure response during treadmill testing as a risk factor for new-onset hypertension. The Framingham Heart Study. *Circulation* 1999; 99(14):1831–1836.

37. Filipovsky J, Ducimetiere P, Safar ME. Prog-nostic significance of exercise blood pressure and heart rate in middle-aged men. *Hyperten-sion* 1992;20(3):333–339.

38. Mundal R, Kjeldsen SE, Sandvik L, et al. Exer-cise blood pressure predicts cardiovascular mortality in middle-aged men. *Hypertension* 1994;24(1):56–62.

39. Mundal R, Kjeldsen SE, Sandvik L, et al. Exer-cise blood pressure predicts mortality from myocardial infarction. *Hypertension* 1996;27 (3 Pt 1):324–329.

40. Fagard RH, Pardoens K, Staessen JA, Thijs L. Prognostic value of invasive hemodynamic measurements at rest and during exercise in hypertensive men. *Hypertension* 1996;28(1): 31–36.

41. Manolio TA, Burke GL, Savage PJ, et al. Exer-cise blood pressure response and 5-year risk of elevated blood pressure in a cohort of young adults: the CARDIA study. *Am J Hyper-tens* 1994;7(3):234–241.

42. Gibbons RJ, Balady GJ, Bricker JT, et al. ACC/ AHA 2002 guideline update for exercise test-ing: summary article. A report of the Ameri-can College of Cardiology/American Heart

Association Task Force on Practice Guidelines (Committee to Update the 1997 Exercise Testing Guidelines). *J Am Coll Cardiol* 2002;40(8):1531–1540.

43. Rodgers GP, Ayanian JZ, Balady G, et al. American College of Cardiology/American Heart Association Clinical Competence statement on stress testing: a report of the American College of Cardiology/American Heart Association/American College of Physicians–American Society of Internal Medicine Task Force on Clinical Competence. *J Am Coll Cardiol* 2000;36(4):1441–1453.

44. Astrand I, Guharay A, Wahren J. Circulatory responses to arm exercise with different arm positions. *J Appl Physiol* 1968;25(5): 528–532.

45. Humphreys PW, Lind AR. The blood flow through active and inactive muscles of the forearm during sustained hand-grip contractions. *J Physiol* 1963;166:120–135.

46. Johnson BL, et al. A comparison of concentric and eccentric muscle training. *Med Sci Sports* 1976;8(1):35–38.

47. Lind AR, McNicol GW. The circulatory effects of sustained voluntary muscle contraction. *Clin Sci* 1964;27:229–244.

48. MacDougall JD, Tuxen D, Sale DG, et al. Arterial blood pressure response to heavy resistance exercise. *J Appl Physiol* 1985;58(3): 785–790.

48. Nieman DC. *Exercise Testing and Prescription*, 5th ed. New York: McGraw-Hill Higher Education; 2003.

50. Jouven X, Empana JP, Schwartz PJ, et al. Heart-rate profile during exercise as a predictor of sudden death. *N Engl J Med* 2005; 352(19):1951–1958. (see comments)

51. Kannel WB, Kennel C, Paffenbarger RS Jr, Cupples LA. Heart rate and cardiovascular mortality: The Framingham Study. *Am Heart J* 1987;113(6):1489–1494.

52. Levine HJ. Rest heart rate and life expectancy. *J Am Coll Cardiol* 1997; 30(4):1104–1106.

53. Arai Y, Albrecht P, Harttey LH, et al. Modulation of cardiac autonomic activity during and immediately after exercise. *Am J Physiol* 1989;256(1 Pt 2):H132–H141.

54. Furlan R, Piazza S, Dell'Orto S, et al. Early and late effects of exercise and athletic training on neural mechanisms controlling heart rate. *Cardiovasc Res* 1993;27(3):482–488. (see comments)

55. Hull SS Jr, Vanoli E, Adamson PB, et al. Exercise training confers anticipatory protection from sudden death during acute myocardial ischemia. *Circulation* 1994;89(2):548–552. (see comments)

56. Kokkinos PF, Narayan P, Papademetriou V. Exercise as hypertension therapy. *Cardiol Clin* 2001;19(3):507–516.

57. Kokkinos PF, Narayan P, Fletcher RD, et al. Effects of aerobic training on exaggerated blood pressure response to exercise in African-Americans with severe systemic hypertension treated with indapamide +/− verapamil +/− enalapril. *Am J Cardiol* 1997;79(10):1424–1426.

58. Bersohn MM, Scheuer J. Effects of physical training on end-diastolic volume and myocardial performance of isolated rat hearts. *Circ Res* 1977;40(5):510–516.

59. Saltin B, Blomqvist G, Mitchell JH, et al. Response to exercise after bed rest and after training. *Circulation* 1968;38(5 Suppl):VII1–78.

60. Scheuer J, Tipton CM. Cardiovascular adaptations to physical training. *Annu Rev Physiol* 1977;39:221–251.

61. Rowell LB. *Human Cardiovascular Control*. New York: Oxford University Press; 1994.

62. Osler W. *The Principles and Practice of Medicine*. New York: Appleton, 1892;635.

63. Puffer JC. Overview of the athletic heart syndrome. In DP Paul, ed. *Exercise and Sports Cardiology*. New York: McGraw-Hill Medical Publishing Division; 2001:30–42.

64. Deutsch F, Kauf E. *Heart and Athletics*. St. Louis, MO: CV Mosby Company; 1927.

65. Pelliccia A, Maron BJ, Culasso F, et al. Athlete's heart in women. Echocardiographic characterization of highly trained elite female athletes. *JAMA* 1996; 276(3):211–215.

66. Pelliccia A, Maron BJ, Spataro A, et al. The upper limit of physiologic cardiac hypertrophy in highly trained elite athletes. *N Engl J Med* 1991; 324(5):295–301.

67. Maron BJ. Structural features of the athlete heart as defined by echocardiography. *J Am Coll Cardiol* 1986;7(1):190–203.

68. Spirito P, Pelliccia A, Proschan MA, et al. Morphology of the "athlete's heart" assessed by echocardiography in 947 elite athletes representing 27 sports. *Am J Cardiol* 1994; 74(8):802–806.

69. Granger CB, Karimeddini MK, Smith VE, et al. Rapid ventricular filling in left ventricular hypertrophy: I. Physiologic hypertrophy. *J Am Coll Cardiol* 1985;5(4):862–868.

70. McLenachan JM, Henderson E, Morris KI, Dargie HJ. Ventricular arrhythmias in patients with hypertensive left ventricular hypertrophy. *N Engl J Med* 1987;317(13):787–792.

71. Martin WH III, Coyle EF, Bloomfield SA, Ehsani AA. Effects of physical deconditioning after intense endurance training on left ventricular dimensions and stroke volume. *J Am Coll Cardiol* 1986;7(5):982–989.

72. Maron BJ, Shirani J, Poliac CC, et al. Sudden death in young competitive athletes. Clinical, demographic, and pathological profiles. *JAMA* 1996;276(3):199–204. (see comments)

73. Maron BJ, Epstein SE, Roberts WC. Causes of sudden death in competitive athletes. *J Am Coll Cardiol* 1986;7(1):204–214.

74. DeSouza CA, Shapiro CF, Clevenger CM, et al. Regular aerobic exercise prevents and restores age-related declines in endothelium-dependent vasodilation in healthy men. *Circulation* 2000;102(12):1351–1357.

75. Hansson GK. Inflammation, atherosclerosis, and coronary artery disease. *N Engl J Med* 2005;352(16):1685–1695.

76. Libby P. Inflammation in atherosclerosis. *Nature* 2002;420(6917):868–874.

77. Ross R. Atherosclerosis is an inflammatory disease. *Am Heart J* 1999;138(5 Pt 2): S419–S4120.

78. Pearson TA, Mensah GA, Alexander RW, et al. Markers of inflammation and cardiovascular disease: application to clinical and public health practice: a statement for healthcare professionals from the Centers for Disease Control and Prevention and the American Heart Association. *Circulation* 2003;107(3): 499–511. (see comments)

Cardiovascular Disease Epidemiology and Physical Activity

This final section of the book, which focuses on the epidemiology of the cardiovascular system and the disease process, is presented in a unique way. In the course of describing each study's findings, the pathophysiology and mechanisms involved in the disease process are explained. Collectively, this information provides the reader with (1) a body of evidence accumulated over decades on the association between physical activity and cardiovascular disease, and (2) an understanding of the mechanisms of disease. In addition, and perhaps most importantly, this information builds on the knowledge accumulated from the previous two sections to provide a more complete understanding of the physiologic pathways by which physical activity can intervene in the prevention of cardiovascular disease. Consequently, it provides a broad platform for those who are interested to probe further into new research and explore new ideas in the associations between physical activity and cardiovascular health.

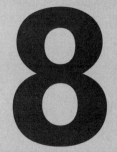

CHAPTER

8

Epidemiology of Cardiovascular Disease

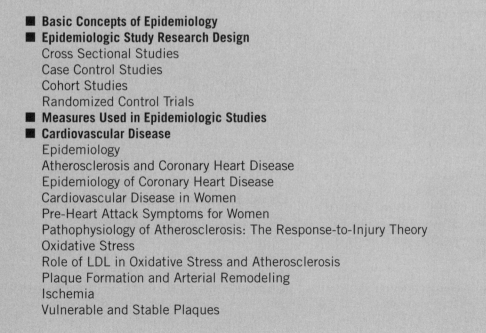

- **Distribution:** Deals with the identification of who is getting the disease as well as when and where the disease is occurring.
- **Determinants:** Identification of factors that influence the occurrence of the disease.

> Epidemiology is based on the assumption that human disease does not occur at random; rather, there are certain factors that cause or favor the occurrence a disease.

■ BASIC CONCEPTS OF EPIDEMIOLOGY

The word **epidemiology** is derived from three Greek words: *epi* (on or upon), *demos* (people), and *logos* (the study of). Epidemiology is the scientific discipline involved in the systematic study of the distribution and determinants of disease or events in specified populations.[1] Epidemiology is based on the assumption that human disease does not occur at random; rather, there are certain factors that cause or favor the occurrence a disease. Subsequently, the identification of these factors can lead to prevention of the disease. Thus, epidemiology has three components: frequency, distribution, and determinants.

- **Frequency:** Quantification of the existence or occurrence of disease. It also involves the rate or risk of the disease in the population.

■ EPIDEMIOLOGIC STUDY RESEARCH DESIGN

Epidemiologic studies are designed to either describe the distribution of disease/events or the determination or elucidation of the determinants of the disease (risk factors). Three research designs are common in epidemiologic research: cross sectional studies, case control studies, and cohort studies. The study design depends mostly on the scientific question to be answered. However, the availability of data, resources, and time also play a role. Each design has its unique strengths and limitations. A brief overview of the aforementioned designs strengths and limitations is provided here.

Cross Sectional Studies

Cross sectional studies are designed to evaluate the frequency of various characteristics, prevalence of risk factors, and to assess relationships between these factors and characteristics with disease outcome at a particular time. They provide a snapshot of the population. No temporal relationships can be assessed by cross sectional studies.

Cross sectional studies are quick, easy, and inexpensive to conduct. However, they provide more limited information than the other two study types.

Case Control Studies

In this type of (retrospective) study, the participants are selected based on the presence of a disease or event of interest (e.g., heart disease). Participants who have the disease are referred to as **cases**. These participants are then matched on several variables that may influence the results (e.g., age weight, gender, etc.) to those who do not have the disease of interest. Comparisons are then made between the two groups to determine potential factors associated with the disease. It is important to emphasize that in case-control studies, the investigator selects individuals on the basis of whether or not they have the disease and then attempts to determine the factors that cause the disease. In other words, the investigator examines relationships between the disease and certain factors the individuals may have been exposed to in the past that may cause the disease.

This type of study is appropriate to study rare events and is also relatively inexpensive and quick to conduct. However, it does not provide information on temporal or causal relationships.

Cohort Studies

The term **cohort** refers to a clearly defined group of individuals to be studied. Cohort studies can be prospective or retrospective.

Prospective cohort studies involve the selection of a group free from the disease of interest. Information about the individuals in the group is collected that includes the habits and factors to which these individuals are exposed. The group then is followed for a period of time and the incidence of disease is tracked. For example, in a group of individuals free of disease, data such as body weight, height, physical activity habits, dietary habits, and a number of clinical and other parameters, etc., can be collected. The group is then followed for a several years with periodic check-ups, and the incidence of coronary heart disease is recorded. Investigators then attempt to assess the factors that might contribute or explain the incidence rate of the disease or its progression. One of these factors can be dietary habits, physical inactivity, or body weight.

Retrospective cohort studies are similar to the prospective studies in that they attempt to assess risk factors that explain the incidence of the disease. However, there is a distinct difference between the two studies. Retrospective studies examine the relationships between disease and risk factors when the disease has already occurred. In contrast, prospective studies begin with a cohort free of disease and follow them until the development of the disease of interest.[1]

Cohort studies are expensive to conduct and time-consuming. Sometimes they suffer from loss of follow-up data that may affect the outcome. However, they provide a true absolute assessment of risk and allow multiple diseases to be studied.

Randomized Control Trials

Randomized control trial design is considered the gold standard of research design for testing the hypothesis of interest.[1] The unique feature of this design is randomization. Participants are selected and randomly assigned to either the experimental group or control group. The trial can be single or double blind. A single-blind trial is one that the participant does not know the group that he or she is assigned (experimental or control group). A double-blind trial is one that neither the investigator nor the participants are aware of which group the participants are assigned. This design assures that the findings are not biased by the investigators. All participants are assessed at baseline and after the intervention. Differences between the groups are then assessed.

Randomized control trials pose several challenges. They are expensive and time-consuming. In addition, they require that the participants must accept that they have a 50-50 chance to be assigned to the intervention group or control group. An additional challenge unique for studies involving physical activity and mortality is that they cannot be blinded. That is, both the participants and the investigator know the group assigned to each participant. Yet, one way to deal with this drawback is to "blind" the individual examining the findings. For example, let us assume that a randomized study is designed to assess blood pressure and heart function changes after 16 weeks of exercise training. The study can be designed so that the individuals assigned to take blood pressure and read the echocardiograms do not know the group to which each individual is assigned. This approach removes potential investigator bias.

■ MEASURES USED IN EPIDEMIOLOGIC STUDIES

Prevalence is defined as the ratio between the number of people who have a disease or a characteristic and the number of all study participants at a given point or period in time.

Incidence is the ratio of new cases of a disease per unit of time. The unit of time is not necessarily 1 year, although incidence is often presented in terms of 1 year.

Absolute risk is the risk ratio of developing a disease over a time period. For example, let us assume that the risk for developing heart disease in the next 10 years is 1 in 10. This can also be expressed as 0.1 (1/10 = 0.1) or as a 10% risk.

Absolute risk reduction is the difference between two event rates. For example, let us assume that an individual has a 10% risk of dying during the next 10 years as a result of untreated diabetes. Let us then assume that this individual is placed on medication and diabetes is managed. By doing so, the individual's risk of death is reduced from 10% to 6%. The absolute risk reduction for the individuals will then be 4% (10% – 6% = 4%). If two groups are compared (e.g., experimental and control group), the absolute risk reduction is the difference in the risk between the two groups. For example, if the risk of developing the disease is 40% in the control group and 30% in the experimental group, the absolute risk reduction is 10% (40% – 30% = 10%).

Relative risk is the comparison of the absolute risks in two different groups of people. For example, one can compare the risk of developing a disease in those who smoke versus non-smokers or physically active individuals versus those who are sedentary.

Relative risk reduction is the difference in even rates between two groups. It is calculated by dividing the absolute risk reduction (i.e., absolute risk at the beginning of the study minus the absolute risk at the end of the study) by the control event rate. In the aforementioned example, the absolute risk reduction for the experimental group was 10%. The event rate for the control group was 40%. Thus, the relative risk reduction will be 25% (10%/40%).[2]

Odds ratio is defined as the ratio of the odds of an event occurring in one group to the odds of it occurring in another group. Odds ratios are usually associated with retrospective or case-control studies but also can be used in prospective studies.

■ CARDIOVASCULAR DISEASE

Cardiovascular disease (CVD) is a general term that includes heart attacks, heart failure, stroke, and peripheral artery diseases. The common factor in all types of CVD is the loss of the natural elasticity of the arteries, a condition referred to as **atherosclerosis**.

Atherosclerosis (the Greek word for accumulation of lipid and hardening of the artery), is the result of a chronic inflammatory response within the walls of large and medium-sized muscular arteries. This leads to series of events that promote the deposits of lipids, cholesterol (specifically, low density lipoprotein [LDL]-cholesterol), calcium, and cellular debris within the inner layer of the arterial wall. This slow and insidious process of deposits leads to the formation of multiple plaques within the inner wall of the arteries. As atherosclerosis progresses, the arteries not only become progressively less flexible, but the diameter of the arteries involved also narrows. Eventually, blood supply to the area beyond the narrowed area is decreases substantially and dangerously.

Atherosclerosis can affect all arteries of the body at different degrees. However, for reasons not completely understood, certain arteries or areas of arteries are more susceptible than others. In addition, certain organs that depend on steady blood flow—the heart and brain—can suffer irreparable damage (heart attack, stroke) if blood flow is disrupted even for a few minutes.

When atherosclerosis afflicts the arteries of the heart (coronary arteries) and consequently the heart muscle, the disease is referred to as **coronary artery disease (CAD) or coronary heart disease (CHD)**. When vessels of the periphery are involved, the outcome can either be a stroke (if arteries supplying blood to the brain are involved) or pain of the lower legs when walking, a condition known as **peripheral vascular disease (PVD),** or a more precise term, **low extremity arterial disease (LEAD)** (discussed later in this chapter).

Epidemiology

CVD presents an enormous global health problem. According to the 2009 report from the American Heart Association Statistics Committee and Stroke Statistics Subcommittee, an estimated 80,000,000 American adults (1 in 3) have one or more types of CVD (**Table 8.1**).[3-5] CVD has accounted for more deaths than any other single cause or group of causes of death in the United States every year since 1900, with the exception of 1918.[3-5] The prevalence and incidence of CVD increase with age (**Figures 8.1** and **8.2**).

Approximately 2,400 Americans die each day from CVD (**Figure 8.3**). This translates to an average of one death every 37 seconds. This death toll is almost double that of cancer (**Figure 8.4**) and as high as the next three leading causes of death (cancer, accidents, and chronic lower respiratory disease) combined in men and even higher than the next four leading causes of death (cancer, accidents, chronic lower respiratory disease, and Alzheimer's) in women (**Figure 8.5**). In 2006, CVD accounted for approximately 34.2% of all deaths or 1 of every 2.9 deaths.[3-5] The estimated direct and indirect cost of CVD for 2007 was $431.8 billion, $448.5 billion in 2008, and $475.3 billion for 2009.[3-6]

Among these dismal reports, there is some good news. According to recent statistics, CVD mortality declined every year from 1980 to 2002. The average reduction in CVD mortality was 52% among men and 49% among women 65 years and older. However, in women ages 35 to 54, a trend towards higher CVD mortality was noted between 2000 and 2002. The increase was more prevalent and significant in women ages 35 and 44 years.[3,7]

Approximately 2,400 Americans die each day from CVD or an average of one death every 37 seconds. This death toll is almost double that of cancer.

Table 8.1 Cardiovascular Disease

Population Group	Prevalence 2006 Age 20+	Mortality 2005 All Ages*	Cost for 2008	Cost for 2009
Both sexes	80,000,000 (36.3%)	864,480	448.5 billion	475.3 billion
Men	38,700,000 (37.6%)	409,867 (47.4%)	—	—
Women	41,300,000 (34.9%)	445,613 (52.6%)	—	—
Non-Hispanic white men	37.8%	329,607	—	—
Non-Hispanic white women	33.3%	372,191	—	—
Non-Hispanic black men	45.9%	47,384	—	—
Non-Hispanic black women	45.9%	52,401	—	—
Mexican-American men	26.1%	—	—	—
Mexican-American women	32.5%	—	—	—

Sources: Lloyd-Jones D, Adams R, Carnethon M, et al. Heart disease and stroke statistics—2009 update: a report from the American Heart Association Statistics Committee and Stroke Statistics Subcommittee. *Circulation* 2009;119:480–486.

Rosamond W, Flegal K, Friday G, et al. Heart disease and stroke statistics—2008 update: a report from the American Heart Association Statistics Committee and Stroke Statistics Subcommittee. *Circulation* 2008;117(4): e25–e146.

Rosamond W, Flegal K, Furie K, et al. Heart disease and stroke statistics—2007 update: a report from the American Heart Association Statistics Committee and Stroke Statistics Subcommittee. *Circulation* 2007;115(5): e69–e171.

Figure 8.1 Prevalence of CVD.

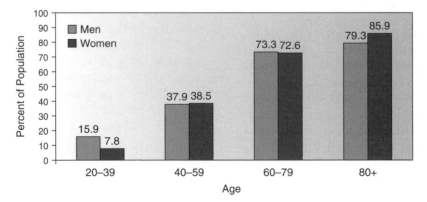

Source: From Lloyd-Jones D, et al. Heart disease and stroke statistics—2009 update. A report from the American Heart Association Statistics Committee and Stroke Statistics Subcommittee. *Circulation* 2009;119:e21–e181.

Figure 8.2 Incidence of CVD.

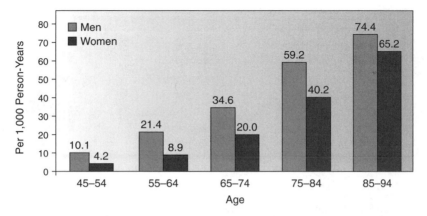

Source: From Lloyd-Jones D, et al. Heart disease and stroke statistics—2009 update. A report from the American Heart Association Statistics Committee and Stroke Statistics Subcommittee. *Circulation* 2009;119:e21–e181.

Atherosclerosis and Coronary Heart Disease

Atherosclerosis of the arteries that supply blood to the heart (coronary artery disease) is a major concern. Because the heart requires a constant supply of blood to perform its work, without it the heart is damaged irreparably. This is the case with myocardial infarction (MI; also known as a heart attack).

The atherosclerotic plaque does not occur within a few days or weeks. Rather, it is a process that begins in early adolescence. It continues silently and (in most cases) undetected for decades without symptoms. Evidence of early stages of atherosclerosis (fatty streaks) was found in healthy young men (autopsies) who died during the Korean and Vietnam Wars.[8,9] Significant atherosclerotic lesions in the coronary artery were found in over 77% of the young

Figure 8.3 Deaths from cardiovascular disease (United States: 1900–2006 preliminary).

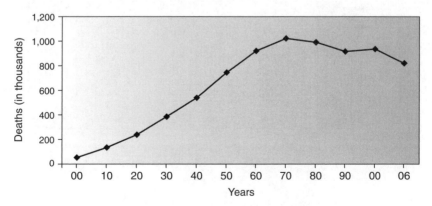

Source: NCHS and NHLBI; Lloyd-Jones D, et al. *Circulation* 2009;119:e11–e161.

Figure 8.4 CVD deaths versus cancer deaths by age.

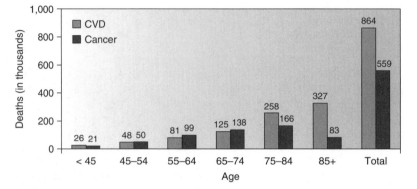

Source: NCHS and NHLBI; Lloyd-Jones D, et al. *Circulation* 2009;119:e11–e161.

soldier killed in the Korean War and in 45% of those killed in the Vietnam War.

In general, when the diameter of one or more of the coronary arteries is reduced (blocked) by 70% or more, atherosclerosis reaches a degree of clinical significance. At this point, the coronary circulation is compromised and the delivery of blood rich with oxygen and other nutrients to the parts of the heart beyond the blockage is inadequate. This condition can lead to symptoms and MI. However, it is important to point out that symptoms prior to a heart attack may or may not be present. According to U.S. data for the year 2004, for about 65% of men and 47% of women, the first symptom of atherosclerotic cardiovascular disease is a MI or sudden cardiac death.[10,11]

Figure 8.5 CVD and other major causes of death for all males and females (United States: 2004).

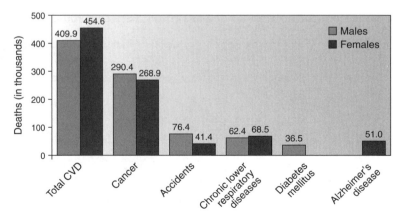

Source: From Lloyd-Jones D, et al. Heart disease and stroke statistics—2009 update. A report from the American Heart Association Statistics Committee and Stroke Statistics Subcommittee. *Circulation* 2009;119:e21–e181.

Figure 8.6 Percentage breakdown of deaths from CVDs.

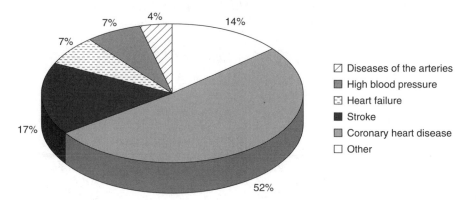

- ☒ Diseases of the arteries
- ▨ High blood pressure
- ⊟ Heart failure
- ■ Stroke
- ▨ Coronary heart disease
- ☐ Other

Source: From Lloyd-Jones D, et al. Heart disease and stroke statistics—2009 update. A report from the American Heart Association Statistics Committee and Stroke Statistics Subcommittee. *Circulation* 2009;119:e21–e181.

Epidemiology of Coronary Heart Disease

According to American Heart Association (AHA) statistics, CHD comprises more than half of all cardiovascular events and death in men and women under age 75 (**Figure 8.6**). An estimated 785,000 Americans will have a new coronary attack in 2009 and about 470,000 will have a recurrent event. An additional 195,000 will have a silent myocardial infarction each year.[3] This translates to one coronary event for every 25 seconds and one death each minute.[3] The average age of a person having a first heart attack is 65.8 for men and 70.4 for women.[3,4,12] The prevalence and incidence of CHD increase with age for both men and women (**Figure 8.7** and **8.8**).

CHD is the single largest killer of American males and females. In 2005, CHD caused 445,687

Figure 8.7 Prevalence of CVD by age and sex (NHANES: 2005–2006).

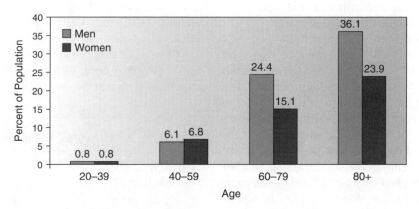

Source: From Lloyd-Jones D, et al. Heart disease and stroke statistics—2009 update. A report from the American Heart Association Statistics Committee and Stroke Statistics Subcommittee. *Circulation* 2009;119:e21–e181.

Figure 8.8 Annual number of American having diagnosed heart attack by age and sex (Atherosclerosis Risk in Communities study [ARIC]:1987–2000).

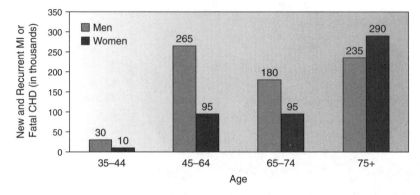

Source: From Rosamond W, et al. *Circulation* 2007;115:e69–e171.

deaths (1 in every 5) in the United States with men having slightly higher rates than women (**Table 8.2**). According to the AHA computations, approximately 38% of the people who experience a coronary event in a given year will die from it.[4] The annual incidence of sudden cardiac deaths is three to four times higher in men than in women. Between 70% and 89% sudden cardiac deaths occur in men. However, this disparity decreases with advancing age. Symptoms prior to a heart attack may or may not be manifested. Fifty percent of men and 64% of women who died suddenly of a heart attack had no previous symptoms of this disease.

Here again, there is evidence that progress is made. Overall CHD death rates decreased by 59% from 1950 to 1999. Sudden cardiac death fell by 49% and non-sudden CHD death decreased by 64%. These trends were seen in men and women, in subjects with and without a prior history of CHD, and in smokers and non-smokers.[11,12] From 1994 to 2004, the death rate from CHD declined 33% and the actual number of deaths declined only 14.7%.[12] However, there is some concern for younger women ages 34 to 45 years. Mortality rates among these women have been increasing on an average of 1.3%

since 1997.[7] The estimated direct and indirect cost of CHD for 2008 was 156.4 billion and 165.4 for 2009 (**Table 8.2**).[3,4]

Cardiovascular Disease in Women

There is a widespread misconception in the United States, Europe, and the rest of the world that CVD and particularly CHD is a "male disease." In fact, CVD is the largest single cause of death among women and accounts for one third of all deaths worldwide, with more women than men dying annually from CHD.[5,12,13] In addition, CVD and CHD accounts for more deaths in women than any other cause, including all types of cancer combined (**Figure 8.9** and **8.10**).[14] Furthermore, outcomes after a heart attack are worse in women than men.[15]

CVD is the largest single cause of death among women. It accounts for more deaths in women than any other cause, including all types of cancer combined.

Outcomes after a heart attack are worse in women than men.

Table 8.2 Coronary Heart Disease

Population Group	Prevalence CHD 2006 Age ≥ 20	Prevalence MI 2006 Age ≥ 20	New and Recurrent MI and Fatal CHD Age ≥ 35	Mortality CHD 2005 All Ages	Mortality MI 2005 All Ages	Cost CHD 2007	Cost CHD 2008	Cost CHD 2009
Both sexes	16,800,000 (7.6%)	7,900,000 (3.6%)	1,255,000	445,687	151,004	$151.6 billion	$156.4 billion	$165.4 billion
Men	8,700,000 (8.6%)	4,700,000 (4.7%)	740,000	232,115 (52.1%)	80,079 (53%)	—	—	—
Women	8,100,000 (6.8%)	3,200,000 (2.7%)	515,000	213,572 (47.9%)†	70,925 (47%)†	—	—	—
Non-Hispanic white men	8.8%	4.9%	675,000	203,924	70,791	—	—	—
Non-Hispanic white women	6.6%	3.0%	445,000	186,497	61,573	—	—	—
Non-Hispanic black men	9.6%	5.1%	70,000	22,933	7,527	—	—	—
Non-Hispanic black women	9%	2.2%	65,000	23,094	8,009	—	—	—
Mexican-American men	5.4%	2.5%	—	—	—	—	—	—
Mexican-American women	6.3%	1.1%	—	—	—	—	—	—

Sources: Lloyd-Jones D, Adams R, Carnethon M, et al. Heart disease and stroke statistics—2009 update: a report from the American Heart Association Statistics Committee and Stroke Statistics Subcommittee. *Circulation* 2009;119:480–486.
Rosamond W, Flegal K, Friday G, et al. Heart disease and stroke statistics—2008 update: a report from the American Heart Association Statistics Committee and Stroke Statistics Subcommittee. *Circulation* 2008;117(4):e25-e146.

Figure 8.9   CVD and other major causes of death in women, United States, 2005.

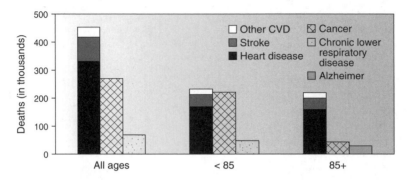

Source: From Lloyd-Jones D, et al. Heart disease and stroke statistics—2009 update. A report from the American Heart Association Statistics Committee and Stroke Statistics Subcommittee. *Circulation* 2009;119:e21–e181.

Several factors have been identified as contributors for this epidemic in women. First, women and many of their healthcare providers are not aware of the extent of the threat heart disease imposes to women. This often leads to a less aggressive approach in diagnosis and treatment and consequently worse outcomes.[16–18]

It is also becoming evident that heart attack symptoms present differently in women than men. In fact, women are less likely than men to feel chest pain during a heart attack. Studies suggest that the traditional chest pain experienced by men during a heart attack may be absent in women. Instead, women are more likely to experience the so-called "atypical" symptoms. Atypical symptoms include but are not limited to:

- Back, neck, or jaw pain
- Nausea

Figure 8.10   Age-adjusted death rates for CHD, stroke, and lung and breast cancer for white and black females (United States, 2005).

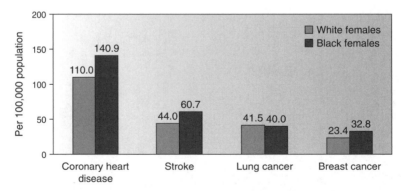

Source: From Lloyd-Jones D, et al. Heart disease and stroke statistics—2009 update. A report from the American Heart Association Statistics Committee and Stroke Statistics Subcommittee. *Circulation* 2009;119:e21–e181.

- Vomiting
- Indigestion
- General weakness or fatigue
- Dizziness or lightheadedness

According to one study, shortness of breath as a heart attack symptom is more common in women, whereas sweating is more common in men.[15] In another study of 515 women who had heart attacks, 78% experienced at least one pre-heart attack symptom for more than 1 month, either daily or several times a week, before their heart attack. About 70% of these women experienced unusual fatigue and about 50% experienced sleep disturbance; many women (about 40%) rated both of these symptoms as severe (**Table 8.3**).[19–22] Women are also more than twice as likely as men to experience nausea, vomiting, or indigestion as heart attack symptoms.[19]

Pre-Heart Attack Symptoms for Women

Pre-heart attack or **prodromal** symptoms are usually experienced by more women than men, and generally occur from about 4 to 6 months to 1 week before a heart attack.[20] The most common of these pre-heart attack symptoms are listed in **Table 8.4**.

Evidence also supports that the development and progression of CVD may be different in women from men. In men, plaque formation within the coronary arteries often builds up in one or two areas. In some women, the process of atherosclerosis does not form localized plaques. Instead, the plaques are more diffuse, involving to some degree the entire circumference of the artery. These women, in response to atherosclerosis, "remodel" the entire artery so that the lining of the artery becomes thickened throughout, making the plaques flush with the wall of the artery. Because localized plaques are absent, the discrete narrowing of the vessel that is visualized by cardiac catheterization is also absent. In other words, the entire coronary arteries appear smooth-walled and normal, though they may look "small" in diameter.[13] Of course, this can lead to misdiagnosis.

The clinical implications of the aforementioned perceptions and factors are serious. Heart attack therapies, such as clot dissolving medications and balloon angioplasty, work best if given within the first hour of the onset of a heart attack. A heart attack symptom that is dismissed or misdiagnosed will surely delay life-saving intervention. This delay can result in death or long-lasting heart damage, and it is one of the reasons why women tend to experience worse outcomes after a heart attack than men.

Table 8.3 Signs and Symptoms of a Heart Attack in Men and Women

Classic Symptoms in Men	More Likely Symptoms in Women
• Chest pain, tightness, or pressure	• Indigestion or gas-like pain
• Shortness of breath	• Dizziness, nausea, or vomiting
• Sweating	• Unexplained weakness, fatigue
• Recurring chest discomfort	• Discomfort/pain between shoulder blades
• Pain spreading to shoulders, neck, or arm	• Sense of anxiety or impending doom
• Clammy skin or paleness	

Table 8.4 Common Prodromal Symptoms Experienced by Women Prior to a Heart Attack

Symptoms	Percent of Women Reporting These Symptoms
Unusual fatigue	70%
Sleep disturbance	48%
Shortness of breath	42%–58%
Indigestion	39%
Anxiety	35%
Weakness	55%
Cold sweat	39%
Dizziness	39%

Source: McSweeney JC, Cody M, O'Sullivan P, et al. Women's early warning symptoms of acute myocardial infarction. *Circulation* 2003;108(21):2619–2623.

Finally, certain cardiac medications may not benefit women and in some cases may even increase the risk of death.[21]

Pathophysiology of Atherosclerosis: The Response-to-Injury Theory

The common factor in CVD is atherosclerosis. In the 1970s, the thinking among clinicians was that high blood cholesterol levels were the culprit in the development of the atherosclerotic lesions and later plaques.[22] However, since the 1980s, attention has been focused on possible link of an inflammatory process of the endothelial layer of small and medium vessels.

Although the mechanisms of atherosclerosis are still not completely understood, it is now accepted that atherosclerosis is a chronic inflammatory disease of the arterial wall referred to as the **response-to-injury** theory.[23–25] The theory states that atherosclerosis develops as a result of repetitive injury and ongoing inflammatory process of the inner arterial wall (endothelial layer) of large and medium-sized arteries. This inflammation is caused by a number of agents including high blood cholesterol and more specifically low-density lipoprotein (LDL)-cholesterol; toxins, including the byproducts of cigarette smoking, hyperglycemia, hypertension, obesity, and infections.

Inflammation of the endothelial layer leads to endothelial dysfunction. A compromised endothelial cell layer is the initial step that allows the infiltration of oxidized LDL-cholesterol (LDL that has lost one of its electrons) within the sub-endothelial spaces (located underneath the intima layer of the vessel). This triggers a number of responses by the endothelium, including monocyte (macrophages) infiltration into the intima. Macrophages are "scavenger cells" that take up LDL-cholesterol. In a sense, macrophages are the "repair crew" of the arteries.

This action is a normal response by the system to remove the oxidized LDL-cholesterol from the site and repair the damage. However, large quantities of oxidized LDL-cholesterol infiltrating the intima can overwhelm this scavenger mechanism. As a result, substantial LDL-cholesterol accumulates, leading to an ingestion of more and more of the invading LDL-cholesterol by the macrophages and the formation of foam cells that are characteristic of early atherosclerosis.[23,24,26,27] If the factors responsible for endothelial dysfunction are not removed (i.e., LDL-cholesterol is not lowered), a progressive buildup of LDL-cholesterol, calcium, and cellular debris within the intima of the arterial wall continues, resulting in plaque formation, remodeling of the arterial wall, a reduction in diameter of the vessel, obstruction of blood flow, and diminished oxygen supply to target organs.

> The response-to-injury theory states that atherosclerosis develops as a result of repetitive injury and ongoing inflammatory process of the inner arterial wall (endothelial layer) of large and medium-sized arteries.

Oxidative Stress

Oxidative stress is a general term used to describe the potential damage in a cell, tissue, or organ that may be caused when highly active molecules formed during aerobic metabolism overwhelm the natural antioxidant defense mechanisms.[28] These molecules, known as *free radicals*, are the by-products of biochemical reactions known as **oxidation-reduction reactions** or **redox**. Such reactions involve an electron gain by one reaction species (reduction) and an electron loss (oxidation) by the other species involved in the reaction. These highly active molecules can react with various cellular components including DNA, proteins, and lipids. Reactions between cellular components and free radicals can lead to DNA damage, mitochondrial malfunction, cell membrane damage, and eventually cell death.

> Oxidative stress is a general term used to describe the potential damage in a cell, tissue, or organ that may be caused when highly active molecules known as free radicals, overwhelm the natural antioxidant defense mechanisms.

It is important to emphasize that these reactions are absolutely critical to life and the basis of all aspects of metabolism. Most of these oxygen-derived species are produced at a low level by normal aerobic metabolism. Under normal conditions, these pro-oxidant free radicals pose no harm to the system. Their formation is balanced by a similar rate of antioxidant activity and the potential damage they cause is constantly prevented or repaired by these antioxidants. *Antioxidants* are molecules or compounds (electron donors) within the cells that act with free radicals and form innocuous end products. Consequently, antioxidants neutralize the deleterious effects that free radicals have on cells.

Disruption of the balance between the formation and neutralization of pro-oxidants results in increased oxidative stress. The level of oxidative stress and the resulting oxidative damage to the organism depend upon the size of these changes. Although the cells can usually overcome small disturbances in this balance, more severe oxidative stress can lead to cell death.[29,30]

Role of LDL in Oxidative Stress and Atherosclerosis

It is well-established that elevated LDL-cholesterol levels in blood play a major role in the development of atherosclerosis and CVD.[31,32] As discussed in Chapter 4, LDL-cholesterol binds to LDL receptors. It is then internalized and transported through the endothelium. During this process, LDL undergoes a low-level oxidation in the subendothelial layer and possibly in the blood.[33] This oxidized form of LDL-cholesterol is now more atherogenic than the native form.[34,35] As a normal response, the antioxidant properties of the healthy endothelium protect against damage and the injurious oxidized LDL is ingested by the macrophages and any damage to the arterial wall is repaired.

However, the natural protective antioxidant properties of the healthy endothelium are overwhelmed by elevated blood levels of LDL-cholesterol. As a result, excessive amounts of oxidized LDL are accumulated. There is strong evidence that oxidized LDL is the largest component of the atherosclerotic plaque.[36] In addition to the actual formation of the plaque, evidence suggests that oxidized LDL is involved in the early stages of atherosclerosis. Oxidized LDL promotes a wide range of toxic effects and arterial cell wall dysfunctions that favor the development of the atherosclerotic plaque: These dysfunctions include:

1. Impaired endothelium-dependent dilation and paradoxical vasoconstriction known as endothelial dysfunction.
2. Monocyte attraction and adhesion of these molecules to the arterial wall.
3. Formation of foam cells.

Thus, oxidative stress is now recognized as the most significant contributor to atherosclerosis. Evidence supports that elevated LDL-cholesterol is a major contributor of endothelial dysfunction and oxidative stress.[37]

Oxidized LDL play a major role in the development of atherosclerosis and CVD. It is involved in the early stages of atherosclerosis by promoting conditions within the arterial wall that favor the formation of the plaque. It also becomes the prominent component of the atherosclerotic plaque.

Plaque Formation and Arterial Remodeling

The end result of the atherosclerotic process is the formation of atherosclerotic plaques within the arterial wall. Plaque formation is a dynamic process and also a compensatory response to maintain blood flow through the artery. Initially, plaque formation was considered to be the only determinant of arterial luminal narrowing, as it progressively claimed more of the lumen (diameter) of the artery. However, studies revealed that changes occur within the artery (remodeling process) to compensate for the loss of luminal size and maintain adequate blood flow.[38–41] More specifically, the arteries initially enlarge in relation to the plaque area and the size of the lumen remains constant. This arterial remodeling compensates for arterial stenosis until the lesion occupies up to 40% of the internal lamina area.[38] Naturally, as the atherosclerotic process progresses, the lumen is progressively compromised and the severity of CAD increases (**Figure 8.11**).

Arterial remodeling refers to changes within the artery to compensate for the loss of luminal size (the result of plaque formation) and maintain adequate blood flow.

Ischemia

It is important to emphasize that the manifestation of cardiac symptoms (chest pressure, tightness, pain, nausea, etc.) indicate that blood flow to the myocardium is not adequate, a condition known as **ischemia** (Greek for inadequate blood flow). Ischemia at rest does not occur until the diameter of at least one of the major coronary arteries is over 80% blocked. However, ischemia is more likely to occur when the heart is challenged, as is the case during physical work or emotional stress.

Figure 8.11 An illustration of possible sequence of changes in atherosclerotic arteries. Note that the artery enlarges initially to compensate for loss in lumen size resulting from plaque formation. However, as the plaque formation continues and at approximately 40% of lumen stenosis, the artery no longer can enlarge sufficiently to compensate for the progressive narrowing of the lumen.

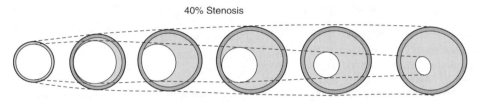

40% Stenosis

Source: Adapted from Glagov S, et al. *NEJM* 1987;316:1371–1375.

In fact, ischemia during physical work or exercise is likely to occur when the diameter of at least one of the major coronary arteries is about 60% or more blocked (**Figure 8.12**).[42]

This is the rationale for the standardized exercise tolerance test (ETT) or graded exercise test (GXT) described in Chapter 2. Briefly, the test consists of walking/jogging on a treadmill while the workload increases by progressively increasing the speed and elevation of the treadmill. As the leg muscles are progressively challenged during the test, the demand for blood also increases. In turn, the heart works harder to meet the demands of the working leg muscles. With increased workload, the heart's demand for blood (oxygen) also increases. To meet the increased demand, the coronary blood vessels dilate and blood flow to the heart increases. A healthy heart can easily provide the necessary blood flow to the working muscles. In other words, oxygen demand is always equal to oxygen supply.

However, when the diameter of one of the coronary arteries is compromised (reduced), the following occurs. As the workload increases and oxygen demand (blood flow) increases, the coronary arteries again dilate to increase blood flow. When one of the coronary arteries is compromised significantly (the result of plaque formation), then dilation of

Figure 8.12 Coronary blood flow at rest and during maximal exercise as affected by the percent blockage in a major coronary artery. Note that coronary blood flow at rest is compromised when the lesion claims about 90% of the diameter. During exercise, coronary blood flow is compromised when the lesion claims more than 60% of the diameter.

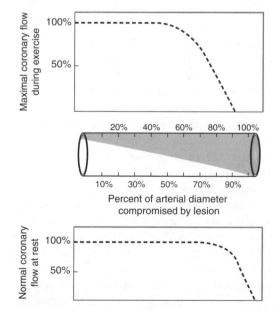

Source: Modified from Gould KL, Lipscomb K. Effects of coronary stenoses on coronary flow reserve and resistance. *Am J Cardiol* 1974;34(1):48–55.

the artery is also compromised. Thus, blood flow beyond the plaque is impaired and ischemia ensues. At this point, symptoms are likely to manifest.

Vulnerable and Stable Plaques

Another compensatory response that takes place within the artery is the attempt to "cure" the evolving plaque and preserve blood flow to the myocardium. Thus, a fibrous cap or shell forms around the cholesterol deposits. This shell acts as a wall to separate the flowing blood from the debris that is accumulated.

However, it is important to realize that this is only a compensatory response designed to delay the inevitable. Plaques can rupture. This rupture usually occurs in the shoulder regions of the plaque where the shear stress is high. When plaques rupture, a series of events occurs that results in the formation of thrombus. Then chest pain, myocardial infarction, and even death (often sudden) will ensue if medical intervention does not take place. The majority of these clinical events occur with the rupture of plaques that claim less than 70% of the initial lumen of a major coronary artery.

Evidence is still accumulating to more accurately define the characteristics of plaques that are likely to rapture. The vulnerability of the plaque to rupturing depends on a number of factors that include the LDL-cholesterol content of the plaque (large lipid core), inflammatory processes, and the thickness of the fibrous cap.[43] The thinner the cap is, the more vulnerable the plaque will be to rupturing. An analogy for this can be made with a raw egg inside of its shell. The shell is thin so a raw egg is relatively more likely to crack and its contents spilled out than one that is boiled. But as the raw egg is boiled, the contents inside the shell become thicker and thicker. In the process, the egg is now less and

less vulnerable to cracking. So it is with the plaque formation.

> The vulnerability of the plaque to rupturing depends on a number of factors including the LDL-cholesterol content of the plaque (large lipid core), inflammatory processes, and the thickness of the fibrous cap.

The body's goal is to "cure" the plaque or contain it so that it is less likely to rupture. To accomplish this end, the artery needs time to cure from the injury. Keep in mind that the vulnerability of the plaque depends in part on the amount of LDL-cholesterol entering the wall of the artery and consequently forming the plaque. When the amount of cholesterol entering the arterial wall overwhelms the body's ways to deal with it, the plaque remains active and formation of the fibrous cap is thin and vulnerable to rupture. When blood cholesterol is reduced and therefore less is entering the arterial wall, the artery has time to deal with the existing plaque and the process of "curing" it can take place (**Figure 8.13**).[44]

■ CVD RISK FACTORS

Over the years, data acquired from the Framingham Heart Study have allowed scientists to identify several factors that predispose an individual to a higher risk for future cardiovascular events. Thus, the term **risk factors** has been introduced in medicine. The term generally applies to a parameter that can predict a future cardiovascular event with some degree of accuracy.

> The term *risk factors* generally applies to a parameter that can predict a future event.

Figure 8.13 A schematic representation of two approximately same size plaques. Note that the cap of the vulnerable plaque is thinner and the lipid core larger when compared to the more stable plaque.

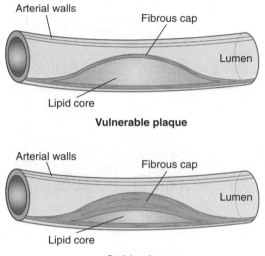

Vulnerable plaque

Stable plaque

Risk factors are used by physicians as a tool to assess an individual's risk for developing heart disease. For example, the presence or absence of risk factors will categorize an individual as having a high or low risk, respectively, for a cardiovascular event within a certain time frame.

Risk assessment methods are available from a number of sources. Data from the Framingham Heart Study allowed the development of the Framingham Risk Score (FRS).[45] The FRS is designed to predict the 10-year risk of developing coronary heart disease based on an individual's gender, age total cholesterol or LDL-cholesterol, HDL-cholesterol, blood pressure, and smoking (**Figure 8.14** and **8.15**).

As expected, the risk of CHD increases progressively with the constellation of risk factors (**Figure 8.16**).

A similar risk assessment method was developed by the European Society of Cardiology known as the Systematic Coronary Risk Estimation (SCORE) project.[46] This project was initiated to develop a risk scoring system for the clinical management of cardiovascular risk in European clinical practice. The 10-year risk for fatal cardiovascular disease was calculated for populations having a high risk for cardiovascular heart disease and for those having low risk for cardiovascular disease. Two risk estimation models were developed. One was based on total cholesterol and the other on the total cholesterol/HDL cholesterol ratio.

Risk Factors for Heart Disease

Several risk factors for heart disease can be modified either by changing the individual's lifestyle or by medical interventions. For example, quitting smoking is an approach one can take to modify the risk factor and therefore lower the risk for heart disease. Factors that can influence risk are known as **modifiable**. Other factors, however, such as aging, cannot be changed and are known as **non-modifiable risk factors**. A list of non-modifiable and modifiable risk factors is presented in **Table 8.5** and **8.6**, respectively.

The FRS (United States) and SCORE (Europe) are risk assessment methods designed to predict the 10-year risk of developing coronary heart disease based on an individual's gender, age, and risk factors.

Several investigators have focused on defining the potential health benefits associated with the modification of cardiovascular risk factors. Survival in these studies was associated with the absence of major risk factors.[43–48] Risk

(*text continues on page 206*)

Figure 8.14 The Framingham CHD risk assessment score sheet for men. Note the 10-year CHD risk is estimated (step 8) based on the total score accumulated (step 7).

Step 1

Age Years	LDL Pts	Chol Pts
30-34	-1	[-1]
35-39	0	[0]
40-44	1	[1]
45-49	2	[2]
50-54	3	[3]
55-59	4	[4]
60-64	5	[5]
65-69	6	[6]
70-74	7	[7]

Step 2

LDL-C (mg/dl)	(mmol/L)	LDL Pts
<100	<2.59	-3
100-129	2.60-3.36	0
130-159	3.37-4.14	0
160-190	4.15-4.92	1
>/=190	>4.92	2

Cholesterol (mg/dl)	(mmol/L)	Chol Pts
<160	<4.14	[-3]
160-199	4.15-5.17	[0]
200-239	5.18-6.21	[1]
240-279	6.22-7.24	[2]
>/=280	>/=7.25	[3]

Step 3

HDL-C (mg/dl)	(mmol/L)	LDL Pts	Chol Pts
<35	<0.90	2	[2]
35-44	0.91-1.16	1	[1]
45-49	1.17-1.29	0	[0]
50-59	1.30-1.55	0	[0]
>/=60	>/=1.56	-1	[-2]

Step 4

Blood Pressure Systolic (mmHg)	Diastolic (mmHg)				
	<80	80-84	85-89	90-99	>/=100
<120	0 [0] pts				
120-129		0 [0] pts			
130-139			1 [1] pts		
140-159				2 [2] pts	
>/=160					3 [3] pts

Note: When systolic and diastolic pressures provide different estimates for point scores, use the higher number

Step 5

Diabetes	LDL Pts	Chol Pts
No	0	[0]
Yes	2	[2]

Step 6

Smoker	LDL Pts	Chol Pts
No	0	[0]
Yes	2	[2]

Step 7
(sum from steps 1-6)

Adding up the points	
Age	
LDL-C or Chol	
HDL-C	
Blood Pressure	
Diabetes	
Smoker	
Point total	

Step 8 (determine CHD risk from point total)

CHD Risk			
LDL Pts Total	**10-Yr CHD Risk**	**Chol Pts Total**	**10-Yr CHD Risk**
<-3	1%		
-2	2%		
-1	2%	[<-1]	[2%]
0	3%	[0]	[3%]
1	4%	[1]	[3%]
2	4%	[2]	[4%]
3	6%	[3]	[5%]
4	7%	[4]	[7%]
5	9%	[5]	[8%]
6	11%	[6]	[10%]
7	14%	[7]	[13%]
8	18%	[8]	[16%]
9	22%	[9]	[20%]
10	27%	[10]	[25%]
11	33%	[11]	[31%]
12	40%	[12]	[37%]
13	47%	[13]	[45%]
>/=14	>/=56%	[>/=14]	[>/=53%]

Step 9 (compare to average person your age)

Comparative Risk			
Age (Years)	**Average 10-Yr CHD Risk**	**Average 10-Yr Hard* CHD Risk**	**Low** 10-Yr CHD Risk**
30-34	3%	1%	2%
35-39	5%	4%	3%
40-44	7%	4%	4%
45-49	11%	8%	4%
50-54	14%	10%	6%
55-59	16%	13%	7%
60-64	21%	20%	9%
65-69	25%	22%	11%
70-74	30%	25%	14%

* Hard CHD events exclude angina pectoris

** Low risk was calculated for a person the same age, optimal blood pressure, LDL-C 100-129 mg/dl or cholesterol 160–199 mg/dl, HDL-C 45 mg/dl, for men or 55 mg/dl for women, non-smoker, no diabetes.

Risk estimates were derived from the experience of the Framingham Heart Study, a predominantly Caucasian population in Massachusetts.

Key	
Color	**Relative Risk**
	Very low
	Low
	Moderate
	High
	Very high

Source: From Wilson PW, et al. Prediction of coronary heart disease using risk factor categories. *Circulation* 1998;97(18):1837–1847.

Figure 8.15 The Framingham CHD risk assessment score sheet for women. Note the 10-year CHD risk is estimated (step 8) based on the total score accumulated (step 7).

Step 1

Age		
Years	**LDL Pts**	**Chol Pts**
30-34	-9	[-9]
35-39	-4	[-4]
40-44	0	[0]
45-49	3	[3]
50-54	6	[6]
55-59	7	[7]
60-64	8	[8]
65-69	8	[8]
70-74	8	[8]

Step 2

LDL-C		
(mg/dl)	**(mmol/L)**	**LDL Pts**
<100	<2.59	-2
100-129	2.60-3.36	0
130-159	3.37-4.14	0
160-190	4.15-4.92	2
>/=190	>4.92	2

Cholesterol		
(mg/dl)	**(mmol/L)**	**Chol Pts**
<160	<4.14	[-2]
160-199	4.15-5.17	[0]
200-239	5.18-6.21	[1]
240-279	6.22-7.24	[1]
>/=280	>/=7.25	[3]

Step 3

HDL-C			
(mg/dl)	**(mmol/L)**	**LDL Pts**	**Chol Pts**
<35	<0.90	5	[5]
35-44	0.91-1.16	2	[2]
45-49	1.17-1.29	1	[1]
50-59	1.30-1.55	0	[0]
>/=60	>/=1.56	-2	[-3]

Step 4

Blood Pressure					
Systolic	**Diastolic (mmHg)**				
(mmHg)	**<80**	**80-84**	**85-89**	**90-99**	**>/=100**
<120	-3 [-3] pts				
120-129		0 [0] pts			
130-139			0 [0] pts		
140-159				2 [2] pts	
>/=160					3 [3] pts

Note: When systolic and diastolic pressures provide different estimates for point scores, use the higher number

Step 5

Diabetes		
	LDL Pts	**Chol Pts**
No	0	[0]
Yes	4	[4]

Step 6

Smoker		
	LDL Pts	**Chol Pts**
No	0	[0]
Yes	2	[2]

Step 7
(sum from steps 1-6)

Adding up the points	
Age	
LDL-C or Chol	
HDL-C	
Blood Pressure	
Diabetes	
Smoker	
Point total	

Step 8 (determine CHD risk from point total)

CHD Risk			
LDL Pts Total	**10-Yr CHD Risk**	**Chol Pts Total**	**10-Yr CHD Risk**
</=-2	1%	[</=-2]	[1%]
-1	2%	[-1]	[2%]
0	2%	[0]	[2%]
1	2%	[1]	[2%]
2	3%	[2]	[3%]
3	3%	[3]	[3%]
4	4%	[4]	[4%]
5	5%	[5]	[4%]
6	6%	[6]	[5%]
7	7%	[7]	[6%]
8	8%	[8]	[7%]
9	8%	[9]	[8%]
10	11%	[10]	[10%]
11	13%	[11]	[11%]
12	15%	[12]	[13%]
13	17%	[13]	[15%]
14	20%	[14]	[18%]
15	24%	[15]	[20%]
16	27%	[16]	[24%]
>/=17	>/=32%	[>/=17]	[>/=27%]

Step 9 (compare to average person your age)

Comparative Risk			
Age (Years)	**Average 10-Yr CHD Risk**	**Average 10-Yr Hard* CHD Risk**	**Low** 10-Yr CHD Risk**
30-34	<1%	<1%	<1%
35-39	<1%	<1%	1%
40-44	2%	1%	2%
45-49	5%	2%	3%
50-54	8%	3%	5%
55-59	12%	7%	7%
60-64	12%	8%	8%
65-69	13%	8%	8%
70-74	14%	11%	8%

* Hard CHD events exclude angina pectoris

** Low risk was calculated for a person the same age, optimal blood pressure, LDL-C 100-129 mg/dl or cholesterol 160–199 mg/dl, HDL-C 45 mg/dl, for men or 55 mg/dl for women, non-smoker, no diabetes.

Risk estimates were derived from the experience of the Framingham Heart Study, a predominantly Caucasian population in Massachusetts.

Key	
Color	**Relative Risk**
	Very low
	Low
	Moderate
	High
	Very high

Source: From Wilson PW, et al. Prediction of coronary heart disease using risk factor categories. *Circulation* 1998;97(18):1837–1847.

Figure 8.16   Estimated 10-year CHD risk in 55-year-old adults according to levels of various risk factors (Framingham Heart Study).

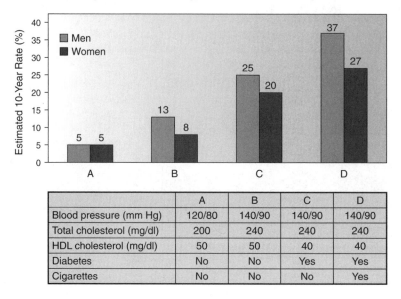

	A	B	C	D
Blood pressure (mm Hg)	120/80	140/90	140/90	140/90
Total cholesterol (mg/dl)	200	240	240	240
HDL cholesterol (mg/dl)	50	50	40	40
Diabetes	No	No	Yes	Yes
Cigarettes	No	No	No	Yes

Source: From Rosamond W, et al. *Circulation* 2007;115:e69–e171.

factors were classified as optimal, elevated, or major (**Table 8.7**).

In general, these studies reported that individuals with optimal risk factors had a significantly lower risk for cardiovascular events and mortality. The median life expectancy was 6 to 10 years longer than those with two or more risk factors.[43–48]

The association of each of the aforementioned cardiovascular risk factors with cardiovascular disease is discussed in their respective chapters. At this point, it is worth mentioning that increased physical activity protects against cardiovascular risk even in the presence of one or multiple risk factors. It also provides protection by positively modifying each and every one of the cardiovascular risk factors.

Stroke or Cerebrovascular Disease

Inadequate blood (oxygen) supply to the brain or parts of the brain for only a few minutes results in the death of brain cells and perhaps death of the individual. This is known as stroke, cerebrovascular accident, or brain attack.

Table 8.5   Non-Modifiable Risk Factors for CHD

Aging
Gender (men are at greater risk than women)
Heredity

Table 8.6 Modifiable Risk Factors for CHD

Major (Established) Risk Factors

Smoking

High blood pressure (SBP ≥ 140 or DBP ≥ 90)

Diabetes

Dyslipidemia (high total cholesterol/LDL-cholesterol or low HDL-cholesterol)

Obesity

Physical inactivity

As discussed previously, *stroke* is a form of cardiovascular disease that affects the blood vessels supplying blood and nutrients to the brain. It is the third most common cause of death in the United States. It strikes over 500,000 persons per year and is fatal in approximately one-half of these individuals.

The chances for complete recovery following a stroke depend on how quickly the circulation returns to normal and the size of the brain

Table 8.7 Classification of Risk Factors

Optimal Status of Risk Factors

BP < 120/80 mm Hg

Total cholesterol < 180 mg/dl

Absence of diabetes

Absence of smoking

30 minutes of more moderate to vigorous physical activity per day

About 1 glass of wine per day

Low body fat (BMI < 25 kg/m^2)

Adherence to Mediterranean diet

Elevated Risk Factors

Stage 1 hypertension (SBP 140–159 mm Hg or DBP 90–99 mm Hg)

Borderline cholesterol levels (200–230 mg/dl)

Major Risk Factors

Stage 2 hypertension (SBP 160 mm Hg or DBP 100–110 mm Hg)

Elevated blood cholesterol (≥ 240 mg/dl)

BP < 120/80 mm Hg

Diabetes

Current smoking

area affected. However, the outcome of stroke survivors is poor. Approximately one-half of the patients who survive a stroke remain permanently disabled, about 9% of stroke survivors suffer another stroke within the first year, 5% will die within 1 year, and 80% will die within 10 years.

■ Transient Ischemic Attack

Transient ischemic attack (TIA) (also referred to as a *mini stroke*) is a brief neurologic dysfunction that can persist for a few seconds to less than 24 hours. It is caused by the changes in the blood supply to a particular area of the brain. The most common cause of a TIA is an embolus (Greek for blockage) that occludes (blocks) an artery in the brain. An embolus can be formed from a dislodged atherosclerotic plaque in one of the carotid arteries or from a thrombus (blood clot) formed in the heart.

■ Epidemiology

The estimated annual rate of stoke is about 795,000, about 610,000 of which are new attacks

and 185,000 recurrent attacks. This is approximately one stroke for every 40 seconds in the United States. The prevalence and incidence of stroke for both men and women increase with age (**Figures 8.17** and **8.18**).[3,4]

The incidence is higher in young women than men and in blacks than whites. The age-adjusted stroke incidence rates of first-ever stroke for both black men and women are almost twice that of whites or Hispanics of the same age.[12] This is believed to be the result of increased prevalence of hypertension in blacks.[49]

Stroke is the third leading cause of death in the United States behind diseases of the heart and cancer. In 2005, stroke accounted for about 1 of every 17 deaths in the United States. On average, someone dies of a stroke every 3 to 4 minutes.[3,4,50] The recurrence of stroke is also high. Among persons 45 to 64 years of age, 8% to 12% of ischemic strokes and 37% to 38% of hemorrhagic strokes result in death within 30 days, according to the Atherosclerotic Risk in Communities (ARIC) study of the National Heart, Lung, and Blood Institute (NHLBI).[3,4,50] Both the incidence of stroke and mortality

Figure 8.17   Prevalence of stroke by age and sex (NHANES: 2005–2006).

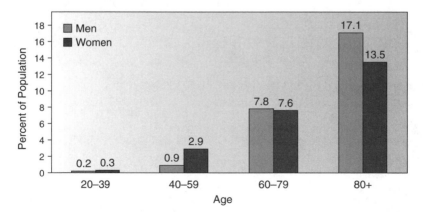

Source: From Lloyd-Jones D, et al. *Circulation* 2009;119:e1–e161.

Figure 8.18 Annual rate of first cerebral infarction by age, sex, and race.

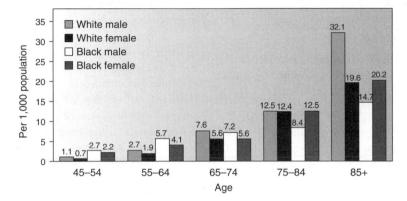

Source: From Lloyd-Jones D, et al. *Circulation* 2009;119:e1–e161.

rates for blacks is almost twice the rates of whites (see Figure 8.18). In addition, more women than men die of stroke each year. Women accounted for 60.6% of U.S. stroke deaths in 2005.[3,4] According to the AHA, women have a higher mortality than men because they live longer than men (**Figure 8.19**). The annual direct and indirect cost for stroke care for 2008

Figure 8.19 Estimated 10-year stroke risk.

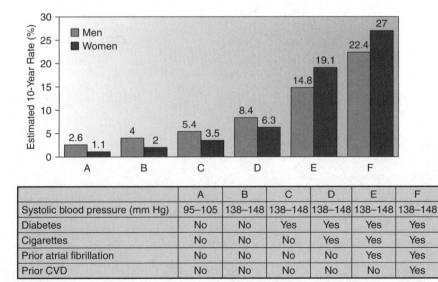

	A	B	C	D	E	F
Systolic blood pressure (mm Hg)	95–105	138–148	138–148	138–148	138–148	138–148
Diabetes	No	No	Yes	Yes	Yes	Yes
Cigarettes	No	No	No	Yes	Yes	Yes
Prior atrial fibrillation	No	No	No	No	Yes	Yes
Prior CVD	No	No	No	No	No	Yes

Note: The risk of stroke increases as cardiovascular risk factors are accrued at a SBP of 138–148 mm Hg.
Source: From Rosamond W, et al. *Circulation* 2007;115:e69–e171.

is estimated to be about $65.5 billion and $68.9 in 2009 (**Table 8.8**).[3,4]

■ Types of Stroke

Strokes are classified as ischemic (from the Greek word meaning inadequate blood supply) or hemorrhagic (Greek for bleeding).

Ischemic Strokes Ischemic strokes are the most common type, comprising 87% of all strokes.[12] They can further be classified as thrombotic or embolic.

Thrombotic stroke is the most common type of stroke. They are caused by a *thrombus*

(blood clot) formed within the vessels of the brain. The thrombus blocks blood flow to critical areas of the brain and deprives brain cells of oxygen and nutrients. Atherosclerosis, hypertension, smoking, and diabetes are the most likely culprits.

Embolic stroke is the second most common type of stroke. An *embolus* (blood clot) formed outside the brain is carried by the bloodstream to the brain where it lodges in a small artery. As just mentioned, oxygen deprivation even for a few minutes leads to brain cell death. Blood clots are likely to form in the heart during prolonged *atrial fibrillation*, a

Table 8.8 Stroke Statistics

Population Group	Prevalence 2006 Age ≥ 20 y	New and Recurrent Attacks All Ages	Mortality 2005	Cost 2008	Cost 2009
Both sexes	6,500,000 (2.9%)	795,000	143,579	65.5 billion	68.9 billion
Men	2,600,000 (2.6%)	370,000 (46.5%)	56,586 (39.4%)	—	—
Women	3,900,000 (3.2%)	425,000 (53.5%)	86,993 (60.6%)	—	—
Non-Hispanic white men	2.3%	325,000	47,194	—	—
Non-Hispanic white women	3.2%	365,000	74,674	—	—
Non-Hispanic black men	3.9%	45,000	7,519	—	—
Non-Hispanic black women	4.1%	60,000	10,022	—	—
Mexican-American men	2.1%	—	—	—	—
Mexican-American women	3.8%	—	—	—	—

Sources : Lloyd-Jones D, Adams R, Carnethon M, et al. Heart disease and stroke statistics—2009 update: a report from the American Heart Association Statistics Committee and Stroke Statistics Subcommittee. *Circulation* 2009;119:480–486.

Rosamond W, Flegal K, Friday G, et al. Heart disease and stroke statistics—2008 update: a report from the American Heart Association Statistics Committee and Stroke Statistics Subcommittee. *Circulation* 2008;117(4): e25–e146.

condition characterized by the loss of regular contraction of the atria (quivering of the atria). Other likely clot sites are the aorta and common carotid artery.

This type of stroke also can occur when plaque formed within the circulatory system is dislodged and travels to the brain where it is lodged in a vessel too small to pass. As in the situation with the blood clot, blood flow to the area of the brain beyond the blockage is obstructed and those brain cells that depend on this blood flow die. The arteries in the neck that supply blood to the brain (carotid arteries) are the most likely place for a plaque to dislodge and travel to the brain.

Hemorrhagic Strokes   Hemorrhagic strokes account for about 13% of all strokes. They occur when a blood vessel in the surface of the brain or within the brain ruptures. The accumulated blood and the typical inflammation that ensues around the injury tissue cause compression in the surrounding blood vessels and blood flow to the area is diminished.

■ Stroke Risk Factors

As with an MI, several risk factors have been identified that predispose an individual to stroke. Some of these risk factors are modifi-able and others are not. A list of non-modifiable and modifiable risk factors is presented in **Tables 8.9** and **8.10** respectively.

The top three risk factors of stroke are hypertension, diabetes mellitus, and current smoking.[54]

■ Prevention

Fortunately, prevention of the premature occurrence of CVD is possible. Strategies to prevent a heart attack and stroke are listed in **Table 8.11**.

Heart Attack

As previously mentioned, the heart requires a constant supply of blood (and oxygen) to work. Unlike any other muscles of the body that can survive without blood for relatively long time, the heart muscle will suffer irreversible damaged if it is deprived of blood for only a few minutes.

Blockages or plaques in one or more of the major arteries of the heart can form over a period of decades without the individual having any symptoms. When the blockage covers about 50% to 70% of the diameter of the artery, a significant reduction in the blood supply to the heart beyond the area of the blockage

Table 8.9 Non-Modifiable Risk Factors for Stroke

Factor	Risks
Age	Stroke doubles with each decade after 55 years of age.
Gender	Women suffer more incidents of stroke than men.
Race	African Americans suffer twice as many strokes as whites.
Family history	The risk for stroke increases if parental history of stroke is present.

Source: Used with permission from: Goldstein LB, et al. Primary prevention of ischemic stroke: a statement for healthcare professionals from the Stroke Council of the American Heart Association. *Circulation* 2001;103:163–182.

Table 8.10 Modifiable Risk Factors for Stroke

Risk Factor	Description
Cigarette smoking	The relative risk of stroke in heavy smokers (> 40 cigarettes/day) is twice that of light smokers (< 10 cigarettes/day). Stroke risk decreases significantly 2 years after cessation of cigarette smoking and is at the level of nonsmokers by 5 years.[48]
Hypertension	Subjects with BP less than 120/80 mm Hg have about half the lifetime risk of stroke of subjects with hypertension.[49]
History of transient ischemic attacks (TIA)	TIAs are mini strokes. In one study, about 10% of patients who experience a TIA developed stroke within 90 days. Ninety-one patients, or 5%, did so within 2 days. Predictors of stroke included: age > 60 years; having diabetes mellitus; focal symptoms of weakness or speech impairment; and TIA lasting longer than 10 minutes.[50]
Heart disease	Including arrhythmias, coronary artery disease, acute myocardial infarction, dilated cardiomyopathy, and valvular disease. AF is an independent risk factor for stroke, increasing risk about fivefold.[48]
Diabetes	Ischemic stroke patients with diabetes are younger, more likely to be African American, and more likely to have hypertension, MI, and high cholesterol than are non-diabetic patients, according to data from the Greater Cincinnati/Northern Kentucky Stroke Study (GCNKSS). Age-specific incidence rates and rate ratios show that diabetes increases ischemic stroke incidence at all ages, but this risk is most prominent before age 55 in African Americans and before age 65 in whites.[51]
Sedentary lifestyle	A study of more than 37,000 women age 45 or older participating in the Women's Health Study suggests that a healthy lifestyle (consisting of abstinence from smoking, low BMI, moderate alcohol consumption, regular exercise, and healthy diet) was associated with a significantly reduced risk of total and ischemic stroke but not of hemorrhagic stroke.[52]
Oral contraceptives	In the Women's Health Initiative trial of estrogen alone, among 10,739 women with hysterectomy, it was found that conjugate equine estrogen alone increased risk of ischemic stroke by 55% and there was no significant effect on hemorrhagic stroke. The excess risk of total stroke conferred by estrogen alone was 12 additional strokes per 10,000 person-years.[53]

Table 8.11 CVD Prevention Strategies
Stop smoking.
Engage in physical activity.
Use diet therapy.
Maintain/reduce weight.
Control blood pressure.
Undergo cholesterol control/statin therapy.
Control blood sugar.
Limit alcohol intake.
Take aspirin as advised*
*For women who have at least a 20% chance of a heart attack or stroke over the next 10 years. *Source:* Used with permission from Becker RC. Heart attack and stroke prevention in women. *Circulation* 2005;112:e273–e275.

occurs during physical work (Figure 8.12). At this point, the patients usually have symptoms when they are engaging in physical work. When the artery is nearly or totally blocked, the area of the heart beyond the blockage is deprived from the necessary oxygen to sustain life even at rest.

A heart attack can occur any time that the blockage is severe enough to deprive a major area of the heart of blood and oxygen. This does not only happen when the blockage slowly fills the diameter of a major artery, but also when a plaque ruptures. In the case of plaque rupture, the artery can totally close within minutes to hours and result in a heart attack.

Heart Failure

Heart failure or congestive heart failure is a complex syndrome characterized by progressive deterioration of ventricular function. The term *heart failure* in some ways is deceiving because it suggests more of a catastrophic condition (failure of the heart) than a progressive deterioration of cardiac function. A term that would reflect the progressive deterioration of

cardiac function would be *cardiac incompetence*. In any case, heart failure is the term to describe this action used in this book.

Heart failure can involve systolic or diastolic dysfunction or both. Systolic dysfunction is characterized by a decrease in the ejection fraction of the left or right ventricle or both. It is assessed by measuring ejection fraction and wall motion abnormalities by an echocardiogram. Diastolic dysfunction is defined as an impaired filling of either or both ventricles. This is the result of impaired relaxation of the myocardium caused by either ischemia or hypertrophy. Consequently, there is a significant decrease in cardiac output, dyspnea at relatively low workloads and diminished physical work capacity. In addition to limitations in the functional capacity of the heart, the 8-year mortality rate is 80% in men and 70% in women less than 65 years of age [3]

Heart failure is rapidly becoming one of the most common heart diseases. Approximately 5 million Americans and 15 million individuals worldwide have had a heart failure. It is also estimated that 670,000 Americans each year develop heart failure.[3] The prevalence of heart failure increases with age (**Figure 8.20**). In the

Figure 8.20 Prevalence of heart failure by age and sex (NHANES: 2005–2006).

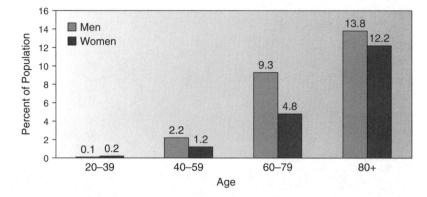

Source: NCHS and NHLBI; Lloyd-Jones D, et al. *Circulation* 2009;119:e11–e161.

past 10 years, the number of patients with heart failure has increased by 70%. According to data from the Framingham Study,[56] the incidence of new heart failure cases approximately doubles with each decade of age (**Figure 8.21**). This trend is expected to continue and even increase in the years to come. In a 1995 national survey, heart failure was the primary cause for 875,000 hospital admissions. The estimated annual cost was $10 billion.[57] From 1979 to 2004, hospital discharge for those with heart failure rose by 175%. In 2004, there were 292,214 deaths from heart failure.[3,4] The estimated direct and indirect cost for 2008 was $34.8 billion and $37.2 billion (**Table 8.12**).[3,4]

Figure 8.21 Incidence of heart failure by age and sex (Framingham Heart Study 1980–2003).

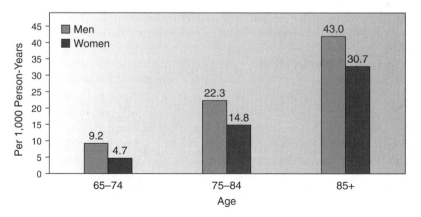

Source: From Lloyd-Jones D, et al. Heart disease and stroke statistics—2009 update. A report from the American Heart Association Statistics Committee and Stroke Statistics Subcommittee. *Circulation* 2009;119:e21–e181.

Table 8.12 Heart Failure

Population Group	Prevalence 2006 Age ≥ 20 y	Incidence (New Cases) Age ≥ 45 y	Mortality 2004* All Ages	Cost 2008	Cost 2009
Both sexes	5,700,000 (2.5%)	670,000	292,214	34.8 billion	37.2 billion
Men	3,200,000 (3.2%)	350,000	126,163 (43.2%)	—	—
Women	2,500,000 (2 %)	320,000	166,051 (56.8%)	—	—
Non-Hispanic white men	3.1%	—	112,550	—	—
Non-Hispanic white women	1.8%	—	148,582	—	—
Non-Hispanic black men	4.2%	—	11,276	—	—
Non-Hispanic black women	4.2%	—	14,928	—	—
Mexican-American men	2.1%	—	—	—	—
Mexican-American women	1.4%	—	—	—	—

Sources: Lloyd-Jones D, Adams R, Carnethon M, et al. Heart disease and stroke statistics—2009 update: a report from the American Heart Association Statistics Committee and Stroke Statistics Subcommittee. *Circulation* 2009;119:480–486.

Rosamond W, Flegal K, Friday G, et al. Heart disease and stroke statistics—2008 update: a report from the American Heart Association Statistics Committee and Stroke Statistics Subcommittee. *Circulation* 2008;117(4): e25–e146.

Heart failure is characterized by a progressive deterioration of ventricular function.

■ Physiology and Pathophysiology

Cardiac cells work in synchrony to produce the intended result: to pump blood throughout the body. The death of cardiac cells as a result of an MI, chronic hypertension, chronic and excessive alcohol use, viral infections, and a number of other known and some yet unknown factors, leads to the deterioration of this concerted work of the left ventricle. As a result, the ability of the heart to pump adequate blood and meet the needs of the body diminishes. This dimin-

ished ability of the heart and specifically of the left ventricle is referred to as heart failure.

In certain cases, heart failure occurs in two phases, an acute and a chronic phase. The acute phase comes suddenly, as is the case during a heart attack. The chronic phase progresses slowly over a period of long time, usually years. In some cases, the acute phase does not take place at all. There is only a progressive deterioration of heart function (chronic heart failure).

Acute Phase The acute phase begins immediately after a heart attack. Within seconds, cardiac output is cut in half. This is life threatening and cannot go on for too long. The system is now on a "Red Alert" situation. In an attempt to increase cardiac output, blood vessels constrict. This increases the blood volume returning from the body to the heart. As more blood enters the left ventricle is stretched. Consequently, the contractions are more forceful when the blood is pumped out of the ventricle and to the body (Frank-Starling mechanism of the heart; see Chapter 7). This raises the cardiac output and the immediate danger is prevented.

Chronic Phase Although the cardiac output usually doubles within a few minutes, this is still not enough to maintain normal body functions. Thus, another system is already activated to correct the situation. The kidneys begin to retain salt and, with it, water. This raises the volume of blood. Higher blood volume means more blood returning to the heart and therefore, more blood is pumped out. This raises the cardiac output to normal or near normal within 7 to 10 days. This is the beginning of the chronic phase.

The initial actions of the system are necessary and designed to evade a catastrophic situation. However, as you will see later, these actions come with a price. As initial phase ends, the heart begins to heal and the second phase begins, known as chronic heart failure. This phase can last from months to years (chronic). This chapter deals only with the chronic heart failure and will simply refer to it as heart failure.

■ Heart Failure and Heart Remodeling

The following key characteristics are unique to the pathophysiology of heart failure:

1. Ejection fraction is reduced.
2. End diastolic volume and end systolic volume increase.

3. Left ventricular pressure increases.
4. Left ventricular mass increases initially (compensated stage).
5. Gradually, the walls of the ventricles become thinner and the chambers are dilated (de-compensated stage).
6. Sodium retention in increases leading to water retention and edema.
7. Sympathetic activity increases while parasympathetic activity decreases.

These and other factors lead to changes in the shape of the left ventricle from an elliptical to the more spherical contour.

■ Who Develops Heart Failure and Why

There are primarily two reasons for the increase in heart failure. The first reason is the advances in the medical treatment improved the survival of patients with coronary heart disease, myocardial infarction of patients, and the treatment of hypertension and other risk factors. These patients—if they live long enough—eventually will develop heart failure. The second reason is that more and more Americans live over the age of 70. Death from heart failure increases dramatically over the age of 74 years.[3,58]

There are a number of factors that contribute to heart failure. Some we know, others we do not. Some cause heart failure directly; others indirectly. One thing we know for certain is that the occurrence of heart failure increases with age.[3,56,58] The main causes are:

1. A previous heart attack
2. Disease of the arteries that supply the heart with blood (coronary arteries)
3. High blood pressure

High blood pressure and coronary heart disease (disease of the blood vessels that feed the heart muscle with blood) were the most common causes from 1950 to mid-1980. Then, in the last decade or so, coronary heart disease has become the primary cause of heart failure. This is probably due great successes in treating high blood pressure.

There are also other causes of heart failure. They claim only small percentage of the incidence. These include viral infections, alcohol abuse, and certain medications (especially when the patient is over-medicated), damaged heart valves, vitamin deficiencies, and other causes not yet known.

From Heart Attack to Heart Failure Heart failure is not a direct consequence of the damage to the heart muscle following myocardial infarction. In fact, patients who suffer an acute myocardial infarction involving relatively large areas of the left ventricle may still recover spontaneously. Heart failure symptoms and signs are evident months later even if they suffer no further damage to the myocardium.

Damage to the heart as a result of a heart attack often leads to heart failure.

How does a heart attack lead to heart failure? Following an extensive MI, the damage to the left ventricle is substantial. Because some of the cardiac cells are dead or injured and no longer able to perform work, cardiac output decreases. In order to compensate for the reduced cardiac output, feedback mechanisms are activated. Certain hormones are secreted that are designed to constrict the arterial resistance vessels and increase contractility of the myocardium. This leads to the maintenance of normal arterial pressure and increased venous return to the heart. Consequently, cardiac output increases (the Frank-Starling mechanism; see Chapter 7).

Although these actions are necessary to maintain cardiac output, in the long term they are detrimental to the heart. The reduction in the number of viable cardiac cells that can work and the increased wall stress leads to two events: (1) hypertrophy of the non-infarcted area of the myocardium to compensate for the lost cells and (2) thinning and dilation of the infarcted area (**Figures 8.22–8.25**). Both of these condition lead to further myocardial dysfunction, further remodeling, and consequently heart failure.

Coronary Artery Disease and Heart Failure In the presence of significant coronary artery disease, especially when the plaque formation compromises about 70% or more of the arterial diameter, the area beyond this blockage under certain conditions during the course of a day becomes ischemic. An example may be the situation when the individual is walking fast, climbing stairs, rushing through

Figure 8.22 Myocardial infarction leads to death of cardiac cells.

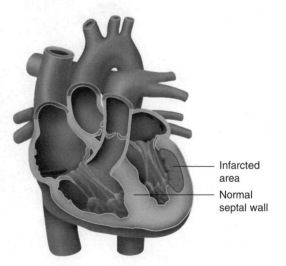

Infarcted area

Normal septal wall

Figure 8.23 The infracted area becomes progressively thinner while the remaining healthy myocardium hypertrophies to compensate for the loss of the cardiac cells. This is the compensated stage in heart failure.

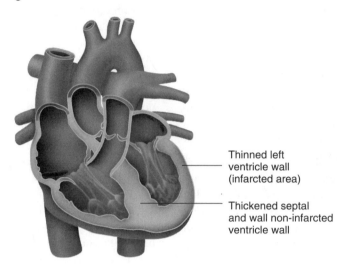

Thinned left
ventricle wall
(infarcted area)

Thickened septal
and wall non-infarcted
ventricle wall

Figure 8.24 Eventually, the entire myocardium gets progressively thinner and the cavity is enlarged (decompensated stage).

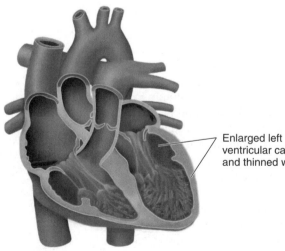

Enlarged left
ventricular cavity
and thinned walls

Figure 8.25 Myocardial remodeling following myocardial infarction.

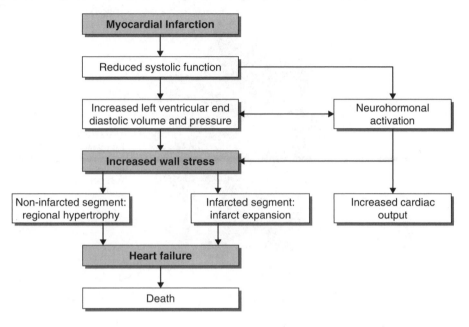

the airport, or getting angry and upset, etc. This leads to myocardial hypoxia and impaired myocardial function. As a result, cardiac output is diminished. A number of events to compensate for the diminished cardiac output follow. These events include the secretion of a number of hormones, hypertrophy of the myocardium, and hemodynamic changes. Although these events compensate for the reduced cardiac output, in the long run they are detrimental to the heart and eventually lead to heart failure in a similar fashion to the process of developing a myocardial infarction.

High Blood Pressure and Heart Failure
Hypertension is the most common risk factor and a cardinal precursor of heart failure.[59–61] It is associated with a two- to threefold increase in risk for developing heart failure.[60] Several

mechanisms exist through which hypertension contributes to the development of heart failure. The relative contribution of these mechanisms is not yet fully understood. The prevailing theory is that the left ventricle adapts to the chronic increase in wall stress as a result of increased total peripheral resistance consequent to hypertension.[62] Based on this concept, the following events occur and are depicted in **Figures 8.26–8.28**.

1. Ventricular wall thickness increases in proportion to blood pressure to maintain normal wall stress. This is referred to as *concentric hypertrophy*. Patients with concentric hypertrophy usually have elevated peripheral resistance. It is a compensatory response to maintain normal stroke volume.[63–65]

Figure 8.26   Normal heart.

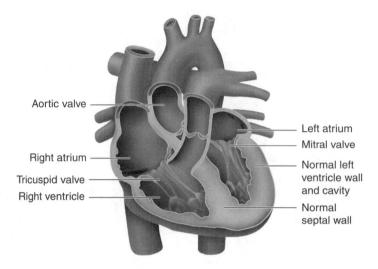

Figure 8.27   Compensated stage where persistent hypertension has led to an increase in peripheral resistance and ventricular wall stress. To maintain normal wall stress and stroke volume, the ventricles are thickened. This is referred to as concentric hypertrophy.

Figure 8.28   De-compensated stage. A progressive thinning of the ventricular walls and enlargement of the ventricular cavity ensues. This is referred to as eccentric hypertrophy.

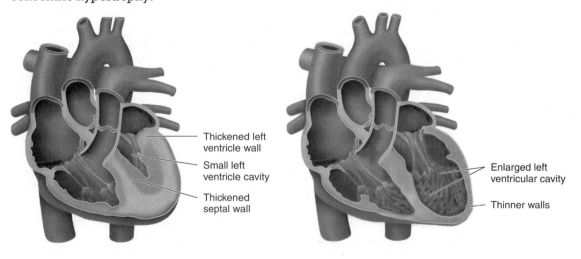

2. However, despite these adaptive changes and benefits, cardiac hypertrophy carries a substantial risk in the long run.[66-68] Hemodynamic changes as a result of the concentric left ventricle remodeling, end diastolic volume, and end systolic volume increase. The increased blood volume in the ventricle causes a greater distension of the ventricle.[60]

3. Enlargement of the left chamber leads to an increase in the radius and a decrease in wall thickness. This is referred to as *eccentric left ventricular hypertrophy*. This type of hypertrophy is considered a late transition to heart failure.[62,69]

■ Classification of Heart Failure

Heart failure individuals are classified based on how much work they can perform. According to the New York Heart Association classification, there are four classes of heart failure.

Class I: Patients can perform ordinary daily activities such as walking and climbing stairs without any symptoms such as chest pressure/pain, extreme fatigue, fast heart rate, or shortness of breath.

Class II: Such patients are comfortable at rest. However, they have slight limitations in performing ordinary daily activities such as walking and climbing stairs. These activities result in symptoms such as chest pressure/pain, extreme fatigue, fast heart rate, or shortness of breath.

Class III: These patients are also comfortable at rest. However, they have marked limitations in performing less than ordinary daily activities. Such activities result in symptoms such as chest pressure/pain, extreme fatigue, fast heart rate, or shortness of breath.

Class IV: Symptoms in these patients are even present at rest. They are not able to carry on any physical activity without discomfort.

Lower Extremity Arterial Disease or Peripheral Artery Disease

Peripheral artery disease (PAD) or peripheral vascular disease is characterized by the atherosclerotic, inflamatory process of the large peripheral arteries. The progressive development of atherosclerotic lesions ultimately leads to significant stenosis of the arteries involved. Consequently, blood flow distal to lesions is significantly impaired, leading to leg pain, numbness, cold legs or feet, and muscle pain in the thighs, calves, or feet. The term *peripheral* implies to all peripheral arteries (other than the arteries of the heart and brain) are involved. Indeed, multiple arteries can be and are usually involved. However, PAD is usually referred to the arteries of the lower extremities. In fact, the symptoms of the disease are manifested in the legs as a result of the inadequate blood supply to the leg muscles (**Figure 8.29**). For this reason, the term that describes the disease more exactly is *lower extremity arterial disease (LEAD)*. For this reason, LEAD will be adopted throughout this book.

LEAD is common among men in their 40s or older and women older than 50 years of age. The prevalence increases with age, affecting only 3% of the population younger than 60 years and over 20% of those 75 years or older (**Figure 8.30**).[70] LEAD co-exists with CAD and the prevalence of CAD in patients with LEAD is 92%.[71]

In the early stages of the disease, patients are asymptomatic when performing low-intensity daily activities. As the severity of the disease progresses, arterial blood flow distal to

Figure 8.29 Low extremity arterial disease (LEAD) resulting from plaque formation in the leg artery.

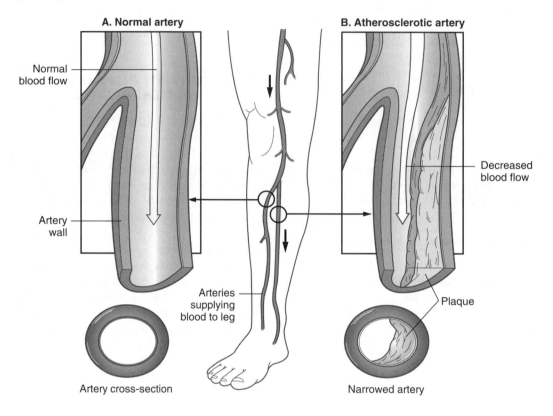

the lesions is progressively impaired. Symptoms occur when blood flow requirements to meet the metabolic demand of the lower extremity musculature are not met. The earliest and most frequent presenting symptom is intermittent claudication (aching or cramping) primarily of the calf and thigh muscles during daily activities requiring walking.[72] The ischemic pain inhibits walking and causes limping unilaterally or bilaterally. The pain discourages patients from walking or participation in any form of exercise. Consequently, muscular and cardiovascular capacities deteriorate, fostering an even more sedentary lifestyle, and further deterioration of muscular and cardiorespiratory functions. Limitations in the walking ability of the patients become more evident as the disease progresses and the patient's capacity to perform occupational, leisure, or social activities is severely limited.[73] It is estimated that the maximal walking distance on a flat surface at 4 km/hr is less that 1,000 meters for about 84% of LEAD patients without pain at rest.[74] Eventually, patients develop pain at rest.

Figure 8.30 The increased prevalence of LEAD in men and women with advancing age.

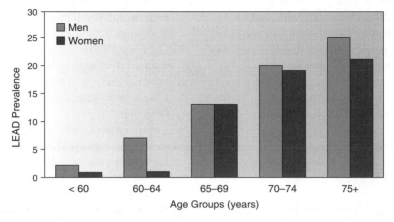

Source: From Criqui MH, et al. The prevalence of peripheral arterial disease in a defined population. *Circulation* 1985;71(3):510–515.

Classification of the disease is based on symptoms and is as follows:

Class I: Blood flow reduction does not produce visible symptoms and patients are asymptomatic.

Class II: Intermittent claudication is precipitated by moderate exertion; that is, walking fast, uphill, or distances longer than 200 meters.

Class III: Claudication occurs when walking a short distance of approximately 50 to 100 meters.

Class IV: Ischemic pain occurs at rest.

■ Risk Factors

Several risk factors have been identified to contribute a role in the development of LEAD. These risk factors are similar to those discussed for CVD and include smoking, diabetes, abnormal blood lipids and lipoprotein levels, and elevated blood pressure.[74] These risk factors are discussed in some detail here.

Smoking The single most important modifiable cause of LEAD is smoking, exposure to second-hand smoke, or tobacco use in any form. Smokers have up to a tenfold increase in relative risk for LEAD in a dose-related effect. Smoking promotes endothelial dysfuction, which is a precursor to atherosclerosis.[75,76]

Diabetes Mellitus LEAD is 20 times more likely to occur in type 2 diabetics than age- and sex-matched control subjects. Diabetics with LEAD also have higher mortality than those without LEAD. Diabetics account for up to 70% of nontraumatic amputations performed, and a known diabetic who smokes runs an approximately 30% risk of amputation within 5 years.[74,77–79]

Hypertension Elevated blood pressure is correlated with an increase in the risk of developing LEAD, as well as in associated coronary and cerebrovascular events (heart attack and stroke).[80]

Dyslipidemia Elevation of total cholesterol, LDL-cholesterol, and triglyceride levels each have been correlated with accelerated LEAD. There is convincing evidence that correction of dyslipidemia by diet and/or medication can benefit LEAD patients greatly.[81]

In addition, other risk factors being studied include levels of various inflammatory mediators such as C-reactive protein, homocysteine, and fibrinogen.

■ SUMMARY

- Epidemiology is the scientific discipline involved in the systematic study of the distribution and determinants of disease or events in specified populations.
- Epidemiology is based on the assumption that human diseases are caused or fostered by certain factors.
- Study designs applied in epidemiologic research include: cross-sectional studies, case-control, retrospective and prospective cohort trial, and randomized control trials.
- Some of the common measures used in epidemiologic research include: prevalence, incidence, absolute risk, absolute risk reduction, relative risk, relative risk reduction, and odds ratio.
- Cardiovascular disease (CVD) is a general term that includes heart attacks, heart failure, stroke, and peripheral artery diseases.
- Atherosclerosis (hardening of the artery) is the result of a chronic inflammatory response within the walls of large and medium-sized muscular arteries.
- Cardiovascular disease presents an enormous global health problem. An estimated 80,700,000 American adults have one or more types of CVD.

- Coronary heart disease (CHD) comprises more than half of all cardiovascular events and death in men and women under age 75.
- CVD and CHD accounts for more deaths in women than any other cause, including all types of cancer combined. The outcomes after a heart attack are worse in women than men.
- Contributing factors for the this epidemic in women include the misconceptions that heart disease poses an insignificant threat to women, and that heart attack symptoms are the same in women as in men.
- Women are less likely than men to feel chest pain during a heart attack and more likely to have so-called "atypical" symptoms, such as shortness of breath, nausea, and fatigue.
- It is believed that atherosclerosis is a chronic inflammatory disease of the arterial wall known as the response-to-injury theory. The theory states that the atherosclerosis develops as a result of repetitive injury and ongoing inflammatory process of the inner arterial wall (endothelial layer) of large and medium-sized arteries.
- The inflammation is caused by a number of agents including high blood cholesterol and more specifically LDL-cholesterol, cigarette smoking, hyperglycemia, hypertension, obesity, and infections.
- Oxidative stress describes the potential damage in a cell, tissue, or organ when highly active molecules formed during aerobic metabolism.
- Elevated LDL-cholesterol is a major contributor of endothelial dysfunction and oxidative stress.
- Oxidative stress is now recognized as the most significant contributor to atherosclerosis.

- The end result of the atherosclerotic process described is the formation of atherosclerotic plaque arterial wall and arterial remodeling.
- Plaques can rupture and cause series health problems including death. The vulnerability of a plaque to rupture depends on a number of factors such as the LDL-cholesterol content of the plaque (large lipid core), inflammatory processes, and the thickness of the fibrous cap.
- The term *risk factors* in medicine generally applies to a parameter that predisposes an individual to a higher risk for future cardiovascular events. Several risk factors have been identified over the years and are classified as modifiable or non-modifiable.
- Stroke or cerebrovascular accident is a form of cardiovascular disease that affects the blood vessels supplying blood and nutrients to the brain. Stroke is the third most common cause of death in the United States. It strikes over 500,000 persons per year and is fatal in approximately one-half of these individuals.
- Strokes are classified as ischemic (most common) or hemorrhagic.
- Heart failure or congestive heart failure is a complex syndrome characterized by progressive deterioration of ventricular function. It can involve systolic or diastolic dysfunction or both.
- Systolic dysfunction is characterized by a decrease in the ejection fraction of the left or right ventricle or both. Diastolic dysfunction is defined as an impaired filling of either or both ventricles.
- The incidence of new heart failure cases approximately doubles with each decade of age. This trend is expected to continue and even increase in the future.

- Primary factors contributing to heart failure are: a previous heart attack, coronary artery disease, and high blood pressure.
- Atherosclerotic inflamatory processes of the large peripheral arteries lead to the progressive development of atherosclerotic lesions and significant stenosis of the arteries involved. Consequently, blood flow distal to lesions is significantly impaired.
- When the arteries carrying blood to the legs are involved (lower extremity arterial disease), symptoms include leg pain, numbness, cold legs or feet, and muscle pain in the thighs, calves, or feet.
- Several risk factors have been identified that contribute to the development of LEAD. These risk factors are similar to those discussed for CVD and include smoking, diabetes, abnormal blood lipids and lipoprotein levels, and elevated blood pressure.

■ REFERENCES

1. Hennekens C, Buring J. *Epidemiology in Medicine.* Boston/Toronto: Little Brown; 1987.
2. Barratt A, Wyer PC, Hatala R, et al. Tips for learners of evidence-based medicine: 1. Relative risk reduction, absolute risk reduction and number needed to treat. *CMAJ* 2004; 171(4):353–358.
3. Lloyd-Jones D, Adams R, Carnethon M, et al. Heart disease and stroke statistics—2009 update: a report from the American Heart Association Statistics Committee and Stroke Statistics Subcommittee. *Circulation* 2009; 119:480–486.
4. Rosamond W, Flegal K, Friday G, et al. Heart disease and stroke statistics—2008 update: a report from the American Heart Association Statistics Committee and Stroke Statistics Subcommittee. *Circulation* 2008;117(4)e25–e146.

5. Rosamond W, Flegal K, Furio K, et al. Heart disease and stroke statistics—2007 update: a report from the American Heart Association Statistics Committee and Stroke Statistics Subcommittee. *Circulation* 2007;115(5): e69–e171.

6. Minino AM, Heron MP, Smith BL. Deaths: preliminary data for 2004. *Natl Vital Stat Rep* 2006;54(19):1–49.

7. Ford ES, Capewell S. Coronary heart disease mortality among young adults in the U.S. from 1980 through 2002: concealed leveling of mortality rates. *J Am Coll Cardiol* 2007;50(22): 2128–2132.

8. Enos WF, Holmes RH, Beyer J, et al. Coronary disease among United States soldiers killed in action in Korea. *JAMA* 1953;152(12): 1090–1093.

9. McNamara JJ, Molot MA, Stremple JF, Cutting RJ. Coronary artery disease in combat casualties in Vietnam. *JAMA* 1971;216(7):1185–1187.

10. National Center for Health Statistics. Health United States 2005. Hyattsville, MD: National Center for Health Statistics; 2005. Available at www.cdc.gov/nchs/data/hus/hus05 .pdf. Accessed March 4, 2009.

11. Fox CS, Evans JC, Larson MG, et al. Temporal trends in coronary heart disease mortality and sudden cardiac death from 1950 to 1999: the Framingham Heart Study. *Circulation* 2004; 110(5):522–527.

12. Incidence and Prevalence: *2006 Chart Book on Cardiovascular and Lung Diseases*. Bethesda MD: National Heart, Lung and Blood Institute; 2006. Available at: www.nhlbi .nih.gov/resources/docs/06a_ip_chtbk.pdf. Accessed March 4, 2009.

13. Lerman A, Sopko G. Women and cardiovascular heart disease: clinical implications from the Women's Ischemia Syndrome Evaluation (WISE) Study. Are we smarter? *J Am Coll Cardiol* 2006;47(3 Suppl):S59–S62.

14. The National Coalition for Women with Heart Disease. *Facts and Figures*. Available at: www .womenheart.org/resources/factsfigs.cfm. Accessed March 4, 2009.

15. Goldberg RJ, O'Donnel C, Yarzebski J, et al. Sex differences in symptom presentation associated with acute myocardial infarction: a population-based perspective. *Am Heart J* 1998;136(2):189–195.

16. Mosca L, Mochari H, Christian A, et al. National study of women's awareness, preventive action, and barriers to cardiovascular health. *Circulation* 2006;113(4):525–534.

17. Mosca L, Linfante AH, Benjamin EJ, et al. National study of physician awareness and adherence to cardiovascular disease prevention guidelines. *Circulation* 2005;111(4): 499–510.

18. Christian AH, Rosamond W, White AR, Mosca L. Nine-year trends and racial and ethnic disparities in women's awareness of heart disease and stroke: an American Heart Association national study. *J Womens Health* 2007;16(1):68–81.

19. McSweeney JC, Cody M, O'Sullivan P, et al. Women's early warning symptoms of acute myocardial infarction. *Circulation* 2003; 108(21):2619–2623.

20. McSweeney JC, Cody M, Crane PB. Do you know them when you see them? Women's prodromal and acute symptoms of myocardial infarction. *J Cardiovasc Nurs* 2001;15(3): 26–38.

21. Rathore SS, Wang Y, Krumholz HM. Sex-based differences in the effect of digoxin for the treatment of heart failure. *N Engl J Med* 2002;347(18):1403–1411.

22. Ross R, Harker L. Hyperlipidemia and atherosclerosis. *Science* 1976;193(4258):1094–1100.

23. Hansson GK. Inflammation, atherosclerosis, and coronary artery disease. *N Engl J Med* 2005;352(16):1685–1695.

24. Libby P. Inflammation in atherosclerosis. *Nature* 2002;420(6917):868–874.

25. Ross R. Atherosclerosis is an inflammatory disease. *Am Heart J* 1999;138(5 Pt 2): S419–S420.

26. Libby P, Ridker PM, Maseri A. Inflammation and atherosclerosis. *Circulation* 2002;105(9): 1135–1143.

27. Jialal I, Devaraj S. The role of oxidized low density lipoprotein in atherogenesis. *J Nutr* 1996;126(4 Suppl):1053S–1057S.

28. Maritim AC, Sanders RA, Watkins JB III. Diabetes, oxidative stress, and antioxidants: a review. *J Biochem Mol Toxicol* 2003;17(1):24–38.

29. Lelli JL Jr, Becks LL, Dabrowska MI, Hinshaw DB. ATP converts necrosis to apoptosis in oxidant-injured endothelial cells. *Free Radic Biol Med* 1998;25(6):694–702.

30. Lennon SV, Martin SJ, Cotter TG. Dose-dependent induction of apoptosis in human tumour cell lines by widely diverging stimuli. *Cell Prolif* 1991;24(2):203–214.

31. The Lipid Research Clinics Coronary Primary Prevention Trial results. II. The relationship of reduction in incidence of coronary heart disease to cholesterol lowering. *JAMA* 1984; 251(3):365–374.

32. Murray CJ, Lopez AD. Global mortality, disability, and the contribution of risk factors: Global Burden of Disease Study. *Lancet* 1997;349(9063):1436–1442.

33. Chisolm GM, Steinberg D. The oxidative modification hypothesis of atherogenesis: an overview. *Free Radic Biol Med* 2000;28(12): 1815–1826.

34. Berliner JA, Territo MC, Sevanian A, et al. Minimally modified low density lipoprotein stimulates monocyte endothelial interactions. *J Clin Invest* 1990;85(4):1260–1266.

35. Frostegård J, Nilsson J, Haegerstrand A, et al. Oxidized low density lipoprotein induces differentiation and adhesion of human monocytes and the monocytic cell line U937. *Proc Natl Acad Sci USA* 1990;87(3):904–908.

36. Gleissner CA, Leitinger N, Ley K. Effects of native and modified low-density lipoproteins on monocyte recruitment in atherosclerosis. *Hypertension* 2007;50(2):276–283.

37. Al-Benna S, Hamilton CA, McClure JD, et al. Low-density lipoprotein cholesterol determines oxidative stress and endothelial dysfunction in saphenous veins from patients with coronary artery disease. *Arterioscler Thromb Vasc Biol* 2006;26(1):218–223.

38. Glagov S, Weisenberg E, Zaring CK, et al. Compensatory enlargement of human atherosclerotic coronary arteries. *N Engl J Med* 1987;316(22):1371–1375.

39. Pasterkamp G, Hillen B, Borst C. Arterial remodelling by atherosclerosis. *Semin Interv Cardiol* 1997;2(3):147–152.

40. Pasterkamp G, Schonveld AH, von Wolferen W, et al. The impact of atherosclerotic arterial remodeling on percentage of luminal stenosis varies widely within the arterial system. A postmortem study. *Arterioscler Thromb Vasc Biol* 1997;17(11):3057–3063.

41. Eefting FD, Pasterkamp G, Claijs RJ, et al. Remodeling of the atherosclerotic arterial wall: a determinant of luminal narrowing in human coronary arteries. *Coron Artery Dis* 1997;8(7):415–421.

42. Gould KL, Lipscomb K. Effects of coronary stenoses on coronary flow reserve and resistance. *Am J Cardiol* 1974;34(1):48–55.

43. Davies MJ. The contribution of thrombosis to the clinical expression of coronary atherosclerosis. *Thromb Res* 1996;82(1):1–32.

44. Lilly LS. *Pathophysiology of Heart Disease*, 2nd ed. Baltimore: Williams and Wilkins; 1998.

45. Wilson PW, D'Agostino RB, Levy D, et al. Prediction of coronary heart disease using risk factor categories. *Circulation* 1998;97(18): 1837–1847. (see comments)

46. Conroy RM, Pyörälä K, Fitzgerald AP, et al. Estimation of 10-year risk of fatal cardiovascular disease in Europe: the SCORE project. *Eur Heart J* 2003;24(11):987–1003.

47. Goldstein LB, Adams R, Becker K, et al. Primary prevention of ischemic stroke: a statement for healthcare professionals from the Stroke Council of the American Heart Association. *Circulation* 2001;103(1):163–182.

48. Wolf PA, D'Agostino RB, Kannel WB, et al. Cigarette smoking as a risk factor for stroke. The Framingham Study. *JAMA* 1988;259 (7):1025–1029.

49. Seshadri S, Beiser A, Kelly-Hayes M, et al. The lifetime risk of stroke: estimates from the

Framingham Study. *Stroke* 2006;37(2):345–350. (see comments)

50. Johnston SC, Gress DR, Browner WS, Sidney S. Short-term prognosis after emergency department diagnosis of TIA. *JAMA* 2000; 284(22):2901–2906.

51. Kissela BM, Khoury J, Kleindorfer D, et al. Epidemiology of ischemic stroke in patients with diabetes: the Greater Cincinnati/Northern Kentucky Stroke Study. *Diabetes Care* 2005;28:355–359.

52. Hu FB, Stampfer MJ, Colditz GA, et al. Physical activity and risk of stroke in women. *JAMA* 2000;283:2961–2967.

53. Hendrix SL, Wassertheil-Smoller S, Johnson KC, et al. Effects of conjugated equine estrogen on stroke in the Women's Health Initiative. *Circulation* 2006;113(20):2425–2434.

54. Ohira T, Shahar E, Chambless LE, et al. Risk factors for ischemic stroke subtypes: the Atherosclerosis Risk in Communities study. *Stroke* 2006;37(10):2493–2498.

55. Becker RC. Cardiology patient page: heart attack and stroke prevention in women. *Circulation* 2005;112(17):e273-e275.

56. Kannel WB, Ho K, Thom T. Changing epidemiological features of cardiac failure. *Br Heart J* 1994;72(2 Suppl):S3–S9.

57. Graves EJ. National Hospital Discharge Survey: annual summary, 1993. *Vital Health Stat 13* 1995;13(121):1–63.

58. Centers for Disease Control and Prevention. Mortality from heart failure—United States 1980–1990. *Morbid Mortal Wkly Rep MMWR* 1994;5(7):77–81.

59. Kannel WB, Castelli WP, McNamara PM, et al. Role of blood pressure in the development of congestive heart failure. The Framingham Study. *N Engl J Med* 1972;287(16):781–787.

60. Lawrence T, McKee PA, Castelli WP, et al. Heart failure and hypertension. *N Engl J Med* 1972;286(12):667–668.

61. Levy D, Larson MG, Vasan RS, et al. The progression from hypertension to congestive heart failure. *JAMA* 1996;275(20):1557–1562. (see comments)

62. Devereux RB, Savage DD, Sachs I, Laragh JH. Relation of hemodynamic load to left ventricular hypertrophy and performance in hypertension. *Am J Cardiol* 1983;51(1):171–176.

63. Lorell BH, Grossman W. Cardiac hypertrophy: the consequences for diastole. *J Am Coll Cardiol* 1987;9(5):1189–1193.

64. Strauer BE. Ventricular function and coronary hemodynamics in hypertensive heart disease. *Am J Cardiol* 1979;44(5):999–1006.

65. Swynghedauw B, Schwartz K, Apstein CS. Decreased contractility after myocardial hypertrophy: cardiac failure or successful adaptation? *Am J Cardiol* 1984;54(3):437–440.

66. Levy D, Anderson KM, Savage DD, et al. Echocardiographically detected left ventricular hypertrophy: prevalence and risk factors. The Framingham Heart Study. *Ann Intern Med* 1988;108(1):7–13.

67. McLenachan JM, Henderson E, Morris KI, Dargie HJ. Ventricular arrhythmias in patients with hypertensive left ventricular hypertrophy. *N Engl J Med* 1987;317(13):787–792.

68. Messerli FH, Ventura HO, Elizardi DJ, et al. Hypertension and sudden death. Increased ventricular ectopic activity in left ventricular hypertrophy. *Am J Med* 1984;77(1):18–22.

69. Frohlich ED, Apstein C, Chobanian AV, et al. The heart in hypertension. *N Engl J Med* 1992;327(14):998–1008.

70. Criqui MH, Fronek A, Barrett-Connor E, et al. The prevalence of peripheral arterial disease in a defined population. *Circulation* 1985;71 (3):510–515.

71. Hertzer NR, Beven EG, Young JR, et al. Coronary artery disease in peripheral vascular patients. A classification of 1000 coronary angiograms and results of surgical management. *Ann Surg* 1984;199(2):223–233.

72. Zatina MA, Berkowitz HD, Gross GM, et al. 31P nuclear magnetic resonance spectroscopy: noninvasive biochemical analysis of the ischemic extremity. *J Vasc Surg* 1986;3(3): 411–420.

73. Ekroth R, Dahllöf AG, Grundevall B, et al. Physical training of patients with intermittent

claudication: indications, methods, and results. *Surgery* 1978;84(5):640–643.

74. Beach KW, Bedford GR, Bergelin RO, et al. Progression of lower-extremity arterial occlusive disease in type II diabetes mellitus. *Diabetes Care* 1988;11(6):464–472.

75. Bell AG, Mavridis AN. Smoking and smoking cessation. In: *Lower Extremity Arterial Disease*, DG Caralis, GL Bakris, eds. Totowa, NJ: Humana Press Inc; 2005:39–52.

76. Levy LA. Smoking and peripheral vascular disease. Podiatric medical update. *Clin Podiatr Med Surg* 1992;9(1):165–171.

77. Beach KW, Brunzell JD, Conquest LL, Strandness DE. The correlation of arteriosclerosis obliterans with lipoproteins in insulin-dependent and non-insulin-dependent diabetes. *Diabetes* 1979;28(9):836–840.

78. Beach KW, Brunzell JD, Strandness DE Jr. Prevalence of severe arteriosclerosis obliterans in patients with diabetes mellitus. Relation to smoking and form of therapy. *Arteriosclerosis* 1982;2(4):275–280.

79. Beach KW, Strandness DE Jr. Arteriosclerosis obliterans and associated risk factors in insulin-dependent and non-insulin-dependent diabetes. *Diabetes* 1980;29(11):882–888.

80. Bakris GL. Peripheral Arterial Disease and Diabetes. In: *Lower Extremity Arterial Disease*. DG Caralis, GL Bakris, eds. Totowa, NJ: Humana Press; 2005.

81. Babu A, Kannan CR, Mazzone T. Hyperlipidemia in peripheral arterial disease. ed. In: *Lower Extremity Arterial Disease*. DG Caralis, GL Bakris, eds. Totowa, NJ: Humana Press; 2005.

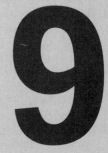

Cardiovascular Diseases and Physical Activity

The association between physical activity and health, vitality, and longevity has been recognized since antiquity. Over 2,500 years ago, the Greek physician Hippocrates (460–377 BC) succinctly and accurately summed up the benefits of exercise and physical activity as follows:

> Speaking generally, all parts of the body which have a function, if used in moderation and exercised in labors to which each is accustomed, become thereby healthy and well developed and age slowly; but if unused and left idle, they become liable to disease, defective in growth, and age quickly.

The quest to define the role of physical activity in human health, disease, and mortality began in the early 1950s. In their landmark study, Morris and coworkers reported that those with physically demanding occupations (London mail carriers and double-decker bus conductors) had approximately 50% lower rates of CHD when compared to the more sedentary bus drivers and desk clerks.[1] Despite the fact that the investigators did not control for confounding factors such as body weight, blood pressure, and blood cholesterol, which are likely to be more abnormal in the sedentary cohort, these findings stimulated worldwide interest in the relationship between physical activity and cardiovascular mortality.

Subsequent leisure time physical activity studies and occupational studies from variety of industries included postal, railroad, and farm workers; employees of utility companies; civil servants; longshoremen; police officers and firefighters; all designed to examine the physical activity–mortality relationship. Most of these studies reported that the most active individuals had one third to three fourths fewer cardiovascular events and deaths when compared to the least active.[2]

A most influential review regarding physical activity and coronary heart disease was by Powell and coworkers in 1987.[3] To assess the relationship between physical activity and mortality, the authors identified 121 studies and carefully evaluated the quality of each. Of the 121 studies, 43 were found to be well-conducted and were included in the final analysis (meta-analysis). Their conclusion was that physical activity is inversely related to the risk of coronary heart disease (CHD). The association was independent of other confounding factors and was as robust as that of established risk factors such as smoking, hypercholesterolemia, and hypertension (**Figure 9.1**).

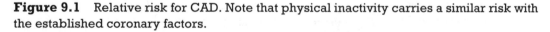

Figure 9.1   Relative risk for CAD. Note that physical inactivity carries a similar risk with the established coronary factors.

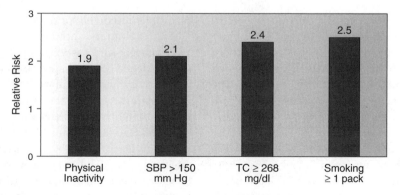

Source: Modified from Powell, et al. *Ann Review Public Health* 1987;8:253–287.

This chapter presents the most influential studies examining the association between physical activity, fitness and cardiovascular disease, and all-cause mortality. In addition, potential mechanisms of exercise-related protection against cardiovascular disease are discussed.

■ OCCUPATIONAL AND LEISURE TIME PHYSICAL ACTIVITY STUDIES

Occupational and leisure time activity studies utilized questionnaires to assess the physical activity habits of the participants. Despite the subjective nature of such surveys, the overall findings of these studies support a graded reduction in mortality risk with increased level of physical activity. This association is similar for men and women regardless of age. Several of these studies are discussed in some detail because of their unique aspects.

The study by Paffenbarger and Hale[4] followed 6,351 longshoremen for 22 years. The unique feature of this study is that the level of energy output for each participant was estimated based on the energy requirements of 49 longshoring jobs. Accordingly, workers who loaded and unloaded ships were classified as heavy activity, clerks as light activity, and those in between as moderate activity workers. The age-adjusted coronary death rate was 70% higher in the moderate activity and 80% higher in the light activity work group. Because there was little difference in the death rates between moderate and heavy activity workers, the investigators suggested the existence of a protective threshold of physical activity or caloric expenditure.[4]

Fatal and non-fatal coronary events were assessed in 5,288 men and 5,229 women who lived in 58 Israeli settlements called kibbutzim.[5] Participants were classified as physically active or sedentary based on data collected by a physical activity questionnaire. One unique aspect of this study is that these kibbutzim provided communal dining facilities and similar medical care for a relatively homogeneous group. Thus, many of the confounding factors present in epidemiologic studies were eliminated. In addition, risk factors were similar in between physically active and sedentary groups. The other unique aspect is that the study provided information on a large number of women.

The investigators reported that the 15-year relative risk value for fatal and non-fatal coronary events was 2.5 times higher in men engaged in sedentary occupations compared to the men who performed with more physically demanding jobs. For women, the risk was 3.1 times greater for the corresponding occupations.[5]

Not all studies came to similar conclusions. In a Finnish study, the rate of coronary heart disease mortality was greater among lumberjacks compared to less active farmers of the same region.[6] However, this finding must be interpreted with caution for two reasons. Although farmers were less active than lumberjacks, they were not sedentary. Thus, the study compared highly active (lumberjacks) to somewhat less active (farmers) individuals. This along with the higher fat consumption and smoking rates among lumberjacks is likely to have attenuated the positive effects of physical activity in the lumberjacks and showed more favorable outcomes for the farmers.

The landmark epidemiologic work by Paffenbarger and associates provided persuasive evidence on the association between physical activity and mortality. In 1978, the same investigators assessed the association between leisure time physical activity and heart attacks in 16,963 Harvard alumni who entered Harvard between 1916 and 1950 and responded to a questionnaire.[7] The cohorts were categorized based on weekly caloric expenditure based on leisure time activities, ranging from < 500 to more than 4,000 kcal/week. The data revealed that the risk of first heart attack was related inversely to the level of energy expenditure during leisure time. A sharp reduction in fatal and non-fatal heart attacks rates with increase in weekly energy expenditure was noted at the energy expenditure of 2,000 kcal per week. Those who expended less than 2,000 kcal per week had a 64% higher risk for a heart attack.

Another important finding of this study was that the reduction in risk was only evident if physical activity was maintained throughout the study participant's life. Those who played varsity sports but did not maintain a physically active lifestyle had a higher mortality rate compared to those who maintained a physically active lifestyle in adulthood. Conversely, those who avoided athletics in college but subsequently took up a more active lifestyle also had similarly low rates of mortality.[7]

In the next two reports that followed on the same cohort,[8,9] the investigators reported a consistent, inverse, and graded trend towards a lower all-cause mortality rate; as physical activity-related caloric expenditure increased form 500 to 2,000 kcal per week, the mortality rate decreased. More specifically, the mortality risk for men whose weekly energy expenditure from leisure time activities total 2,000 kcal or more had about 25% to 33% lower mortality rate compared to those with a caloric expenditure of less than 2,000 kcal per week. Paffenbarger et al. speculated that physical activity accounted for approximately 1 to 2 years of additional life. An interesting observation of the study was that the mortality risk tended to increase slightly in those expending more than 3,500 kcal per week.[8] This is equivalent to about 30 to 35 miles of jogging per week.

In the more recent study, Paffenbarger et al.[9] examined the relative risk of death based on different types of physical activity that included walking (miles/week), stair-climbing (floors), and playing sports in 10,269 Harvard alumni over a 9-year period. The inverse and graded association between mortality risk and volume of physical activity was again evident and in accord with their previous findings. In addition, and particularly noteworthy, was the 30% to 40% reduction in mortality risk, evident in those individuals engaging in moderate-to-vigorous activity levels (≥ 4.5 METs; see Chapter 2) with only minimal additional benefits achieved by engaging in activities of greater intensity. The reduction was similar when physical activity was expressed as kilocalories per week (the sum of walking, stair climbing, and sports participation), suggesting that a 40% reduction in mortality occurs by engaging in modest levels of activity (1,000 to 2,000 kcal/week, equivalent to three to five 1-hour sessions of activity).

Collectively, the findings of these studies[4,7,9] provided evidence in support of an exercise intensity threshold of about 5 to 6 METs and an exercise volume threshold somewhere between 1,000 and 2,000 kcal per week for a significant reduction in mortality risk. Furthermore, the findings suggest that most of the benefits occur at moderate exercise volumes and moderate intensities.

Similar results have been reported from large studies that have followed cohorts for coronary heart disease (CHD) morbidity and mortality in the range of 10 to 20 years among British civil servants, U.S. railroad workers, San Francisco longshoremen, nurses, physicians, other healthcare workers, and other cohorts. The findings of these studies are summarized in two comprehensive reviews.[10,11]

Clearly, the accumulated epidemiological evidence provided strong support for the existence of a strong inverse relationship between physical exercise and risk of CHD. As stated by Paffenbarger and Hyde, ". . . the questions to be addressed are not whether exercise is a real element for cardiovascular health, but what kind of exercise is needed, and how much, i.e., with what frequency, intensity, timing, and duration.

An understanding of the ways and means by which exercise alters coronary heart disease risk is only beginning to emerge, but there is wide acceptance that its benefits are vitally needed in the sedentary Western world."[12]

According to a recent review that included 44 observational studies from 1966 to 2000,[13] the collective findings support the following: First, there is strong evidence of an inverse linear dose-response relationship between volume of physical activity and all-cause mortality. Second, an exercise volume threshold can be defined beyond which a significant reduction in mortality risk occurs. This threshold appears to be at a caloric expenditure of approximately 1,000 kcal per week for an average reduction of 20% to 30% in mortality risk. Further reductions in risk are observed with higher volumes of energy expenditure. Third, the independent contribution of the exercise components of intensity, duration, and frequency to the reduction of mortality risk was not clear. The authors emphasized the need for more research to better understand the contribution of each component.[13] Indeed, efforts to define the intensity, duration, frequency, volume, and type of exercise necessary for cardiovascular health and longevity continue. Although progress has been made, much more work is needed.

The influence of genetic factors in the reduction of the mortality risk cannot be dismissed. Furthermore, the argument can be made that it is not the physical activity that provides protection but the genetic composition of these individuals.

In this regard, the independent association of physical activity and mortality and the influence of genetic and other familial factors were assessed in a cohort of same-sex twins born in Finland before 1958 and with both alive in 1967.[14] In 1975, healthy men (n = 7,925) and healthy women (n = 7,977) responded to a questionnaire on physical activity, occupation, smoking habits, body weight, alcohol use, and physician-diagnosed diseases. Individuals who reported engaging in brisk walk for a mean duration of 30 minutes, at least six times per month were classified as physically active. Those who reported no leisure time activity were classified as sedentary. The remaining individuals were classified as occasional exercisers. When compared to the sedentary twins, the adjusted risk of mortality was 33% lower among the twins who exercised occasionally and 44% lower among the physically active twins. The investigators concluded that physical activity is associated with lower mortality independent of genetic and other confounding factors.

> Epidemiological evidence supports a strong inverse relationship between physical exercise and coronary heart disease risk.

Physical Fitness Studies

Physical activity questionnaires provide valuable information and are useful in assessing physical activity levels. However, by nature, they are not objective. A shift from assessing physical activity by questionnaires to a more objective assessment was provided by Steve Blair and his co-investigators in their landmark study.[15] The investigators assessed physical fitness of 10,224 men and 3,120 women by a maximal exercise test at the Institute of Aerobic Research. The cohort was grouped into five fitness categories based on the MET level achieved and were followed for a period of over 8 years. After adjusting for age, blood pressure, smoking habits, fasting blood glucose levels, and family history of coronary heart disease, there was an inverse, strong, and graded association between physical fitness and cardiovascular and all-cause mortality for both men and women. The most striking finding of the study was that the major reduction in mortality risk occurred when moving from the least fit (< 7

Figure 9.2   Age-adjusted all-cause mortality in men according to exercise capacity.

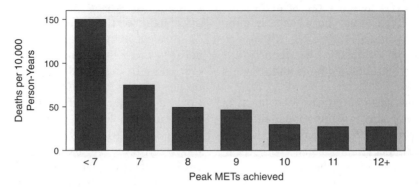

Source: From Blair, et al. *JAMA* 1989;262:2395–2401.

METs) to the next fit category of 7 METs. The risk continued to decline with higher fitness levels and appears to plateau at approximately 9 to 10 METs for women and men, respectively (**Figure 9.2**). The investigators emphasized that the MET levels of 7 to 10 achieved for optimal health benefits are attainable by a brisk walk of 30 to 60 minutes each day.

Despite the objectivity of the maximal exercise test and its greater accuracy in the classification of fitness categories, it still represents a single baseline assessment of fitness. With a single exposure assessment at baseline, it is difficult to discount the influence of genetic factors, underlying diseases, and other confounding variables on the association between fitness and mortality. For example, the low exercise capacity at baseline and the cause of death within the follow-up period of the study may be due to underlying disease and not the low fitness level. In this case, the mortality risk for the low fitness categories will be over-inflated and the association spurious.

To address this issue, Blair and coworkers controlled for some of these confounding variables by assessing the fitness of the cohort with two maximal exercise tests. The investigators reported that men who were unfit at

both examinations had the highest mortality rate. Those who increased their physical activity and moved from the unfit to fit category within the first and subsequent examinations had a 44% reduction in adjusted mortality risk when compared to men who remained unfit at both examinations (**Figure 9.3**). In addition, the

Figure 9.3   Survival curves for fit and unfit men. A 44% reduction in adjusted mortality risk was noted in the unfit who became fit compared to the unfit men who stayed unfit.

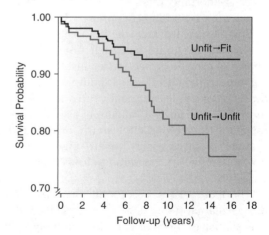

Source: From Blair, et al. *JAMA* 1995;273:1093–1097.

investigators estimate a 7.9% reduction in mortality risk for every minute increase in the peak treadmill exercise time between examinations.[16] This finding also provides evidence to support that the association between fitness and mortality is independent and beyond genetic factors.

The inverse association between physical activity and mortality remains robust after statistical adjustments of potential confounders. However, the impact of physical activity within groups in the presence of known risk factors such as hypertension, diabetes, or smoking has not been assessed. In this regard, Blair and coworkers[17] assessed the impact of fitness within groups who possess specific risk factors. The cohort consisted of 25,241 men and 7,080 women with baseline evaluations that included a maximal exercise test. Low, moderate, and high-fit categories were established based on the peak exercise time.

The findings of this study lead to three principal conclusions. First, an inverse and graded association between fitness and mortality was evident and consistent within the various subgroups examined. For men who smoked, had high blood cholesterol and elevated systolic blood pressure, or were unhealthy, the adjusted all-cause mortality rates were 17% to 39% lower if they were moderately fit compared to low fit. For the fit men, the risk was 32% to 50% lower.

Second, moderate and high fitness levels appear to provide protection against the cumulative detrimental effect of multiple risk factors. For example, the death rates in high-fit individuals with two or three risk factors (smoking, high blood cholesterol, or elevated systolic blood pressure) were significantly lower (15%) when compared to low-fit individuals with no risk factors.

Third, the relative risk for all-cause and cardiovascular mortality due to physical inactivity was similar to those of cigarette smoking and elevated cholesterol levels.

Although the physical activity–mortality relationship was well established by now, information on the intensity, duration, and type of physical activity was still speculative. To address these questions, Lakka and coworkers[18] directly assessed the maximal oxygen uptake by a standardized exercise test. In addition, they collected information by questionnaires on the leisure time physical activity habits of 1,453 healthy men. The cohort was followed for an average of 4.9 years and myocardial infarctions were recorded.

The association between the risk of myocardial infarction and both leisure time physical activity and oxygen uptake was inverse and graded. After adjusting for a number of coronary risk factors, men with an oxygen uptake of more that 34 ml/kg/min (the highest one third of the cohort) had a 55% lower risk of myocardial infarction compared to the risk of the least fit man (the lowest one third). Similarly, men engaging in leisure time activity for more than 2 hours per week had a 60% lower risk than the least fit men. The investigators also reported that a mean intensity of about 6 METs may be the threshold for a reduction in risk.

The unique aspect of this study is that both oxygen uptake and leisure time activity were assessed. Because oxygen uptake was directly measured and not estimated, fitness level is more accurately assessed. Collectively, the oxygen consumption of 34 ml/kg/min, the hours of physical activity per week, and the very similar decrease in risk (55% and 60%) support the contention that physical activity of moderate intensity (about 6 METs as stated by the investigators) is required for risk reduction.

Similar findings were reported in a study of 1,960 middle-aged, Norwegian men whose physical fitness was assessed at baseline by an exercise tolerance test using a bicycle ergometer. During a 16-year follow-up period, the relative risk for cardiovascular mortality was inversely related to physical fitness. Once again, the major reduction in mortality risk (41%) occurred when moving from the least fit (quintile 1) to the next fit category (quintile 2). The risk continued to decline with higher fitness levels reaching 55% and 59% for quintiles 3 and 4, respectively.[19]

The independent effects of exercise type and intensity on the risk for coronary heart disease were assessed in a large cohort of 44,452 men enrolled in the Health Professionals' Follow-up Study.[20] The MET level for each activity performed was calculated and the cohort was categorized into fitness quintiles based on the MET-hours per week of total physical activity.

The findings of this study support an inverse and graded association between the risk of coronary heart disease and the weekly volume of exercise or physical activity. In this regard, the findings of the study are in accord with previous findings and strengthen the contention that physical activity is protective against premature heart disease. In addition, the study provided information on the type, volume, and intensity of several physical activities and their respective efficacy on coronary heart disease risk reduction. It is also important to mention that this was the first study that provided evidence on the efficacy of weight training or resistance training on coronary heart disease risk reduction. The risk reduction achieved by

weight training was similar to that observed by brisk walking and rowing, and approximately half of that observed by running. These findings are summarized in **Table 9.1**.

Because walking was the most frequent form of exercise (58% of men reported walking at least 1 hour per week), the investigators examined the independent effects of intensity and duration of walking on the risk for coronary heart disease. They found that walking pace (intensity) was inversely related to the risk of coronary heart disease independent of walking volume (**Figure 9.4**). A 4% reduction in coronary risk was observed for every 1-MET increase in exercise intensity. The duration of walking was also inversely related to the risk. However, the much stronger association between intensity and risk suggests that walking intensity has a stronger effect on risk reduction than duration.

Evidence supports that both exercise intensity and duration are associated with a reduction in mortality risk. However, the stronger association between intensity and risk suggests that additional health benefits may be possible with relatively higher exercise intensities. There is also limited evidence that weight training may be as effective in lowering mortality risk as aerobic exercise.

Table 9.1 Activity Performed and Coronary Heart Disease Relative Risk Reduction in Men

Activity Performed per Week	Relative Risk Reduction
Running ≥ 1 hour	42%
Rowing ≥ 1 hour	18%
Brisk walk ≥ 30 minutes	18%
Weight training ≥ 30 minutes	23%

Figure 9.4 Adjusted risk for coronary heart disease according to walking pace.

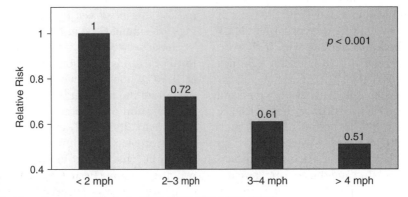

Source: Modified from Tanasescu M, et al. *JAMA* 2002;288:1994–2000.

Quantifying the Dose-Response Association

Recently, several more studies have reported a more precise quantification of the dose (amount of exercise or degree of fitness) and response (mortality risk-reduction) relationship by expressing exercise capacity in the context of survival benefit per MET (**Table 9.2**). These studies present the change in mortality risk for each 1-MET increase in exercise capacity assessed by a maximal exercise test. The reduction in mortality risk per 1-MET increase in exercise capacity ranges between 10% and 25%.[16,21–27] This is evident in both men and women. There is also evidence to suggest that the strength of exercise capacity in predicting risk of mortality may even be greater among women than men.[22,28]

Information on the association between physical activity, exercise capacity, and mortality among African Americans is lacking. It is well-documented that the age-adjusted all-cause mortality rates in African Americans are as much as 60% higher when compared to American Caucasians. To address this issue, Kokkinos et al.[27] assessed the association between exercise capacity and mortality risk in 6,749 African-American and 8,911 Caucasian men. The investigators found exercise capacity to be a more powerful predictor of risk for all-cause mortality than established risk factors (smoking, dyslipidemia, diabetes, and hypertension) among both African Americans and Caucasians after adjusting for cardiac medications. The risk for mortality was 13% lower for every 1-MET increase in exercise capacity for the entire cohort, with similar reductions observed for those with and without CVD.

In addition, when fitness groups were considered, the relative risk for all-cause mortality was approximately 20% lower in those with an exercise capacity of 5 to 7 METs (moderate fit category) when compared to those achieving < 5 METs. The mortality risk was 50% lower for those with an exercise capacity of 7.1 to 10 METs and 70% lower for those with an exercise capacity of more than 10 METs. This gradient for a reduction in mortality with increasing fitness was similar in African Americans and Caucasians in the entire cohort (**Figure 9.5**) and in individuals with and without CVD (**Figures 9.6** and **9.7**). These findings are very

Table 9.2 Survival Benefit per 1-MET Increase in Studies Using Maximal Exercise Testing as a Measure of Fitness

Study	Cohort	N	Mortality Risk Reduction/MET Increase
Blair et al.[16]	Men	9,777	~16%
Dorn et al.[22]	Cardiac rehabilitation	651	8%–14%
Goraya et al.[23]	- Younger	2,593	14%
	- Elderly	514	18%
Myers et al.[26]	Middle-aged men with and without coronary heart disease test	6,213	12%
Gulati et al.[28]	Healthy women	5,721	17%
Mora et al.[24]	Women in the Lipid Research Clinics Trial	2,994	20%
Balady et al.[21]	Framingham Offspring Study:		13%
	- Men	1,431	
	- Women	1,612	
Myers et al.[25]	For every 1,000 kcal/week adulthood activity	6,213	20%
Kokkinos et al.[27]	Middle-aged men with and without coronary heart disease referred for an exercise treadmill test	15,660	13%

Figure 9.5 Adjusted risk for all-cause mortality in African Americans and Caucasians.

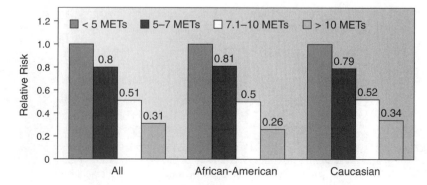

Source: Adapted from Kokkinos, et al. *Circulation* 2008;117:614–622.

Figure 9.6 Adjusted risk for all-cause mortality in African Americans and Caucasians with CVD.

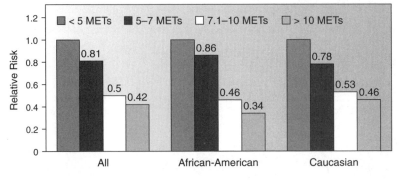

Source: Adapted from Kokkinos, et al. *Circulation* 2008;117:614–622.

similar to the mortality rate reduction reported by Myers et al.[26] in men with and without CVD. Because the cohort of the two studies[26,27] consisted of veterans with very similar health care (the Veterans Affairs Health Care System ensures equal access to care independent of a patient's financial status), the findings strengthen the evidence that higher exercise capacity is associated with lower cardiovascular and all-cause mortality regardless of factors related to socioeconomic strata.

A more precise quantification of the dose (amount of exercise or degree of fitness) and response (mortality risk-reduction) relationship revealed a 10% to 25% reduction in mortality risk for each 1-MET increase in exercise capacity.

These findings have significant public health implications. Mortality risk can be cut in half by just engaging in brisk walk for 2 to 3 hours per week or 30 minutes per session 4 to 5 days

Figure 9.7 Adjusted risk for all-cause mortality in African Americans and Caucasians with no CVD.

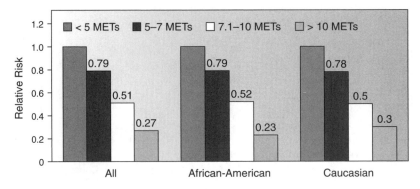

Source: Adapted from Kokkinos, et al. *Circulation* 2008;117:614–622.

per week. This was shown for both African Americans and Caucasians with and without heart disease (see Figures 9.5 to 9.7). Collectively, the findings of the aforementioned studies support the concept that exercise capacity should be given as much attention by clinicians as other major risk factors.

Physical Activity and Mortality in Women

Most of the information on the association between physical activity, fitness, and mortality risk has been derived from studies on men. Extrapolating from the findings of the studies on men and the few studies that included women, the health benefits of exercise are likely to be similar for women. These assumptions were substantiated by a number of relatively large studies published since the late 1990s.

In a study of 10,224 men and 3,120 women, Blair et al.[15] reported similarly lower all-cause and cardiovascular disease mortality rates with increased fitness in men and women. These findings were strengthened by their more recent study that included a substantially larger cohort of women ($n = 7,080$).[17] In addition to the inverse and graded association between physical fitness and mortality, these data revealed differences between men and women, suggesting that the influence of physical activity or fitness on mortality rates may be different in women and men.

First, physical fitness seems to offer a greater degree of protection in women with high blood pressure than men. The reduced risk of mortality in hypertensive but high-fit women was 81% lower when compared to low-fit women. In men, the risk reduction for the comparable groups was only 32%. For the same group comparisons, the risk reduction for elevated blood cholesterol was 50% in men and 23% in women.

Second, the protection against the cumulative detrimental effect of multiple risk factors appears greater for women than men. For example, the death rates in high-fit individuals with two or three risk factors (smoking, high blood cholesterol, or elevated systolic blood pressure) were 15% men and 50% in women when compared to low-fit individuals with no risk factors.

In one of the earlier and largest studies on postmenopausal women (The Iowa Women's Health Study), 40,417 women responded to a survey that included questions related to health habits such as smoking, diet, alcohol consumption, anthropometry, medical history, and leisure time physical activity.[29] Women were classified in three categories (low, moderate and high-fit) based on the frequency and intensity of activity. Physical activities were classified as moderate (those requiring ≤ 6 METs) or vigorous (> 6 METs). Women who participated in moderate activities more than four times per week and those who participated in vigorous activities two or more times per week comprised the high-fit category ($n = 9,919$). Those who reported vigorous activity once a week or moderate activity one to four times a week comprised the moderate-fit category ($n = 10,987$). The remaining women comprised low-fit category ($n = 19,940$). The follow-up period was approximately 7 years.

After adjusting for confounding factors, the investigators reported that high levels of physical activity were associated with decreased risk of mortality.[29] The adjusted risk of mortality was 34% and 48% lower in the moderate- and high-fit women, respectively. Because women who are ill tend to be less active and are likely to die at a higher rate, the mortality rate in the low-fit category may be inflated. To control for this factor, the investigators excluded from the analysis all women who died of cancer or heart disease within the first 3 years of follow-up. When the analysis was repeated, the results did not change substantially.

Another important finding of this study is that the risk appears to be significantly reduced even in those who participated in moderate physical activity once per week to a few per month. This is similar to the findings reported in the Finnish Twin Study.[14] It also supports previous findings of a threshold requirement of about 6 METs for a significant reduction in mortality risk.[18] However, it is in contrast to other studies that reported more vigorous and greater volume of physical activity required for significant risk reduction.[7]

Two reports from the Nurses' Health Study[30,31] provided valuable information on the association between intensity, duration, frequency, and volume of physical activity necessary to reduce the risk of cardiovascular events in women.

The Nurses' Health Study, initiated in 1976, was designed to examine the association between total physical activity (walking and vigorous exercise) and the incidence of cardiovascular events in women. The first study[31] assessed the association between physical activity and the risk of coronary heart disease. The cohort consisted of 72,488 middle-aged women nurses, 40 to 65 years of age, free of cancer and cardiovascular disease at the time of entry into the study who completed a detailed questionnaire about their physical activity habits. Each physical activity (walking, biking, jogging, aerobics, etc.) was expressed in METs and then the total activity level was expressed as MET-hours per week. Five physical activity categories were established as presented in **Table 9.3**. The follow-up period was 8 years.

The large size of the cohort and the long-term follow-up allowed the investigators to address several important questions including the exercise intensity, duration, and volume on the risk for coronary events. By excluding the women who died within the first 2 years of follow-up, the possible overestimation of the mortality rate within the low-fit categories as a result of illness and not low fitness was minimized.

Table 9.3 Relative Risk of Coronary Events According to Weekly Physical Activity (MET-hr/week)

Fitness Category	1	2	3	4	5	*P* value for Trend
(MET-hr/wk)	0–2.0	2.1–4.6	4.7–10.4	10.5–21.7	> 23.7	
Age-adjusted relative risk	1.0	0.77 (0.62–0.96)	0.65 (0.51–0.95)	0.54 (0.50–0.93)	0.46 (0.33–0.67)	< 0.001
Multivariate	1.0	0.83 (0.71–0.95)	0.72 (0.62–0.84)	0.63 (0.54–0.74)	0.55 (0.47–0.65)	< 0.001
Multivariate Excluding first 2 years	1.0	0.89 (0.75–1.04)	0.81 (0.68–0.97)	0.78 (0.66–0.93)	0.72 (0.59–0.87)	< 0.001

Source: Adapted from Manson JE, et al. *N Engl J Med* 1999;341:650–658.
Numbers in parentheses indicate the confidence interval.

A graded reduction in the relative risk of coronary events with increase in the MET-hours per week was noted (see Table 9.3). The association between physical activity and mortality risk was somewhat weaker (mortality risk reduction was attenuated), but still significant, when women who died within the first 2 years of follow-up were excluded (see Table 9.3).

The investigators then sought to assess the attenuating potential effects established risk factors may have on the association between physical activity and coronary events. Thus, the cohort was stratified based on smoking habits, obesity (BMI), and parental history of premature myocardial infarction. For each respective subgroup, physical activity was inversely related to the risk of coronary events in all strata with no substantial differences in the impact of physical activity in the lowering risk (**Figure 9.8**). These findings support that physical activity has a similar attenuating effect on the risk for coronary events even when amplified by the presence of cardiovascular risk factors.

◼ Walking and Coronary Risk Reduction

Approximately 60% of the women in the cohort engaged in at least 1 hour of walking per week and only 26% engaged in vigorous activities requiring ≥ 6 METs and defined vigorous exercise. Thus, the investigators assessed the association between walking and risk of coronary events by excluding the women who reported engaging in vigorous activity. An inverse association was again noted between walking hours per week and the risk for coronary. Women who walked between 1 to 2.9 hours per week at a brisk pace (≤ 20 minutes/mile), the equivalent of 3.9 to 9.9 MET-hours per week had a 30% lower relative risk of coronary events when

compared to the sedentary group (no walk). The risk for the women who walked for 3 or more hours per week (≥ 10 MET hr/wk) was 35% lower.

The investigators then sought to determine if walking pace or exercise intensity was an important determinant of risk of coronary events. In a multiple analyses, walking pace emerged as an independent predictor of risk. The multivariate relative risk for women who walked at an average pace of 2.0 to 2.9 miles per hour (20–30 minutes/mile), was 25% lower risk when compared to women who walked at an easy pace (< 2.0 miles/hour). The risk of those who walked briskly or very briskly was 36% (**Figure 9.9**).

A significant reduction in risk (30%–35%) was also observed when walking more than 60 minutes per week (**Figure 9.10**).

When the investigators examined the combined effect of walking and more vigorous exercise to the coronary event risk reduction, they observed that women who engaged in both walking and vigorous exercise had a greater risk reduction than those participating in either type of activity alone. When the effects of walking and vigorous exercise were examined separately, both were effective in lowering risk. A 14% reduction in risk was noted for every 5 MET-hours per week spent on walking (the equivalent of 1.5 hours of brisk walk per week). For every 5 MET-hours per week spent in vigorous exercise (the equivalent of 45 minutes per week of vigorous activities), the risk was lowered by 6%. This suggests that the exercise duration is more effective in lowering the risk for coronary events than exercise intensity.

In the second report of the Women's Health Study, the investigators assessed the association between physical activity and the risk for cardiovascular disease.[30] The cohort consisted of mostly the same cohort as in the previous

Figure 9.8   Multivariate relative risk of coronary events (nonfatal myocardial infarction or death from coronary causes) according to quintile group for total physical activity within subgroups defined according to smoking status (A), body-mass index (B), and presence or absence of a parental history of premature myocardial infarction (C). For each risk factor, the reference group is the category at highest risk. Relative risks have been adjusted for the variables in the full multivariate model.

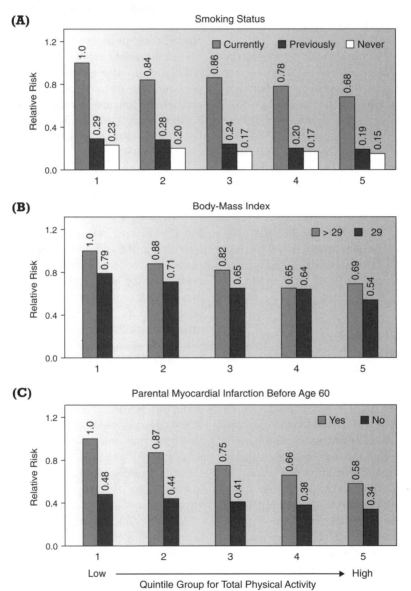

Source: From Manson JE, et al. *N Engl J Med* 1999;341:650–658.

Figure 9.9 Relative risk for coronary events in women ($n = 72,488$) and walking pace.

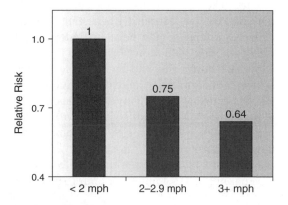

Source: Adapted from Manson JE, et al. *N Engl J Med* 1999;341:650–658.

Figure 9.10 Relative risk for coronary events in women ($n = 72,488$) and minutes of walking at a pace of 3 or more miles per hour.

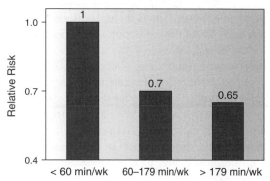

Source: Modified from Manson JE, et al. *N Engl J Med* 1999;341:650–658.

study, but slightly larger ($n = 73,743$) and older (50–79 years of age) and all postmenopausal women.

During the 3.2 years of follow-up, a strong inverse association was noted between the total exercise (MET-hours per week) and the age-adjusted risk of coronary heart disease. Similarly, the age-adjusted risk for cardiovascular disease declined as MET-hours per week increased (**Table 9.4**).

Table 9.4 Relative Risk for Cardiovascular Disease According to Fitness Categories

Fitness Category	1	2	3	4	5	*P* value for Trend
(MET-hr/wk)	0–2.4	2.5–7.2	7.3–13.4	13.5–23.3	≥ 23.4	
CHD Age-Adjusted Relative Risk	1.0	0.73 (0.53–0.99)	0.69 (0.51–0.95)	0.68 (0.50–0.93)	0.47 (0.33–0.67)	< 0.001
CVD Age-Adjusted Relative Risk	1.0	0.83 (0.71–0.95)	0.72 (0.62–0.84)	0.63 (0.54–0.74)	0.55 (0.47–0.65)	< 0.001
Multivariate Relative Risk	1.0	0.89 (0.75–1.04)	0.81 (0.68–0.97)	0.78 (0.66–0.93)	0.72 (0.59–0.87)	< 0.001

Source: Adapted from Manson JE, et al. *N Engl J Med* 2002;347:716–725. Numbers in parentheses indicate confidence intervals.

■ **Walking Versus Vigorous Activity and Cardiovascular Risk**

In the second report of the Women's Health Study,[30] investigators also assessed the independent effects of intensity and volume of physical activity on the reduction of cardiovascular mortality risk. Similar to the previous study, an inverse association was observed between the coronary heart disease and cardiovascular disease mortality with the increase in the MET-hours per week accumulated during brisk walk. More specifically, when compared to the sedentary women, the reduction in risk ranged from approximately 30% to 40% when engaging in either walking or more vigorous exercise for at least 2.5 hours per week (**Table 9.5**).

The reduction in cardiovascular risk was greater (63%) for women engaging in both walking and vigorous exercise, suggesting that the exercise intensity may have an independent effect on risk reduction (**Figure 9.11**). This is supported further by the inverse relationship between walking pace and risk reduction. It also appears that an intensity threshold emerges at the approximate walking pace of 2 to 3 miles per hour. When compared to the women who never or rarely walked, those who walked at the pace of 2 to 3 miles per hour (20 to 30 minutes per mile); 3 to 4 miles per hour (equivalent

Table 9.5 Relative Risk for Cardiovascular Disease According to Energy Expenditure by Walking and Vigorous Exercise

Walking	1	2	3	4	5	P value for Trend
(MET-hr/wk)	0	0.1–2.5	2.6–5.0	5.1–10.0	> 10.0	
CHD Age-Adjusted Relative Risk	1.0	0.71 (0.53–0.96)	0.60 (0.44–0.83)	0.54 (0.39–0.76)	0.61 (0.44–0.84)	< 0.004
CVD Age-Adjusted Relative Risk	1.0	0.88 (0.77–1.01)	0.70 (0.60–0.81)	0.66 (0.57–0.77)	0.58 (0.49–0.68)	< 0.001
Multivariate Relative Risk	1.0	0.91 (0.78–1.07)	0.82 (0.69–0.97)	0.75 (0.63–0.89)	0.68 (0.56–0.82)	< 0.001
Vigorous Exercise						**P value**
Minutes/week	0	1–60	61–100	101–150	> 150	
CHD Age-Adjusted Relative Risk	1.0	1.12 (0.79–1.6)	0.56 (0.32–0.98)	0.73 (0.43–1.25)	0.58 (0.34–0.99)	0.008
CVD Age-Adjusted Relative Risk	1.0	0.87 (0.72–1.04)	0.73 (0.58–0.92)	0.69 (0.53–0.89)	0.60 (0.47–0.76)	< 0.001
Multivariate Relative Risk	1.0	0.91 (0.73–1.12)	0.81 (0.63–1.06)	0.85 (0.64–1.13)	0.76 (0.58–1.0)	0.01

Source: Adapted from Manson JE, et al. *N Engl J Med* 2002;347:716–725. Numbers in parentheses indicate confidence intervals.

Figure 9.11 Relative risk of CVD according to walking and vigorous activity.

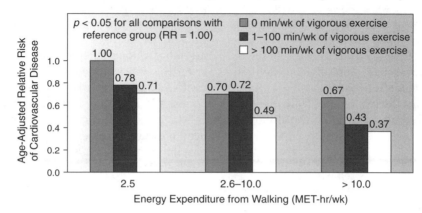

Source: Data from Manson JE, et al. *N Engl J Med* 1999;341:650–658.

to a brisk walk), and more than 4 miles per hour (very brisk walk) had a 14%, 24%, and 42% relative reduction risk of cardiovascular disease (**Figure 9.12**).

Once again, the large size of the cohort allowed the investigators to address several important questions, including the exercise intensity, duration, and volume on the risk for cardiovascular events. In addition, the cohort included a sizable number of African-American women ($n = 5,661$) allowing the opportunity for much needed information in this subgroup.

For the entire cohort, the graded reduction in the relative risk for coronary heart disease and cardiovascular events with an increase in the MET-hours per week was evident for total physical activity or walking alone (see Table 9.5). The risk reduction was similar for Caucasian

Figure 9.12 Relative risk of CVD according to walking pace.

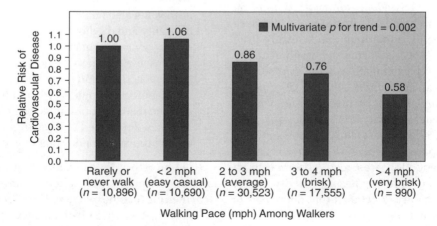

Source: Adapted from Manson JE, et al. *N Engl J Med* 1999;341:650–658.

and African-American women and for different age brackets for total physical activity (**Figure 9.13**) or walking alone (**Figure 9.14**). Similarly, when the cohort was categorized by body mass index (BMI), fitness was also inversely related to the cardiovascular mortality for each subgroup (see Figures 9.13 and 9.14).

In summary, the two reports from the Women's Health Study provided the following information:

1. Both walking and more vigorous forms of exercise are associated with an inverse and graded reduction in the risk for coronary heart disease and cardiovascular disease.
2. The association is evident in lean and obese Caucasian and African-American women of different ages.
3. The exercise duration for a substantial risk reduction in cardiovascular disease and coronary heart disease appears to be approximately 1.5 to 2.5 hours per week.
4. The exercise intensity for similar risk reduction appears to be at the walking pace of approximately 20–30 minutes per mile.

Two other studies examined changes in physical activity status and the mortality risk in women.[32,33] The cohort of the first study consisted of 1,405 Swedish women aged 38 to 60 years who were initially free of major diseases at baseline. Occupational and leisure-time physical activity data from the baseline and 6-year follow-up examinations were evaluated in relation to all-cause mortality.

Moderate levels of leisure time and occupational physical activity were associated with 44% and 72% lower mortality risk respectively, when compared to sedentary women. An insignificant reduction was also observed with higher occupational or leisure activity levels. The investigators concluded that decreases in physical activity as well as low initial levels are strong risk factors for mortality in women. The

effects and predictive value of physical activity persist for several years.[33]

A more recent study[32] examined the relationship of changes in physical activity and mortality among older women. This is a prospective study conducted at four U.S. research centers (Baltimore, MD; Portland, OR; Minneapolis, MN; and Monongahela Valley, PA). The cohort consisted of 7,553 Caucasian women aged 65 years or older who were assessed at baseline (1986–1988) and at a follow-up visit (1992–1994) and followed for about 6 years.

The all-familiar inverse and graded association between increased physical activity and mortality (all-cause and cardiovascular) also was evident in this study. The adjusted all-cause and cardiovascular mortality rate for physically active women who expanded approximately 1,000 to 1,900 kcal per week was approximately 40% lower when compared to the sedentary women. In addition, the following findings are noteworthy:[32]

- Sedentary women who became physically active between baseline and follow-up had a 48% and 36% lower all-cause and cardiovascular mortality rate, respectively, when compared to sedentary women who were sedentary at both visits.
- Women who were physically active at both visits also had 32% lower all-cause mortality and cardiovascular mortality than sedentary women.
- The associations between changes in physical activity and reduced mortality were similar in women with and without chronic diseases but tended to be weaker among women aged at least 75 years and among those with poor health status.

The investigators concluded that increasing and maintaining physical activity levels could lengthen life for older women. The effects appear to be less powerful in women aged at least 75 years and those with poor health status.

Figure 9.13 Relative risk for CVD in women according to total physical activity, by race, age, and BMI.

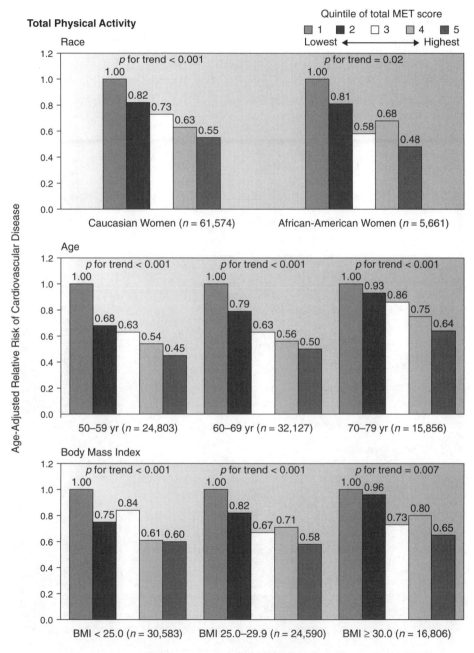

Source: Adapted from Manson JE, et al. *N Engl J Med* 2002;347:716–725.

Figure 9.14 Age-adjusted relative risk for CVD in women according to energy expenditure from walking.

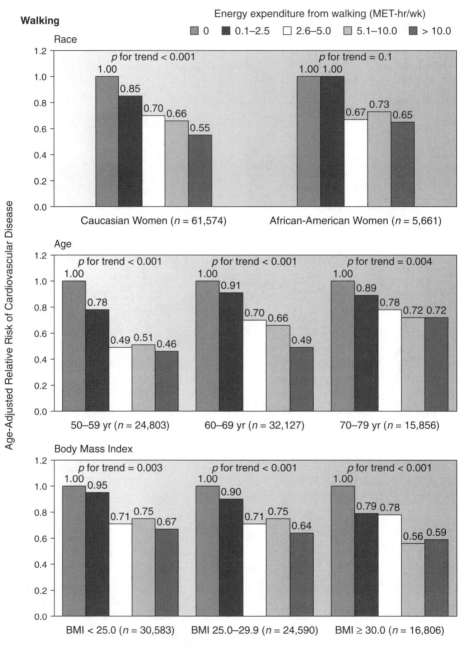

Source: Adapted from Manson JE, et al. *N Engl J Med* 2002;347:716–725.

Two studies in women expressed the mortality risk reduction per 1-MET increase in exercise capacity.[24,28] In both studies, exercise capacity was assessed by exercise stress test. In the study by Gulati et al.[28], the larger of the two, the adjusted mortality risk was 17% lower for each 1-MET increase in exercise capacity. This was a relatively greater reduction than has been reported in men, prompting investigators to speculate that exercise capacity may have an even greater capacity in predicting risk of mortality among women than men.

Similar findings were reported by the Lipid Research Clinic's prevalence study, where nearly 3,000 asymptomatic women were followed for up to 20 years.[24] The age-adjusted risk for cardiovascular death for every 1-MET decrement in exercise capacity was 20% higher.

Studies examining the association between physical activity and mortality in women have yielded similar exercise-related health benefits with those observed in men. There is also some evidence to support a greater dose-response association between exercise and mortality risk reduction for women compared to men. In addition, the recently large studies in women have helped to better define associations between mortality risk and exercise intensity, duration, and frequency.

Physical Activity and Stroke

According to the 1996 *U.S. Surgeon General's Report on Physical Activity and Health*, the relationship between exercise and stroke is inconclusive.[34] Since that report, several large studies have been conducted. Their findings strengthen the suggestion of previous studies that physical activity may protect people against strokes.[35]

The findings from the Physicians' Health Study showed a 14% lower the total risk of stroke among men participating in vigorous exercise five or more times a week.[36] Similarly, in the Harvard Alumni Study total stroke risk in men who were highly physically active was 18% lower when compared to sedentary group.[37] The Northern Manhattan Study (NOMAS) that included Caucasian, African American, and Hispanics, both men and women showed a decrease in ischemic stroke risk associated with physical activity levels across all racial/ethnic and age groups and for each gender.[38] Similarly, in the Atherosclerosis Risk in Communities (ARIC) cohort, physical activity was related to lower risk of ischemic stroke.[39]

In a Japanese cohort of 73,265 men and women, the risk of stroke death in the highest category of walking and sports participation was reduced by 29% and 20%, respectively.[40] Moderate and high levels of leisure-time activity were associated with significant trends toward lower risk of stroke in a study of 4,721 men and women in Finland. A smaller but still significant benefit also was observed with occupational activity.[41]

In the Nurses' Health Study, the risk of total stroke was graded inversely with the level of fitness.[42] The risk was 18%, 26%, and 34% lower for the three highest physical activity categories respectively (**Figure 9.15**). Walking pace and METs were also associated with lower risk in a dose-response manner, independent of the number of hours spent walking (**Figure 9.16**). This finding supports that exercise intensity has an independent effect on risk reduction. Another important finding of the study is that sedentary women who became active in middle to late adulthood had approximately 20% reduction in risk adjusted risk for stroke. This finding suggests that the health benefits of increased physical activity are not attenuated by age. More importantly, the health benefits can be realized even if the individual has been sedentary for some time. However, it is strongly recommended that individuals who have been sedentary for a

Figure 9.15   Relative risk of stroke in women according to total physical activity reported in MET-hours/week.

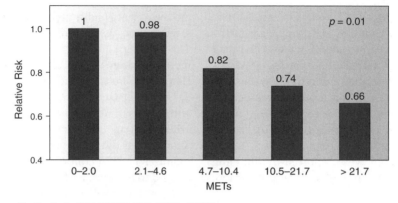

Source: Data from Hu F, et al. *JAMA* 2000;283:2961–2967.

long time consult with a physician prior to embarking on an exercise program.

The association between physical activity and stroke mortality in middle-aged men from the Seven Countries Study (the Corfu cohort), was assessed after taking into account the presence of left ventricular hypertrophy (LVH).[43] The investigators reported that the adoption of even a moderate physically active lifestyle was associated with a significant reduction in the risk of stroke among men with and without LVH. The impact of physical activity on stroke mortality can be appreciated further by the finding that the risk of stroke in physically active men with LVH was 49% lower than the risk observed in sedentary men without LVH. This finding is of particular interest, because LVH is now considered an independent predictor of coronary heart disease and stroke.[44–46]

Finally, the findings of a meta-analysis of 31 observational studies conducted mainly in the United States and Europe support that moderate and high levels of leisure-time and occupational physical activity protected against total stroke, hemorrhagic stroke, and ischemic stroke.[47]

Figure 9.16   Relative risk of stroke in women according to walking pace

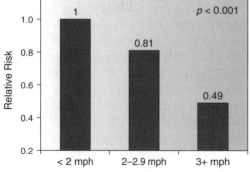

Source: Data from Hu F, et al. *JAMA* 2000;283:2961–2967.

Studies investigating the association between physical activity and stroke are relatively few and their findings are not as compelling as those regarding physical activity and heart diseases. However, most studies support that moderate and high levels of leisure-time and occupational physical activity protected against total stroke. Furthermore, the evidence is likely to strengthen as more studies become available.

Chronic Heart Failure and Exercise Training

Prior to the 1980s, exercise or physical activity was not recommended for individuals with heart failure. The prevailing thinking was that physical exertion would cause further deterioration of the already compromised cardiac function. This notion was challenged by some in the early 1980s. Since then, a systematic scrutiny on the safety and efficacy of exercise as a therapeutic modality for CHF patients was pursued.

The findings of early studies were encouraging. Despite the relatively intense exercise programs (80%–90% of peak oxygen consumption for 50–60 minutes per session), the relatively small number of patients, and lack of a control group in some, significant improvements in exercise capacity and no major complications in patients with moderate or severe left ventricular dysfunction were reported.[48–51]

These findings provided the incentive for several carefully designed, randomized studies, using more moderate exercise intensities. Overwhelmingly, theses studies supported previous findings. Significant improvements in exercise capacity and peak oxygen consumption were shown after just 8 weeks of stationary bicycle exercise.[52,53] A similar program resulted in improvements in exercise capacity, peak oxygen consumption, left ventricular function, and quality of life.[54–56] Several studies used longer training periods at similar intensities. These studies also yielded significant improvements both in exercise capacity and peak oxygen consumption.[57–61] Finally, the safety and efficacy of exercise training for the heart failure patient was confirmed by a relatively large, randomized trial (Chronic Heart Failure and Graded Exercise Study)[62] and a more recent meta analysis comprised of 13 studies that included aerobic and weight training of 2,387 heart failure patients.[63]

> Exercise training studies overwhelmingly support that individuals with heart failure can exercise safely when exercise is carefully tailored to their needs and capacity.

However, exercise implementation in individuals with heart failure was not fully endorsed, especially in patients with heart failure that resulted from a major heart attack. Clinical and experimental evidence suggests that progressive left ventricular dilation occurs in the pathogenesis of CHF, particularly after myocardial infarction.[64] This stretching, thinning, and expanding of the affected myocardium are influenced by several factors including ventricular wall stress.[65–68] Because ventricular wall stress increases during physical exercise, the thinking was that this increased stress may facilitate the remodeling process, exacerbate symptoms, and lead to progressive deterioration of cardiac function. Indeed, the findings of two studies supported that such a remodeling process of the myocardium occurs as a result of exercise.[69,70] However, the exercise programs implemented in these studies were too demanding even for healthy individuals. The programs consisted of morning and evening exercise, five times per week for 4 weeks.

Subsequent well-designed studies that were relatively large and had long training periods revealed that the ejection fraction must be considered when exercise programs are designed for heart failure individuals.[71,72] In a study of 93 individuals who suffered a heart attack, the investigators found no deterioration of ventricular function or changes in ventricular cavity dimensions and significant improvement in ejection fraction after 6 months of exercise training in patients with normal ventricular function and ejection fraction > 40%. Conversely, individuals with initial ejection fraction

< 40% and ventricular dilation had more significant ventricular enlargement, with increased infarct size, and more pronounced distortion in the shape of the ventricle. However, this was evident in both the exercise and no exercise groups. In fact, the exercise group tended to have less ventricular dilation and a substantial increase in ejection fraction from 35% to 39%. Although these findings were not statistically significant, they suggest that exercise training is not responsible for the increased deterioration in myocardial function observed in HF patients with relatively low EF. In fact, exercise may lessen the deterioration of left ventricular function over time.[72] Similar benefits were reported in patients with reduced ventricular function (EF of 26% to 38%) who exercised daily for 2 months at moderate intensities. The program resulted in a 26% increase in exercise capacity and no deleterious effects on left ventricular volume, function, or myocardial wall thinning regardless of the size of the infarct area.[71]

Despite the efficacy and safety of moderate to high exercise intensities, the use of lower exercise intensities may be preferred for several reasons: (1) Low and moderate intensity exercise carry a relatively low risk for cardiac complications and musculoskeletal injuries; (2) patients are more likely to participate and sustain a lower than higher intensity exercise; and (3) physicians may feel more comfortable advising patients to pursue a low-intensity versus a high-intensity exercise program.

The efficacy of low-intensity exercise training for the CHF patient has been demonstrated by several studies. These studies found that improvements in peak oxygen uptake and peak workload were comparable to those reported with much higher exercise intensities. Additionally, the relatively lower left ventricular wall stress during low exercise intensities decreases the risk for left ventricular enlargement that may occur in heart failure individuals.[73,74]

Relatively small exercise training studies provide strong evidence that exercise capacity and cardiac function improve with carefully conducted exercise programs. The limited evidence suggesting that exercise training also can reduce the risk of mortality in individuals with heart failure is encouraging but this theory awaits the confirmation of large clinical trials.

■ MECHANISMS FOR IMPROVEMENT BY EXERCISE TRAINING

The mechanisms for such improvements are not fully understood. The reduction in cardiac output was originally thought to be the determining factor in the exercise capacity of the CHF patient. However, indices of resting cardiac function such as left ventricular ejection fraction and hemodynamic measurements are poorly correlated with peak exercise performance or maximal oxygen consumption.[75,76] Attention shifted to changes in skeletal muscle and vascular pathophysiology to explain the impaired exercise tolerance in such patients. Skeletal muscle atrophy is a common phenomenon in CHF patients occurring early in the course of the disease.[77,78] Improvements in exercise capacity following muscle strength gains[78–80] and positive correlations between muscle mass and peak oxygen uptake in CHF patients[78] support that muscle atrophy may be involve at least in part in the poor exercise capacity of heart failure patients.

In a recent study, Hambrecht et al.[81] noted significant improvements in endothelial-mediated vasodilation of the peripheral vasculature, peripheral blood flow, and peak $\dot{V}O_2$ following 24 weeks of moderate-intensity aerobic exercise training. These favorable findings are attributed to the increased formation and release of endothelial relaxing factors in response to increased shear stress induced by pulsatile blood flow. Similarly, endothelial function was improved after 4 weeks of handgrip exercise. Collectively, these findings suggest that long-term physical training restores impaired endothelial function,[81,82] reverses the neurohormonal activation, and ameliorate the

autonomic derangement observed in CHF patients.[51,53] It is now generally accepted that physical work capacity in these patients is determined by the interaction of cardiovascular and musculoskeletal and hormonal factors (**Figure 9.17**).

Exercise Training and Mortality in Heart Failure

Encouraging findings on the rate of CHF progression, morbidity, and mortality have been

Figure 9.17 Schematic representation of muscular, cardiorespiratory, and neurohormonal changes in heart failure. Patients with heart failure are likely to adopt a sedentary lifestyle. Consequently, there is a deterioration of skeletal muscle and aerobic capacity, fostering an even more sedentary lifestyle and thus further deterioration of muscular and cardiorespiratory functions.

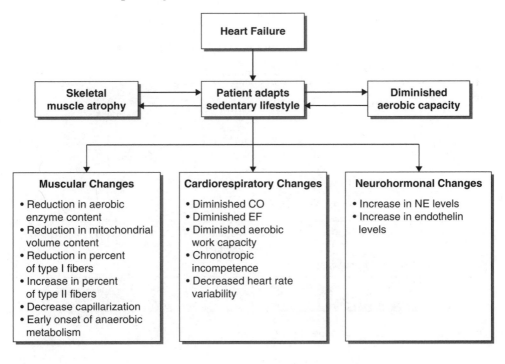

reported by a small randomized and well-controlled trial.[83] Belardinelli et al. randomized 99 middle-aged patients with stable CHF (88 males and 11 women) with EF ≤ 40% into exercise and no exercise groups. After 14 months of aerobic training, the exercise group had lower total and cardiac mortality and hospital readmission for heart failure (**Figure 9.18**). In addition, the quality of life improved in the exercise group. The findings of a meta-analysis of nine randomized trials totaling 801 patients also support a significant reduction in mortality and hospital admissions are significantly reduced after exercise training in HF patients.[84]

Until recently, the impact of exercise training on clinical outcomes in patients with heart failure had not been studied extensively. The findings of a large trial ($n = 2,331$) on exercise and heart failure (HF-ACTION trial) that were recently published support that exercise reduced all-cause mortality and hospitalization by 11% in patients assigned to the exercise group compared to those in the non-exercise group.[85] Although this can be viewed as a modest reduction, several factors should be considered. First, the 11% reduction was in addition to the reduction achieved by the state-of-the-art medical/device management of heart failure patients. Second, in addition to heart failure, a substantial number of the participants in this study had several comorbidities that made their capacity and ability to exercise on a regular basis very difficult. Consequently, the volume of exercise for these individuals was severely compromised. When the investigators examined those who were able to exercise, the findings were more impressive. More specifically, the average reduction in all-cause mortality and hospitalization was 16% and up to 27% for cardiovascular disease mortality and heart failure hospitalization.[85]

Figure 9.18   Exercise training and mortality in heart failure patients.

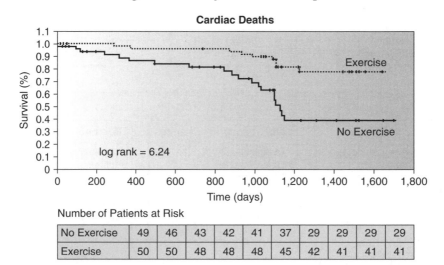

Source: From Belardinelli R, et al. *Circulation* 99:1173–1182.

Conclusions

- The current literature overwhelmingly supports that carefully designed exercise programs are well tolerated and beneficial to patients with stable heart failure.
- Exercise of low to moderate intensity should be preferred because it is equally beneficial, carries a lower risk for muscular and cardiovascular complications, and is better tolerated by the patients than high intensity exercise.
- Both the cardiovascular and muscular systems are inextricably linked in the pathophysiology of CHF. Improvements observed in exercise capacity following exercise training may be the cumulative result of hemodynamic, histological, and biochemical changes.
- Improvement in work performance following aerobic and strength training exercises are similarly impressive. This suggests that decreased blood flow may be the precursor of all the pernicious manifestations of CHF. Future work in this area should consider exercise programs that enhance both aerobic and anaerobic pathways. The benefits of such exercise programs may be additive and therefore more beneficial to the CHF patient than either exercise mode alone.
- Endothelial dysfunction has been implicated in CHF at least in part due to diminished blood flow. Recent trials support that regular physical activity improves endothelial function and work capacity in CHF patients.
- Carefully designed exercise training programs may be the intervention required to reverse the deleterious effects of endothelial dysfunction. The recently

published findings of a large trial (HF-ACTION) support that adequate exercise training increases survival in patients with heart failure.

Low Extremity Arterial Disease and Exercise

As discussed in Chapter 8, the progressive development of atherosclerotic lesions ultimately in the arteries of the lower extremities leads to significant stenosis of the arteries involved. Consequently, blood flow distal to lesions is significantly impaired leading to leg pain, numbness, cold legs or feet, and muscle pain in the thighs, calves, or feet. This is known as *low extremity arterial disease (LEAD)*.

Individuals with this condition lead a sedentary lifestyle. Consequently, the deterioration of cardiorespiratory and muscular functions is accelerated and a decline in the overall health and quality of life for the LEAD patient ensues. In addition, LEAD patients often suffer from comorbidities, including hypertension, diabetes mellitus, dyslipidemia, and coronary artery disease. National health organizations including the American Heart Association, the American College of Sports Medicine, and the Centers for Disease Control and Prevention strongly recommend that increased physical activity alone or as an adjunct to pharmacologic therapy should be implemented for the prevention and management of cardiovascular disease and the aforementioned comorbidities and risk factors.[86,87]

Treatment for intermittent claudication (pain or cramping in legs when walking or exercising) thus should include lifestyle changes for positive modification of the traditional cardiovascular disease risk factors. Exercise training should be an integral part of

Table 9.6 Summary of Select Studies Reporting Improvements in Peak $\dot{V}O_2$ and/or Work Capacity in CHF Patients Following Exercise Training

Reference	N	NYHA Class	Improvements
Esani et al.[49]	15	I	Peak $\dot{V}O_2$; work capacity
Sullivan et al.[51]	12	II, III	Peak $\dot{V}O_2$; work capacity
Lee et al.[50]	18	I–IV	Peak $\dot{V}O_2$; work capacity
Coats et al.[52]	11	II, III	Peak $\dot{V}O_2$; work capacity
Coats et al.[53]	17	II, III	Reduction in NE spillover; sympathetic tone withdrawal and increased vagal tone
Belardinelli et al.[54]	55	II, III	Peak $\dot{V}O_2$; work capacity
Belardinelli et al.[55]	46	II, III	Peak $\dot{V}O_2$; work capacity; LV function; quality of life
Belardinelli et al.[56]	43	II, III	Peak $\dot{V}O_2$; work capacity; LV function
Hambrecht et al.[58]	22	II, III	Improvements in aerobic enzyme and mitochondria content; peak $\dot{V}O_2$; work capacity
Wielenga et al.[62]	81	II–III	Exercise time; anaerobic threshold; quality of life
Demopoulos et al.[74]	16	II–IV	Aerobic work; peak $\dot{V}O_2$
Belardinelli et al.[73]	27	II, III	Improvements in aerobic enzymes and mitochondria content
Kiilavuori et al.[61]	20	II–III	Aerobic work capacity; heart rate variability
Koch et al.[79]	25	N/A	Muscle strength; work capacity; quality of life
Minnotti et al.[80]	5	II–III	Forearm muscle strength and endurance
Mancini et al.[78]	8	I–IV	Respiratory muscle endurance and strength
Hambrecht et al.[81]	20	II–III	Endothelial function; peripheral blood flow; work capacity; peak $\dot{V}O_2$
Hornig et al.[82]	19	III	Endothelial function; peripheral blood flow; work capacity; peak $\dot{V}O_2$
Belardinelli et al[83]	99	II–IV	Improved survival, peak $\dot{V}O_2$ and quality of life
Jugdutt et al.[70]	13	15 wks post-MI; not randomized	Deterioration in global and regional ventricular function
Jette et al.[69]	39	10 wks post-MI; EF < 30%	Aerobic work capacity; peak $\dot{V}O_2$; EF improved in some but not all patients and worsened in one
Giannuzi et al.[72]	95	I, II	Aerobic work capacity; peak $\dot{V}O_2$ improved in patients with EF > 40%; no changes in ventricular cavity dimensions; exercise patients with EF < 40% had less deterioration than controls
Dubach et al.[71]	25	N/A	Aerobic work capacity and peak $\dot{V}O_2$ improved; no deterioration in ventricular performance

Source: Data are from Kokkinos, et al. *American Heart Journal* 2000;140:21–28.

such therapeutic approach. An exercise training program of low to moderate intensity can attenuate the deleterious effects of the aforementioned comorbidities associated with LEAD. It is an attractive and conservative alternative therapy for these patients. For example, walking, the preferred form of exercise for LEAD patients, has a relatively low risk–benefit ratio; it is also relevant to daily living, inexpensive, easily implemented to large populations, contributes to the overall health, can be used alone or as an adjunct to pharmacotherapy, and does not interfere with the surgical possibility that may be deemed necessary in the future. In addition, the well-recognized local vasodilatory effects of exercise and the preservation of lean body tissue can only be of benefit to these patients.

■ Exercise Therapy Findings

The well-known local vasodilation and the consequent increase in blood flow that occurs in the exercising muscle encouraged investigators to assess the possible therapeutic effects of structured exercise programs for LEAD patients. Scientific assessment in patients with mild and moderate claudication began in the 1960s.

Primarily, two exercise training protocols have been used extensively. One requires the patient to walk to the onset of pain (claudication), rest until the pain subsides, and repeat this intermittent walking several times. The other protocol is similar with the exception that the patients walk until near-maximal or maximal claudication is reached.

Without exception, exercise training studies involving LEAD patients yielded substantial and clinically significant improvements in walking distance to the onset of pain or maximal pain.[88–102] A meta-analysis of 21 studies revealed that following exercise rehabilitation, the average walking distance to onset of clau-

dication increased by 179% and the distance to maximal claudication by 122%.[90] Significant increases in peak oxygen uptake along with improvements in maximal and pain-free walking time also have been reported.[91]

There is evidence of a synergistic effect when exercise is combined with pharmacologic therapy. After 6 months of either antiplatelet therapy, exercise therapy, or a combination of antiplatelet therapy plus exercise, walking distance improved in all groups. However, the greatest improvements were observed in the combined therapy group. Pain-free and maximal walking distances increased by 120% and 105% in the combined therapy group, 90% and 86% in the exercise alone group, and only 35% and 38% in the antiplatelet-only group.[98]

Exercise training following reconstructive arterial surgery also merits special attention. In one study, patients were randomized to reconstructive surgery, exercise alone, or reconstructive surgery plus exercise. Performance was assessed at baseline and 48 weeks following intervention. The symptom-free and maximal walking distance in the exercise alone group increased by 179% and 151%, respectively. In the surgery-only group, the increase was 376% in the symptom-free distance and 173% in the maximal walking distance. In the group with a combination of surgery with exercise, symptom-free and maximal walking distance increased by 698% and 263%, respectively.[97]

The findings of the two studies presented (arterial reconstructive surgery and the antiplatelet therapy) support that the implementation of a well-designed exercise program as an adjunct to either therapy can significantly improve the outcome for the LEAD patient. Exercise rehabilitation is now recommended and implemented as the first line of therapy for LEAD patients in stage I and II alone, or in conjunction with medical therapy and after reconstructive arterial surgery in patients with significant hemodynamic improvements.

Without exception, exercise training studies involving LEAD patients have yielded substantial and clinically significant improvements in walking distance to the onset of pain or maximal pain. There is also string evidence of a synergistic effect when exercise is combined with pharmacologic therapy and/or after reconstructive arterial surgery.

■ Exercise Mode

The mode of exercise for most studies is walking combined with some other forms of leg exercise such as running, cycling, stair climbing, dancing, jumping, and other dynamic and static leg exercises.[90] Two studies used walking alone and two other studies combined and compared walking with resistance (strength) training.[92,100] Walking appears to be superior to other forms of exercise training, especially when the exercise protocol requires that patients perform intermittent bouts of walking to near-maximal or maximal pain.[89] Although both studies reported that resistance training was inferior to walking and no additional benefits to the patient were noted when the walking program was supplemented with resistance training, in some cases, muscle weakness can compromise walking performance. Thus, the possible therapeutic effects of an exercise program that combines aerobic and resistance exercise for the LEAD patient should not be dismissed.

■ Intensity

The intensity of the exercise programs is not well described in any of the studies. It is estimated that only 16% of patients who do not experience pain at rest can walk a distance of 1,000 meters or more on a flat surface at 4 km/hr or 2.5 miles/hr.[103] Collectively, this information from available studies supports an exercise intensity of approximately 2 to 4 mph walking speed on a flat surface.[104]

■ Frequency, Duration, and Length of Training

Most evidence supports that exercising three or more sessions per week yields greater improvements in claudication distance when compared with fewer than three times per week.[90] Most studies also support that the exercise duration should be between 30 to 60 minutes per session. Improvements in the onset of claudication pain and maximal claudication pain walking distances are significant in patients exercising 30 or more minutes per session when compared to those exercising less. It thus appears that most improvements in physical performance for LEAD patients occur when exercising for at least 90 minutes per week. However, the interaction between duration and frequency cannot be discerned from the existing literature.

Noticeable improvements in walking distance can be observed even after 4 weeks of training. However, longer training periods are clearly more successful. Greater improvements in walking distances were associated stronger with the length of training lasting 6 months or longer.[90]

■ Potential Mechanisms

The mechanisms responsible for the exercise-induced improvements in walking distance remain illusive. The compromised blood flow to the lower extremities in LEAD patients and the well-known vasodilation and consequent increase in blood flow in the exercising muscle deserve special attention. However, the decline in physical performance observed in LEAD patients is likely the collective outcome of deterioration on several physiologic systems. Likewise, the exercise-induced improvements in the functional capacity of these patients are the result of favorable changes in several of these systems.

Potential Mechanisms for the Physical Activity–Related Reduction in Cardiovascular Risk

The mechanisms for the inverse association between physical activity and the risk of cardiovascular disease and cardiovascular mortality are not completely understood. It has been long suspected and is likely that the favorable modification physical activity or exercise exerts on several established cardiovascular risk factors translates to the cardioprotection observed. Evidence for this is provided by a recent prospective study that included 27,055 apparently healthy women.[105] The investigators assessed several metabolic and hemodynamic parameters and inflammatory biomarkers. They also recorded the presence of hypertension and diabetes, and the self-reported physical activity levels of these women. After a mean follow-up period of almost 11 years, the investigators noted a linear decrease in risk for CVD events with higher physical activity levels. The relative risk reductions risk for women who expanded 200 to 599 kcal per week was 27% lower when compared to those expanding less that 200 kcal. The relative risk was 32% and 41% lower for those women who expanded 600 to 1,499, and 1,500 or more kcal/wk, respectively.

The same investigators then assessed the contribution of risk factors to lower risk. Differences in known risk factors explained a large proportion (59.0%) of the observed inverse association. They concluded that the inverse association between physical activity and CVD risk is mediated mostly by known risk factors, particularly inflammatory factors and blood pressure, and to a lesser by lipids, body composition (BMI), and diabetes.

Author's Note

Since the early 1950s, a plethora of scientific evidence has accumulated to support that increased physical activity and exercise lower the risk of cardiovascular disease and overall morbidity and mortality. Study findings are eloquently summarized in a 2002 editorial entitled "Survival of the Fittest."[106] In it, Dr. Gary Balady stated, "During the past 15 years, many long-term epidemiologic studies have shown an unequivocal and robust relation of fitness, physical activity, and exercise to reduced mortality overall and from cardiovascular causes and reduced cardiovascular risk."

Our next challenge is no longer to prove that physical activity or exercise protects against premature death. It isn't even to define the kind of exercise needed, how much, or of what intensity. Although research must continue to define these issues for different populations and diseases, the most compelling challenge is to promote a physically activity lifestyle for people of all ages.

■ SUMMARY

- Epidemiologic studies support a strong inverse relationship between physical exercise and coronary heart disease risk. This evidence provided the basis to seek answers as to kind of exercise, duration, intensity, and volume needed to reduce the risk of heart disease.

- Physical fitness assessed by a treadmill or bike test allows a more precise quantification of fitness and its association with mortality. The most striking findings of these studies are: (1) the inverse, graded, and independent association between the volume of physical activity and mortality risk; and (2) the relatively low intensity and volume of physical activity required to achieve substantial reduction in mortality risk.

- The exercise components of intensity and duration are also inversely associated with the risk of coronary heart disease independent of exercise volume.
- Some evidence supports that intensity may be more strongly associated with risk reduction. However, it is more likely that a threshold for exercise intensity and duration must be achieved before health benefits are realized.
- A number of observational studies support that moderate and high levels of leisure-time and occupational physical activity protected against total stroke, hemorrhagic stroke, and ischemic stroke.
- Exercise for the heart failure patients was not recommended until recently for the fear that it may worsen the condition. However, well-designed studies that tailored their exercise programs have proven that heart failure patients can tolerate exercise well.
- A number of these small studies provide strong evidence that well-designed exercise training studies yield significant and favorable changes in cardiac function and structure for the heart failure patients.
- Recent evidence from a large randomized trial supports that exercise training reduces hospitalization and mortality in these patients.
- Well-designed exercise programs can be beneficial for individuals with low extremity arterial disease.
- Walking distance can be improved substantially following such programs. Exercise can be used in adjunct to pharmacologic therapy or surgery. Such approaches provide even greater improvements in walking distance for such individuals.
- Recent evidence supports that the cardiovascular risk reduction observed with increased levels of physical activity is mediated by the favorable effects physical activity exerts on several cardiovascular risk factors. More specifically, most of the reduction is mediated by favorable changes in inflammatory factors and blood pressure and to a lesser by lipids, body composition (BMI), and diabetes.

■ REFERENCES

1. Morris JN, Heady JA, Raffle PA, et al. Coronary heart-disease and physical activity of work. *Lancet* 1953;265(6796):1111–1120.
2. Leon AS Physical activity levels and coronary heart disease. Analysis of epidemiologic and supporting studies. *Med Clin North Am* 1985;69(1):3–20.
3. Powell KE, Thompson PD, Caspersen CJ, Kendrick JS. Physical activity and the incidence of coronary heart disease. *Annu Rev Public Health* 1987;8:253–287.
4. Paffenbarger RS, Hale WE. Work activity and coronary heart mortality. *N Engl J Med* 1975;292(11):545–550.
5. Brunner D, Mandis G, Modan, M, Levin S. Physical activity at work and the incidence of myocardial infarction, angina pectoris and death due to ischemic heart disease. An epidemiological study in Israeli collective settlements (kibbutzim). *J Chronic Dis* 1974;27(4):217–233.
6. Punsar S, Karvonen MJ. Physical activity and coronary heart disease in populations from east and west Finland. *Adv Cardiol* 1976; 18(0):196–207.
7. Paffenbarger RS Jr, Wing AL, Hyde RT. Physical activity as an index of heart attack risk in college alumni. *Am J Epidemiol* 1978; 108(3):161–175.
8. Paffenbarger RS Jr, Hyde RT, Wing AL, Hsieh CC. Physical activity, all-cause mortality, and longevity of college alumni. *N Engl J Med* 1986;314(10):605–613.
9. Paffenbarger RS Jr, Hyde RT, Wing AL, et al. The association of changes in physical-activity level and other lifestyle characteris-

tics with mortality among men. *N Engl J Med* 1993;328(8):538–545. (see comments)

10. Kohl HW 3rd. Physical activity and cardiovascular disease: evidence for a dose response. *Med Sci Sports Exerc* 2001;33(6 Suppl):S472–S483; discussion S493–S494.

11. Lee IM, Paffenbarger RS Jr. Do physical activity and physical fitness avert premature mortality? *Exerc Sport Sci Rev* 1996;24:135–171.

12. Paffenbarger RS Jr, Hyde RT. Exercise in the prevention of coronary heart disease. *Prev Med* 1984;13(1):3–22.

13. Lee IM, Skerrett PJ. Physical activity and all-cause mortality: what is the dose-response relation? *Med Sci Sports Exerc* 2001;33(6 Suppl):S459–S471; discussion S493–S494.

14. Kujala UM, Kaprio J, Sarna S, Koskenvuo M. Relationship of leisure-time physical activity and mortality: the Finnish twin cohort. *JAMA* 1998;279(6):440–444.

15. Blair SN, Kohl HW 3rd, Paffenbarger RS Jr, et al. Physical fitness and all-cause mortality. A prospective study of healthy men and women. *JAMA* 1989;262(17):2395–2401.

16. Blair SN, Kohl HW 3rd, Barlow CE, et al. Changes in physical fitness and all-cause mortality. A prospective study of healthy and unhealthy men. *JAMA* 1995;273(14):1093–1098.

17. Blair SN, Kampert JB, Kohl HW 3rd, et al. Influences of cardiorespiratory fitness and other precursors on cardiovascular disease and all-cause mortality in men and women. *JAMA* 1996;276(3):205–210.

18. Lakka TA, Venäläinen JM, Rauramaoa R, et al. Relation of leisure-time physical activity and cardiorespiratory fitness to the risk of acute myocardial infarction. *N Engl J Med* 1994;330(22):1549–1554.

19. Sandvik L, Erikssen J, Thaulow E, et al. Physical fitness as a predictor of mortality among healthy, middle-aged Norwegian men. *N Engl J Med* 1993;328(8):533–537.

20. Tanasescu M, Leitzmann MF, Rimm EB, et al. Exercise type and intensity in relation to coronary heart disease in men. *JAMA* 2002;288(16):1994–2000. (see comment)

21. Balady GJ, Larson MG, Vasan RS, et al. Usefulness of exercise testing in the prediction of coronary disease risk among asymptomatic persons as a function of the Framingham risk score. *Circulation* 2004;110(14):1920–1925.

22. Dorn J, Naujton J, Imamura D, Trevisan M. Results of a multicenter randomized clinical trial of exercise and long-term survival in myocardial infarction patients: the National Exercise and Heart Disease Project (NEHDP). *Circulation* 1999;100(17):1764–1769.

23. Goraya TY, Jacobsen SJ, Pellikka PA, et al. Prognostic value of treadmill exercise testing in elderly persons. *Ann Intern Med* 2000;132(11):862–870.

24. Mora S, Redberg RF, Cui Y, et al. Ability of exercise testing to predict cardiovascular and all-cause death in asymptomatic women: a 20-year follow-up of the lipid research clinics prevalence study. *JAMA* 2003;290(12):1600–1607. (see comment)

25. Myers J, Kaykha A, George S, et al. Fitness versus physical activity patterns in predicting mortality in men. *Am J Med* 2004;117(12):912–918.

26. Myers J, Prakash M, Froelicher V, et al. Exercise capacity and mortality among men referred for exercise testing. *N Engl J Med* 2002;346(11):793–801. (see comment)

27. Kokkinos P, Myers J, Kokkinos JP, et al. Exercise capacity and mortality in black and white men. *Circulation* 2008;117(5):614–622.

28. Gulati M, Pandey DK, Arnsdorf MF, et al. Exercise capacity and the risk of death in women: the St James Women Take Heart Project. *Circulation* 2003;108(13):1554–1559. (see comment)

29. Kushi LH, Fee RM, Folsom AR, et al. Physical activity and mortality in postmenopausal women. *JAMA* 1997;277(16):1287–1292. (see comment)

30. Manson JE, Greenland P, La Croix AZ, et al. Walking compared with vigorous exercise for the prevention of cardiovascular events in women. *N Engl J Med* 2002;347(10):716–725. (see comment)

31. Manson JE, Hu FB, Rich-Edwards JW, et al. A prospective study of walking as compared with vigorous exercise in the prevention of coronary heart disease in women. *N Engl J Med* 1999;341(9):650–658.

32. Gregg EW, Cauley JA, Stone K, et al. Relationship of changes in physical activity and mortality among older women. *JAMA* 2003; 289(18):2379–2386.

33. Lissner L, Bengtsson C, Bjökelund C, Wendel H. Physical activity levels and changes in relation to longevity. A prospective study of Swedish women. *Am J Epidemiol* 1996;143 (1):54–62.

34. United States Department of Health and Human Services: a report by the Surgeon General, 1996. Historical document (1999) available at www.nku.edu/~lipping/PHE125/A%20Report%20of%20the%20Surgeon%20General.doc. Accessed March 15, 2009.

35. Kiely DK, Wolf PA, Cupples LA, et al. Physical activity and stroke risk: the Framingham Study. *Am J Epidemiol* 1994;140(7):608–620. (see erratum)

36. Lee IM, Henneken CH, Berger K, et al. Exercise and risk of stroke in male physicians. *Stroke* 1999;30(1):1–6.

37. Lee IM, Paffenbarger RS Jr. Physical activity and stroke incidence: the Harvard Alumni Health Study. *Stroke* 1998;29(10):2049–2054.

38. Sacco RL, Gan R, Boden-Albala B, et al. Leisure-time physical activity and ischemic stroke risk: the Northern Manhattan Stroke Study. *Stroke* 1998;29(2):380–387.

39. Evenson KR, Rosamond WD, Cai J, et al. Physical activity and ischemic stroke risk. The atherosclerosis risk in communities study. *Stroke* 1999;30(7):1333–1339.

40. Noda H, Iso H, Toyoshima H, et al. Walking and sports participation and mortality from coronary heart disease and stroke. *J Am Coll Cardiol* 2005;46(9):1761–1767.

41. Hu G, Sarti C, Jousilahti P, et al. Leisure time, occupational, and commuting physical activity and the risk of stroke. *Stroke* 2005; 36(9):1994–1999.

42. Hu FB, Stampfer MJ, Colditz GA, et al. Physical activity and risk of stroke in women. *JAMA* 2000;283(22):2961–2967. (see comments)

43. Pitsavos C, Panagiotakos DB, Crysohoou C, et al. Physical activity decreases the risk of stroke in middle-age men with left ventricular hypertrophy: 40-year follow-up (1961–2001) of the Seven Countries Study (the Corfu cohort). *J Hum Hypertens* 2004;18(7): 495–501.

44. Benjamin EJ, Levy D. Why is left ventricular hypertrophy so predictive of morbidity and mortality? *Am J Med Sci* 1999;317(3): 168–175.

45. Levy D, Garrison RJ, Savage, DD, et al. Prognostic implications of echocardiographically determined left ventricular mass in the Framingham Heart Study. *N Engl J Med* 1990; 322(22):1561–1566. (see comments)

46. Rodriguez CJ, Sacco RL, Sciacca RR, et al. Physical activity attenuates the effect of increased left ventricular mass on the risk of ischemic stroke: the Northern Manhattan Stroke Study. *J Am Coll Cardiol* 2002; 39(9):1482–1488.

47. Wendel-Vos GC, Schuit AJ, Feskens EJ, et al. Physical activity and stroke. A meta-analysis of observational data. *Int J Epidemiol* 2004; 33(4):787–798.

48. Conn EH, Williams RS, Wallace AG. Exercise responses before and after physical conditioning in patients with severely depressed left ventricular function. *Am J Cardiol* 1982;49(2):296–300.

49. Ehsani AA. Adaptations to training in patients with exercise-induced left ventricular dysfunction. *Adv Cardiol* 1986;34:148–155.

50. Lee AP, Ice R, Blessey R, Sanmarco ME. Long-term effects of physical training on coronary patients with impaired ventricular function. *Circulation* 1979;60(7): 1519–1526.

51. Sullivan MJ, Higginbotham MB, Cobb FR. Exercise training in patients with severe left ventricular dysfunction. Hemodynamic and metabolic effects. *Circulation* 1988;78(3): 506–515.

52. Coats AJ, Adamopoulos S, Meyer TE, et al. Effects of physical training in chronic heart

failure. *Lancet* 1990;335(8681):63–66. (see comments)

53. Coats AJ, Adamopoulos S, Radaelli A, et al. Controlled trial of physical training in chronic heart failure. Exercise performance, hemodynamics, ventilation, and autonomic function. *Circulation* 1992;85(6):2119–2131. (see comments)

54. Belardinelli R, Georgiou D, Cianci G, et al. Exercise training improves left ventricular diastolic filling in patients with dilated cardiomyopathy. Clinical and prognostic implications. *Circulation* 1995;91(11):2775–2784.

55. Belardinelli R, Georgiou D, Cianci G, Purcaro A. Effects of exercise training on left ventricular filling at rest and during exercise in patients with ischemic cardiomyopathy and severe left ventricular systolic dysfunction. *Am Heart J* 1996;132(1 Pt 1): 61–70.

56. Belardinelli R, Georgiou D, Ginzton L, et al. Effects of moderate exercise training on thallium uptake and contractile response to low-dose dobutamine of dysfunctional myocardium in patients with ischemic cardiomyopathy. *Circulation* 1998;97(6):553–561.

57. Goebbels U, Myers J, Dziekan G, et al. A randomized comparison of exercise training in patients with normal vs. reduced ventricular function. *Chest* 1998;113(5):1387–1393.

58. Hambrecht R, Fiehn E, Yu J, et al. Effects of endurance training on mitochondrial ultrastructure and fiber type distribution in skeletal muscle of patients with stable chronic heart failure. *J Am Coll Cardiol* 1997;29 (5):1067–1073.

59. Hambrecht R, Niebauer J, Fiehn E, et al. Physical training in patients with stable chronic heart failure: effects on cardiorespiratory fitness and ultrastructural abnormalities of leg muscles. *J Am Coll Cardiol* 1995;25(6):1239–1249.

60. Keteyian SJ, Levine AB, Brawner CA, et al. Exercise training in patients with heart failure. A randomized, controlled trial. *Ann Intern Med* 1996;124(12):1051–1057.

61. Kiilavuori K, Sovijärvi A, Näveri H, et al. Effect of physical training on exercise capacity and gas exchange in patients with chronic heart failure. *Chest* 1996;110(4):985–991.

62. Wielenga RP, Huisveld IA, Bol E, et al. Safety and effects of physical training in chronic heart failure. Results of the Chronic Heart Failure and Graded Exercise study (CHANGE). *Eur Heart J* 1999;20(12): 872–879.

63. Smart N, Marwick TH. Exercise training for patients with heart failure: a systematic review of factors that improve mortality and morbidity. *Am J Med* 2004;116(10):714–716.

64. Gaudron P, Eilles C, Kugler I, Ertl G. Progressive left ventricular dysfunction and remodeling after myocardial infarction. Potential mechanisms and early predictors. *Circulation* 1993;87(3):755–763.

65. Braunwald E. Optimizing thrombolytic therapy of acute myocardial infarction. *Circulation* 1990;82(4):1510–1513.

66. Braunwald E, Pfeffer MA. Ventricular enlargement and remodeling following acute myocardial infarction: mechanisms and management. *Am J Cardiol* 1991;68(14): 1D–6D.

67. Pfeffer MA, Braunwald E. Ventricular remodeling after myocardial infarction. Experimental observations and clinical implications. *Circulation* 1990;81(4):1161–1172.

68. Pfeffer MA, Braunwald E. Ventricular enlargement following infarction is a modifiable process. *Am J Cardiol* 1991;68(14): 127D–131D.

69. Jette M, Heller R, Landry F, Blümchen G. Randomized 4-week exercise program in patients with impaired left ventricular function. *Circulation* 1991;84(4):1561–1567.

70. Jugdutt BI, Michorowski BL, Kappagoda CT. Exercise training after anterior Q wave myocardial infarction: importance of regional left ventricular function and topography. *J Am Coll Cardiol* 1988;12(2):362–372.

71. Dubach P, Myers J, Dziekan G, et al. Effect of exercise training on myocardial remodeling in patients with reduced left ventricular function after myocardial infarction: application of magnetic resonance imaging. *Circulation* 1997;95(8):2060–2067.

72. Giannuzzi P, Tavazzi L, Temporelli PL, et al. Long-term physical training and left ventricular remodeling after anterior myocardial infarction: results of the Exercise in Anterior Myocardial Infarction (EAMI) trial. EAMI Study Group. *J Am Coll Cardiol* 1993;22(7): 1821–1829.

73. Belardinelli R, Georgiou D, Scocco V, et al. Low intensity exercise training in patients with chronic heart failure. *J Am Coll Cardiol* 1995;26(4):975–982.

74. Demopoulos L, Bijou R, Fergus I, et al. Exercise training in patients with severe congestive heart failure: enhancing peak aerobic capacity while minimizing the increase in ventricular wall stress. *J Am Coll Cardiol* 1997;29(3):597–603.

75. Franciosa JA, Park M, Levine TB. Lack of correlation between exercise capacity and indexes of resting left ventricular performance in heart failure. *Am J Cardiol* 1981; 47(1):33–39.

76. Szlachcic J, Massie BM, Kramer BL, et al. Correlates and prognostic implication of exercise capacity in chronic congestive heart failure. *Am J Cardiol* 1985;55(8): 1037–1042.

77. Lipkin DP, Jones DA, Round JM, Poole-Wilson PA. Abnormalities of skeletal muscle in patients with chronic heart failure. *Int J Cardiol* 1988;18(2):187–195. (see comment)

78. Mancini DM, Walter G, Reichek N, et al. Contribution of skeletal muscle atrophy to exercise intolerance and altered muscle metabolism in heart failure. *Circulation* 1992;85(4):1364–1373. (see comment)

79. Koch M, Douard H, Broustet JP. The benefit of graded physical exercise in chronic heart failure. *Chest* 1992;101(5 Suppl):231S–235S.

80. Minotti JR, Johnson EC, Hudson TL, et al. Skeletal muscle response to exercise training in congestive heart failure. *J Clin Invest* 1990;86(3):751–758.

81. Hambrecht R, Fiehn E, Wiegl C, et al. Regular physical exercise corrects endothelial dysfunction and improves exercise capacity in patients with chronic heart failure. *Circulation* 1998;98(24):2709–2715. (see comments)

82. Hornig B, Maier V, Drexler H. Physical training improves endothelial function in patients with chronic heart failure. *Circulation* 1996;93(2):210–214.

83. Belardinelli R, Georgiou D, Cianci G, Purcaro A, et al. Randomized, controlled trial of long-term moderate exercise training in chronic heart failure: effects on functional capacity, quality of life, and clinical outcome. *Circulation* 1999;99(9):1173–1182.

84. Piepoli MF, Davos C, Francis DP, et al. Exercise training meta-analysis of trials in patients with chronic heart failure (ExTraMATCH). *BMJ* 2004;328(7433):189.

85. O'Connor CM, Ehellan DJ, Lee KL, et al. Efficacy and safety of exercise training in patients with chronic heart failure: HF-ACTION Randomized Controlled Trial. *JAMA* 2009;301(14):1439–1450.

86. Fletcher GF, Balady GJ, Amsterdam EA, et al. Exercise standards for testing and training: a statement for healthcare professionals from the American Heart Association. *Circulation* 2001;104(14):1694–1740.

87. Pate RR, Pratt M, Blair SN, et al. Physical activity and public health. A recommendation from the Centers for Disease Control and Prevention and the American College of Sports Medicine. *JAMA* 1995;273(5): 402–407.

88. Alpert JS, Larsen OA, Lassen NA. Exercise and intermittent claudication. Blood flow in the calf muscle during walking studied by the xenon-133 clearance method. *Circulation* 1969;39(3):353–359.

89. Carter SA, Hamel ER, Paterson JM, et al. Walking ability and ankle systolic pressures: observations in patients with intermittent claudication in a short-term walking exercise program. *J Vasc Surg* 1989;10(6): 642–649.

90. Gardner AW, Poehlman ET. Exercise rehabilitation programs for the treatment of claudication pain. A meta-analysis. *JAMA* 1995;274 (12):975–980.

91. Hiatt WR, Regensteiner JG, Hargarten ME, et al. Benefit of exercise conditioning for patients with peripheral arterial disease.

Circulation 1990;81(2):602–609. (see comments)

92. Hiatt WR, Wofel EE, Meier RH, Regensteiner JG, et al. Superiority of treadmill walking exercise versus strength training for patients with peripheral arterial disease. Implications for the mechanism of the training response. *Circulation* 1994;90(4):1866–1874.

93. Hillestad LK. The peripheral blood flow in intermittent claudication. VI. Plethysmographic studies. The blood flow response to exercise with arrested and with free circulation. *Acta Med Scand* 1963;174:671–685.

94. Hillestad LK. The peripheral blood flow in intermittent claudication. V. Plethysmographic studies. The significance of the calf blood flow at rest and in response to timed arrest of the circulation. *Acta Med Scand* 1963; 174:23–41.

95. Hillestad LK. The peripheral blood flow in intermittent claudication. IV. The significance of the claudication distance. *Acta Med Scand* 1963;173:467–478.

96. Larsen OA, Lassen NA. Effect of daily muscular exercise in patients with intermittent claudication. *Lancet* 1966;2(7473):1093–1096.

97. Lundgren F, Dallöf AG, Lundholm K, et al. Intermittent claudication–surgical reconstruction or physical training? A prospective randomized trial of treatment efficiency. *Ann Surg* 1989;209(3):346–355.

98. Mannarino E, Pasqualini L, Innocente S, et al. Physical training and antiplatelet treatment in stage II peripheral arterial occlusive disease: alone or combined? Angiology 1991;42(7):513–521.

99. Regensteiner JG, Meyer TJ, Krupski WC, et al. Hospital vs. home-based exercise rehabilitation for patients with peripheral arterial occlusive disease. *Angiology* 1997;48(4): 291–300.

100. Regensteiner JG, Steiner JF, Hiatt WR. Exercise training improves functional status in patients with peripheral arterial disease. *J Vasc Surg* 1996;23(1):104–115.

101. Skinner JS, Strandness DE Jr. Exercise and intermittent claudication. II. Effect of physical training. *Circulation* 1967;36(1):23–29.

102. Skinner JS, Strandness DE Jr. Exercise and intermittent claudication. I. Effect of repetition and intensity of exercise. *Circulation* 1967;36(1):15–22.

103. Ekroth R, Dahllöf AG, Gundevall B, et al. Physical training of patients with intermittent claudication: indications, methods, and results. *Surgery* 1978;84(5):640–643.

104. Ainsworth BE, Haskell WL, Leon AS, et al. Compendium of physical activities: classification of energy costs of human physical activities. *Med Sci Sports Exerc* 1993;25(1): 71–80. (see comment)

105. Mora S, Cook N, Buring JE, et al. Physical activity and reduced risk of cardiovascular events: potential mediating mechanisms. *Circulation* 2007;116(19):2110–2118.

106. Balady G. Survival of the fittest—more evidence (editorial). *N Engl J Med* 2002;347(4): 288–290.

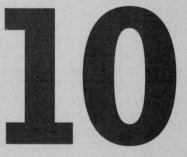

Blood Lipids and Physical Activity

E vidence that blood lipids and lipoprotein levels are associated with coronary heart disease (CHD) has been accumulating for the past five decades or more. Early population studies assessed the association between total cholesterol and CHD.[1–6] As knowledge about cholesterol metabolism expanded, the research emphasis shifted to the role of cholesterol carried by the different lipoproteins. When the early findings emerged suggesting an inverse association between physical activity and mortality from coronary heart disease,[7] researchers focused on the possible favorable effects physical activity may have on lipid and lipoprotein metabolism. This chapter examines the evolution in our understanding of the relationship between physical activity, exercise, and lipoprotein-lipid metabolism.

Figure 10.1 Cholesterol and risk for coronary heart disease.

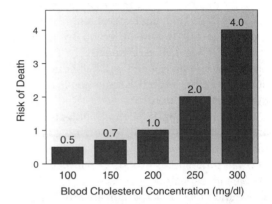

Source: Adapted from Stamler J, et al. (MRFIT) *JAMA* 1986;256(20):2823–2828.

■ TOTAL CHOLESTEROL

Early epidemiologic studies revealed a positive relationship between total blood cholesterol levels and the development of CHD.[1–6] Findings from the Framingham Heart and other studies were similar and suggested that the risk of coronary heart disease increased curvilinearly when blood cholesterol levels exceeded approximately 220 mg/dl. The data suggested an insignificant reduction in risk with cholesterol levels below 220 mg/dl.[1,2,8] However, data from a much larger study of 365,222 men, the Multiple Risk Factor Intervention Trial (MRFIT study), supported that the relationship between cholesterol and heart disease was continuous and graded.[9,10] A significant increase in risk was observed even at cholesterol levels below 200 mg/dl (the increase begins at approximately 180 mg/dL). The risk doubled with every 50 mg/dl increase in blood cholesterol beyond 200 mg/dl (**Figure 10.1**). Based on the results of these studies and for practical reasons, the expert panel of the

Third National Cholesterol Education Program (NCEP) set the standards for desirable blood cholesterol at < 200 mg/dl.[11]

■ LDL-CHOLESTEROL

Low-density lipoprotein (LDL), the "carrier" of cholesterol in the blood, and its association with coronary artery disease (CAD) became the focus of research almost exclusively. During the 1970s and well into the 1980s, the atherogenic nature of LDL-cholesterol (LDL-C), its mechanisms, and significance in predicting CAD were well-documented.[12–16] The results of the Lipid Research Clinics Coronary Primary Prevention Trials (LRC-CPPT) published in the mid-1980s established a cause-and-effect relationship between LDL-C levels and CAD.[17,18]

The LRC-CPPT I and II[17,18] tested the efficacy of cholesterol lowering in reducing risk of coronary heart disease in 3,806 asymptomatic middle-aged men with high blood cholesterol levels. The treatment group received cholesterol-lowering medication and the control group received a placebo for an average of 7.4 years. Both groups followed a moderate cholesterol-lowering diet. Total cholesterol and LDL-C was reduced in the treatment group by approximately 13.4% and 20.3%, respectively. The treatment group experienced a 24% reduction in death from CHD and a 19% reduction in nonfatal myocardial infarction.

When the group receiving medication was analyzed separately, a 19% reduction in CHD risk was also associated with each decrement of 8% in total cholesterol or 11% in LDL-C levels. The investigators estimated approximately a 2% reduction in risk for mortality for every 1% reduction in plasma LDL-C levels.

Desirable levels for LDL-C established by NCEP Adult Treatment Panel III (NCEP-ATP III)[11] depended on the medical history of the individuals; that is, the presence of other risk factors and/or heart disease (**Table 10.1**).

■ TRIGLYCERIDES

Studies examining the association between elevated plasma triglyceride and CAD have yielded conflicting findings. Some found that elevated triglycerides constitute an independent risk factor for CAD[19–22] especially when used in combination with HDL-C and LDL-C.[19] Other studies found no association.[23–28] Despite these inconsistencies, the NCEP-recommended desirable triglyceride levels are < 150 mg/dl (Table 10.1).

■ HDL-CHOLESTEROL AND CAD

Prior to 1975, research on the role of high density lipoprotein (HDL)-cholesterol on CAD was limited despite a 1951 observation by Barr and

Table 10.1 Ideal Levels of Blood Lipids and Lipoproteins

	Desirable	**Moderately High**	**High**
Cholesterol	< 200 mg/dl	200–239 mg/dl	≥ 240 mg/dl
Triglycerides	< 200 mg/dl	200–399 mg/dl	≥ 400 mg/dl
LDL-C	< 130 mg/dl	130–159 mg/dl	≥ 160 mg/dl
LDL-C for those with CHD or CHD equivalent as decided by a physician (high risk)	< 100 mg/dL with optimal goal of < 70 mg/dl		
HDL-C			
Men	≥ 40 mg/dl		
Women	≥ 50 mg/dl		
Cholesterol/HDL-C			
Men	≤ 4.5		
Women	≤ 3.5		

Source: Executive Summary of the Third Report of the National Cholesterol Education Program (NCEP) Expert Panel on Detection, Evaluation, and Treatment of High Blood Cholesterol In Adults (Adult Treatment Panel III). *JAMA* 2001;285(19):2486–2497.

co-workers that healthy men had higher levels of HDL-cholesterol than did men with CAD.[29] Interest about HDL-cholesterol was revived in 1975 when Miller and Miller[30] called attention to existing evidence suggesting an inverse relationship between blood HDL-cholesterol and CAD. Findings from the Framingham Heart Study (**Figure 10.2**) confirmed the protective nature of the HDL lipoprotein by supporting and expanding the original theory proposed by Glomset[31] and then Miller and Miller[30] that the HDL lipoprotein is involved in the transport of cholesterol from peripheral tissues to liver for catabolism. In addition, the Framingham Heart Study findings supported that blood HDL-cholesterol appeared to be the best independent predictor of CAD than any other known risk factor.[32–34]

A cause-and-effect relationship between HDL-cholesterol and the risk of CHD was established in the Helsinki Heart Trial, a randomized, double-blind, 5 year trial involving 4,081 asymptomatic middle-aged men (40–55 years of age) with dyslipidemia.[35] The treatment group (2,051 men) received 600 mg of gemfibrozil twice daily, and the other (2,030 men) received placebo. Gemfibrozil caused a marked increase in HDL-cholesterol and persistent reductions in serum levels of total cholesterol, LDL-C, and triglycerides. The placebo group experienced minimal changes in serum lipid levels.

There was a 34% reduction in the incidence of CHD at the end of the 5-year study. The decline in incidence in the treatment group became evident in the second year and continued throughout the study.

■ TOTAL CHOLESTEROL TO HDL-CHOLESTEROL RATIO

Naturally, the ideal lipid profile is to have low total cholesterol and high HDL-cholesterol levels. However, this is not the case for most people. Because the risk for CHD is influenced by cholesterol and HDL (**Figure 10.3**), to "standardize" the risk for different levels of cholesterol or HDL-cholesterol, the Framingham investigators[34,36] considered the total cholesterol to HDL-cholesterol ratio (TC/HDL-C). According to the Framingham data, if a TC/HDL-C ratio of 5.0 is considered as average risk, then a ratio of 3.5 corresponds to half of that risk.[34] The significance of the TC/HDL-C ratio can best be

Figure 10.2 HDL-cholesterol and mortality risk.

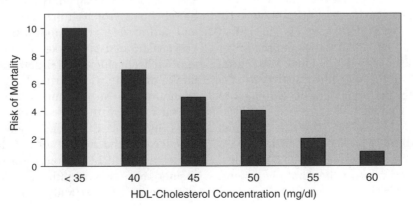

Figure 10.3 Estimated coronary heart disease risk according to total cholesterol and HDL-cholesterol values.

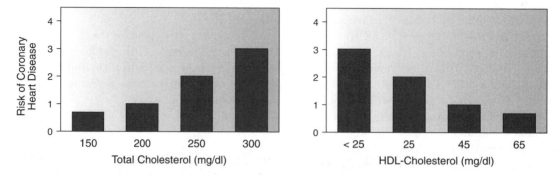

Source: Data from the Framingham Study.

appreciated in the case of an individual who has normal cholesterol levels but a low HDL-cholesterol value. For example, let's assume we have information on individuals A and B (see the following box).

	TC	HDL-C	TC HDL-C
Individual A	245 mg/dl	70 mg/dl	3.5
Individual B	196 mg/dl	28 mg/dL	7.0

As you can see, individual A has substantially higher cholesterol levels than individual B. However, he also has high HDL-cholesterol levels that give a TC/HDL-C of 3.5. This is half of the ratio of individual B, despite the lower cholesterol level of that individual. Most cardiologists will argue that individual B is at a higher risk for the premature development of CHD than individual A.

However, this is not to suggest that high total cholesterol levels or high LDL-C levels are acceptable to have so long as HDL-C levels are high. The lower the total cholesterol value, the lower the risk for CHD. The ideal

situation is a cholesterol value below 200 mg/dl, LDL-cholesterol below 130 mg/dl, and HDL-cholesterol ≥ 40 mg/dl for men and ≥ 50 mg/dl for women. When this combination is disrupted, the coronary risk increases.

The NCEP-ATP III–recommended lipid profiles for healthy individuals and those with cardiac risk factors and heart disease are presented in Table 10.1.

■ DIETS AND BLOOD LIPIDS

The standard recommendations for lowering blood cholesterol are to restrict carbohydrate and saturated fat consumption and to increase polyunsaturated fat intake. This is a prudent approach considering the high saturated fat intake of western countries. In this regard, it is important to keep in mind that several studies have shown that low-fat, low-cholesterol diets, including diets rich in polyunsaturated fats, have a tendency to not only lower blood cholesterol and LDL-cholesterol (a desirable result), but also significantly lower HDL-cholesterol,[37–39] certainly not a desirable outcome. Consequently, the ratios of total cholesterol to HDL-cholesterol or LDL-cholesterol to HDL-cholesterol remain either unchanged or increase slightly.[37–39]

An exception is a diet rich in olive oil. When olive oil (a highly monosaturated oil) is substituted for polyunsaturated oils, total cholesterol and LDL-cholesterol levels decrease to a similar degree observed with the aforementioned diets. However, what is of great interest is that the HDL-cholesterol levels remain unchanged with a diet containing olive oil.[40–43] In summary, it appears that a diet rich in olive oil is at least as effective in lowering plasma cholesterol as a diet low in saturated fat and carbohydrate and high in polyunsaturated fats, but leaves HDL-cholesterol levels unchanged. For this reason and for the safety history of olive oil, it is prudent that olive oil be substituted for other fats in the diet and products rich in olive oil should be preferred.

■ PHYSICAL ACTIVITY AND CAD

As discussed in Chapter 9, early epidemiologic findings supported an inverse relationship between increased physical activity status and the incidence of CAD. In a landmark 1953 study, Morris and co-workers reported that those with physically demanding occupations (i.e., mail carriers) had approximately 50% lower risk of dying from cardiovascular disease than those with sedentary occupations.[7] During the decade of the 1970s, Paffenbarger and coworkers reported that those with physically demanding occupations and those who maintained a physically active lifestyle had significantly lower death rates than their sedentary counterparts.[44,45] These findings sparked interest of a possible association between physical activity and more favorable blood lipids.

■ PHYSICAL ACTIVITY, CHOLESTEROL, AND TRIGLYCERIDES

Epidemiologic Findings

Early epidemiologic studies examined only the association between physical activity and total blood cholesterol and triglyceride values. The findings on cholesterol yielded conflicting evidence. Some studies reported lower blood cholesterol in athletes engaging in competitive aerobic sports than sedentary individuals.[46–49] Most studies, however, showed no relationship between total blood cholesterol levels and physical activity when age and body fat level was considered.[50–61] It is now well accepted that total cholesterol levels are not influenced substantially by increased physical activity.

The findings on the association between physical activity and triglycerides were more favorable. Most early cross-sectional studies examining endurance athletes,[46,49] cross country-skiers,[57] and tennis players[60] support that that physical activity is associated with lower triglyceride levels in physically active individuals compared to sedentary, even when adjustments for body fatness were made.[46,49,55]

Interventional Studies

Exercise training studies confirmed the findings of epidemiologic studies.

Some investigators reported lower total cholesterol levels following exercise training.[62] However, most well-designed studies that controlled for confounding factors such as changes in body composition and weight found that exercise training had no significant effect on total cholesterol concentrations.[63–66]

Triglyceride concentrations are reported by most studies to be reduced significantly following endurance training programs lasting anywhere from 7 weeks to a year.[61–66] The amount of degree of reduction is related to pre-training concentrations and volume of exercise completed during the training period.[66] However, some studies found no changes in triglyceride concentrations after 10 weeks of aerobic exercise.[67,68] Despite these negative findings, the consensus is that exercise training lowers blood triglyceride concentration.

■ PHYSICAL ACTIVITY AND LDL-CHOLESTEROL

As discussed in Chapter 4, the LDL is the lipo-protein responsible for carrying cholesterol (LDL-cholesterol) to the cells. It is the major carrier of cholesterol carrying approximately 60% to 80% of all blood cholesterol. Because the atherogenic properties of elevated LDL-cholesterol concentrations are well documented,[17,18] interest in lowering LDL-cholesterol by increased physical activity was natural.

The reports of observational studies comparing LDL-cholesterol levels of athletes from various sports and sedentary individuals are mixed. Some reported lower LDL-cholesterol in athletes[51,58,69] and others showed no differences.[49,59,70]

Exercise training studies reported no changes in LDL-cholesterol,[65,71,72] while others studies reported relatively small changes of approximately 3% to 8%.[61,62,64,73–78] It is the prevailing consensus that when other factors such as weight reduction and diet are considered, exercise does not have a significant effect on LDL-cholesterol.

The findings from cross-sectional and exercise training studies strongly support that exercise training has little or no effect on LDL-cholesterol.

■ PHYSICAL ACTIVITY AND HDL-CHOLESTEROL

Following the studies by Miller and Miller[30] and Gordon et al.,[33] who emphasized the importance of HDL-cholesterol concentrations in the prediction of CAD, emphasis shifted from LDL-cholesterol to HDL-cholesterol. The protection offered by high blood HDL-cholesterol concentrations against atherosclerosis and CAD is well established. The relationship is strong, inverse, and independent.[79,80] The risk for CAD increases by 2% to 3% for every 1.0 ml/dl decrease in HDL-cholesterol.[80]

Epidemiologic Evidence

Interest on the effects of exercise on HDL-cholesterol metabolism was perpetuated by the significantly higher HDL-cholesterol levels reported by several investigators on elite long distance runners and competitive cross-country skiers when compared to sedentary individuals.[49,53,57,58] Most cross-sectional studies are rather consistent, reporting 20% to 30% higher HDL-cholesterol levels in endurance-trained athletes compared to sedentary groups.[51,52,58,63,69] In addition, a dose-response relationship has been suggested by epidemiological observations studies.[52,81–83]

■ Evidence from Exercise Training Studies

Early exercise training studies conducted during the 1970s and early 1980s reported significant HDL-cholesterol increases following aerobic exercise training.[68,77,84,85] However, a statistical procedure applied to collectively assess the findings of 66 well-conducted exercise training studies (meta-analysis) concluded that HDL-cholesterol concentrations did not change significantly with exercise training.[65] A well-conducted, randomized exercise study disputes this conclusion. After 1 year of exercise training (brisk walking or jogging), the investigators reported significant changes in HDL-cholesterol and overall a more desirable lipoprotein-lipid profile when exercise was combined with a prudent diet.[64] Interestingly, diet alone was not effective in positively changing HDL-cholesterol, especially in women. This further supports observations that lowering fat intake also lowers HDL-cholesterol.[37–39]

What began to emerge from these studies and the epidemiologic evidence was the concept that exercise-induced HDL-cholesterol changes may depend greatly on the intensity and volume of exercise. In fact, these studies combined with the epidemiologic evidence supported the following concepts:

- A certain exercise volume is necessary (i.e., an exercise volume threshold) before HDL-cholesterol changes can occur.
- An exercise intensity threshold may exist.
- A dose-response relationship between exercise volume and HDL-cholesterol changes is likely to exist.
- HDL-cholesterol changes may respond only to a certain type of exercise.

An extensive review of the literature regarding these issues has been published.[86]

■ Exercise Volume Threshold for HDL-Cholesterol Changes

The existence of a minimum exercise volume or exercise volume threshold necessary for HDL-cholesterol changes is very much in accord with the response observed by all biological systems exposed to a stimulus; that is, the stimulus must be of a certain intensity, frequency, and volume to produce the desired outcome. Regarding HDL-cholesterol changes, a certain volume of exercise reached over a

period of weeks, months, or years will trigger the desired changes.

Finding this exercise volume threshold is not an easy task. Because exercise volume is the product of intensity, duration, and frequency of exercise per week plus the length of training (months or years), a number of combinations of these four components can produce varying as well as similar outcomes. It is also likely that a threshold exists for each one of the exercise components. For example, a certain exercise intensity or duration threshold may be necessary regardless of the frequency or length of exercise training.

Work by Kokkinos and colleagues strongly suggested that most changes in HDL-cholesterol occur when jogging for approximately 101 to 124 minutes per week, at distances from 7 to 14 miles.[81] The expected increase in HDL-cholesterol levels is approximately 7% to 11%. HDL-cholesterol changes beyond 14 miles per week are not significant until jogging more than 20 miles per week. At this weekly mileage, HDL-cholesterol levels were 19% higher when compared to the lowest weekly mileage (0–2 miles/week) group (**Figure 10.4**). This suggests that most of the HDL-cholesterol changes can be achieved by a weekly distance of 7 to 14 miles. Therefore, for most people, running more than 14 miles per week for the increase in HDL-cholesterol is not necessary. Others, however, reported about 7% higher HDL-cholesterol levels in those running 18 or more miles per week at exercise intensities of 6 or more METs when compared to sedentary individuals.[82]

Because caloric expenditure encompasses all three exercise components (intensity, duration, and frequency), it allows for more accurate comparisons among several studies. Reporting exercise volume in terms of calories expended (when possible) therefore should be preferred. In this regard, a caloric expenditure of 1,000 to 1,500 kcal/week has also been defined as the threshold dose of exercise to favorably

Figure 10.4 HDL-cholesterol changes according to the weekly distance run.

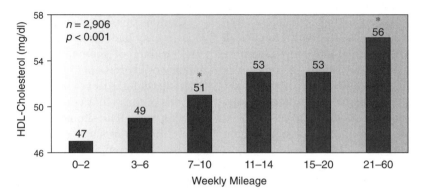

Source: Adapted from Kokkinos P, et al. *Arch Intern Med* 1995;155:415–420.

influence changes in HDL-cholesterol.[87] This is quite similar to the weekly energy expenditure of 1,245 kcal reported for individuals running approximately 7 to 10 miles per week (average 9 miles) and 1,688 kcal for those running 11 to 14 (average 12 miles) miles per week.[81]

Exercise training studies also support a distance threshold of approximately 8 to 10 miles per week. In a randomized, controlled study, men who averaged at least 8 miles per week of running for 1 year increased their HDL-cholesterol levels by 4.4 mg per dl.[74] In a similar study, significant changes in HDL-cholesterol levels were not observed until a threshold of 10 miles per week was maintained for at least 9 months.[88]

In a more recent study designed to answer the question of defining the amount of exercise training required for optimal benefit, Kraus and co-investigators[89] randomly assigned individuals to approximately 8 months in one of four groups:

Group 1: Low-amount–moderate-intensity exercise, the equivalent of walking 12 miles per week at 40% to 55% of peak oxygen consumption.

Group 2: Low-amount–high-intensity exercise, the equivalent of jogging 12 miles per week at 65% to 80% of peak oxygen consumption.

Group 3: High-amount–high-intensity exercise, the caloric equivalent of jogging 20 miles per week at 65% to 80% of peak oxygen consumption.

Group 4: The control group.

The investigators reported that favorable changes in a variety of lipid and lipoprotein variables were observed in all exercise groups when compared to the control group. In addition, higher amount of exercise had the beneficial effects of exercise when compared to the individuals in the control group. The high amount of exercise also resulted in greater improvements than did lower amounts of exercise. The investigators concluded that the improvements in lipid and lipoproteins were related to the amount of activity and not to the intensity of exercise or improvement in fitness.[89]

Collectively, the findings of these studies [74,81,82,87–89] support the notion that both exercise volume and intensity are important in achieving favorable HDL-cholesterol changes. However, there is more support that the volume of exercise is more important than intensity. Studies also support that the exercise volume threshold in the threshold can be achieved by manipulation of the exercise components. As noted earlier, two studies used a length of 12 and 9 months for the exercise training period, respectively.[74,88] Interestingly, lower miles per week (8 vs. 10 miles per week), but longer training periods (1 year vs. 9 months) were required for significant changes. In general, studies of greater than 12 weeks in duration reported some favorable changes in HDL-cholesterol levels. However, not all changes reported were statistically significant and the association was not consistent, suggesting that for shorter periods, the exercise intensity or duration must be higher.[86]

Most studies suggest that a much larger volume of exercise is necessary for HDL-cholesterol changes in women. When compared with a sedentary group, most but not all[90] studies agree that only the most physically active women, such as long distance runners, exhibit significantly higher HDL-cholesterol levels.[52,91–94]

Most exercise training studies in premenopausal women show no effect of exercise training on HDL-cholesterol.[95–97] However, in one study, the findings suggest that the decrease in HDL-cholesterol levels that is usually seen with low fat diet interventions[37–39] was prevented by exercise training.[64]

Most exercise training studies have shown that exercise does not improve HDL-cholesterol levels beyond the improvements seen with hormone replacement therapy.[98–100] Only one study showed a synergistic effect between hormone replacement therapy and exercise training.[101] Interestingly, none of these studies of postmenopausal women receiving hormone replacement therapy were able to show consistent improvements in HDL-cholesterol levels,

despite some of them employing exercise training programs designed to expend 1,000 to 1,200 kcal per week. Again, these results suggest that a high volume of exercise may be required for positive changes in HDL-cholesterol levels in women.

The reasons for exercise being less effective to raise HDL-cholesterol in women have not been investigated. However, one can speculate that the relatively high levels of HDL-cholesterol in women may be one reason.

■ Exercise Intensity Threshold for HDL-Cholesterol Changes

In addition to the exercise volume threshold, it is likely that minimum exercise intensity must be achieved before any changes in HDL-cholesterol occur. The existence of an exercise intensity threshold has been suggested by epidemiologic observations in physically active men.[81,82,87,102] Two of these studies suggest that the habitual physical activity intensity threshold for changes in HDL-cholesterol appears to be at approximately 5 to 6 METs.[82,102] An interesting finding in one of the two studies is that no further improvements in HDL-cholesterol were observed when the intensity of 6 METs was compared with energy expenditure levels between 6 and 9 METs,[102] suggesting no dose-response relationship. In one study of 2,906 men,[81] most changes in HDL-cholesterol occurred in those jogging at exercise intensities of 10 to 11 minutes per mile.

Exercise training studies also supported the presence of an exercise intensity threshold. Researchers found evidence to indicate the existence of an exercise intensity threshold at or above 75% of maximal heart rate.[103] HDL-cholesterol increased by 10% after 16 weeks of aerobic exercise training. The exercise intensity correlated significantly with HDL-cholesterol changed from baseline to 16 weeks, and was the only predictor of these changes. Although the 10% change in HDL-cholesterol was not statistically significant, it suggests that a minimum exercise intensity threshold may be required before favorable HDL-cholesterol changes are realized. Others also reported significant increases in HDL-cholesterol levels in those who exercised at 75% of maximal heat rate for 12 weeks, but no changes in HDL-cholesterol were observed in those who exercised at 65% of maximal heart rate.[76] When the interaction between exercise intensity and duration was considered, a greater increase in HDL-cholesterol levels was noted with a longer duration and low intensity exercise rather than shortened duration and high intensity.[104] However, these findings are based a relatively small number of participants ($n = 6$) and so these data should be interpreted with caution.

Evidence for an exercise intensity threshold necessary for changes in HDL-cholesterol levels in women is limited. In addition, women have approximately 10 to 20 mg/dl higher HDL-cholesterol levels than men. Thus, increases in HDL-cholesterol levels in women may be more difficult to change. In one study on women, the exercise intensity threshold was at approximately 6 METs for women aged over 60 years and 7 METs for younger women.[90]

Exercise training studies attempting to assess the role of exercise intensity on HDL-cholesterol are also few, and their findings are conflicting. For example, Duncan et al.[105] reported similar increases in HDL-cholesterol levels in premenopausal women following 24 weeks of endurance training, regardless of exercise intensity. Interestingly, there was no association between exercise intensity and HDL-cholesterol changes. In contrast to these findings, Santiago et al.[106] reported no changes in HDL-cholesterol levels after a 40-week walking program, employing the same walking distance per session (3 miles) as Duncan et al.[105] One possible explanation for the conflict-

ing findings may be that the baseline HDL-cholesterol levels of the women in this study were relatively high compared to those in the study by Duncan et al. (65 vs. 55 ml/dl), respectively.[105]

Training studies on postmenopausal women also yielded conflicting results and provide no clear evidence on the existence of an exercise intensity threshold. Some who assessed the effect of high and low intensity exercise programs on HDL-cholesterol levels in sedentary women found no significant changes in HDL-cholesterol levels after 12 months, while small but significant increases were noted in both intensity groups after 24 months of exercise training.[107] Although the volume and intensity of exercise was substantially greater in the high intensity group, the changes in HDL-cholesterol were similar.

In contrast, Cauley et al.[98] noted no changes in HDL-cholesterol levels after a 2-year exercise training program utilizing approximately the same training volume as the low intensity group described by King et al.[107] The baseline HDL-cholesterol levels of the women in this study were also substantially higher than those reported by King et al. (62 vs. 55 mg/dl, respectively).[107]

Collectively, the findings of the exercise training studies suggest that relatively low HDL-cholesterol levels may be more amenable to exercise-induced changes in women.

■ A DOSE-RESPONSE RELATIONSHIP

The findings of most studies support the existence of a dose-response relationship between exercise and HDL-cholesterol. In a study of 2,906 middle-aged men, researchers observed a progressive increase in HDL-cholesterol levels, in a dose-response fashion as weekly distance increased.[80] The observed increase was about 0.308 mg/dl in HDL-cholesterol per mile, evident at the lowest mileage group running 3 to 6 miles per week and progressing to the highest mileage group running 21 to 60 miles per week (see Figure 10.4). Similar findings were reported in the National Runners' Health Study of 7,059 men and 1,837 women recreational runners.[108] HDL-cholesterol levels were progressive and significantly higher for every 10-mile incremental increase in weekly mileage up to approximately 50 miles per week.[108] Only one study reported no further improvements in HDL-cholesterol beyond the perceived exercise intensity threshold of 6 METs.[102] An inverse relationship is observed when the ratio of total cholesterol to HDL-C is considered (**Figure 10.5**).

Unfortunately, there is no longitudinal evidence for a dose-response relationship in women. Only limited epidemiologic evidence supports the existence of a dose-response relationship between exercise and HDL-cholesterol levels. Williams et al.[109] reported that weekly running distance was positively related to HDL-cholesterol levels in women. In another study, running distance was more strongly related to HDL-cholesterol than run-ning velocity, suggesting that training volume is a more important contributor to HDL-cholesterol levels than training intensity.[108] Running distance also appears to be related to HDL-cholesterol levels independent of confounding factors such as diet, alcohol intake, and body weight. A positive correlation between training volume and HDL-cholesterol levels has also been reported.[52] Finally, menopausal status does not appear to influence the dose-response relationship.[109]

Author's Note

- The exercise-induced favorable changes in HDL-cholesterol metabolism are likely the result of an interaction between the exercise components of intensity, frequency, duration of each exercise session, and the length of the exercise training period. This interaction between these components comprises an exercise volume.

- Although a threshold for these four exercise components is likely to exist, it is more practical to view changes in HDL-cholesterol as the result of an exercise volume threshold.

Figure 10.5 Total cholesterol to HDL-cholesterol ratio changes according to the weekly distance run.

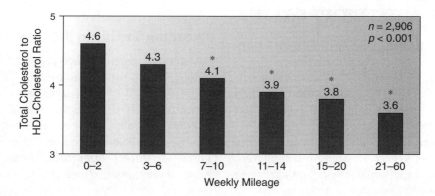

Source: Adapted from Kokkinos P, et al. *Arch Intern Med* 1995; 155:415–420.

- The amount of exercise necessary for favorable HDL-cholesterol changes (exercise volume threshold) appears to be between 7 to 14 miles per week of jogging/running at moderate exercise intensities of approximately 12 minutes per mile. This exercise level is equivalent to approximately 1,200 to 1,600 kcal/week. The expected increase in HDL-cholesterol levels for the aforementioned exercise volume is approximately 7% to 11%.

- It is reasonable to assume that any aerobic activity that meets or exceeds these levels of caloric expenditure and physical demand will result in similar increases in HDL-cholesterol levels.

- The relationship between exercise and HDL-cholesterol levels is less defined in women. Physically fit or highly active women have higher HDL-cholesterol compared with their sedentary counterparts. The volume of exercise required to increase HDL-cholesterol levels in women appears to be substantially more than that required for men. However, the many other health benefits derived from increased physical activity should encourage women to participate in regular exercise regardless of the exercise effects on HDL-cholesterol levels.

■ STRENGTH TRAINING, LIPIDS, AND LIPOPROTEINS

In contrast to the extensive research on the effects of aerobic-type exercise, relatively few studies have examined the effects of strength-type training on lipoprotein-lipid profiles. Recently, however, a number of reports have addressed this topic. The recent surge of training studies resulted from a combination of the increased popularity of strength training and increased emphasis on the association between lipoprotein–lipid profiles and atherosclerosis.

An extensive review of the literature regarding these issues has been published.[110]

■ CROSS-SECTIONAL STUDIES

Epidemiologic studies indicating a low incidence of mortality from heart disease in men engaged in intense muscular activity[111,112] have led to a number of cross-sectional studies focusing on the association between strength training and lipoprotein–lipid profiles.[113–118] Some of these investigators concluded that strength trained athletes have a favorable lipoprotein–lipid profile,[115,117,118] while others reported profiles that were less favorable than those of endurance-trained athletes and/or sedentary controls.[113,114,116] These studies have been reviewed and criticized for lack of adequate controls for body fat, diet, and possible anabolic-androgenic steroid use.[110,117,119,120]

In summary, due to the lack of control for factors that influence lipoprotein–lipid profiles, the small number of subjects used in each study, and the usual limitations of cross-sectional studies, it is not possible to make any valid conclusions regarding the effects of strength training on lipoprotein–lipid profiles from these cross-sectional investigations.[110]

Exercise Training Studies

Several investigators have reported favorable changes in total cholesterol,[121,122] LDL-cholesterol,[121,123–125] and HDL-cholesterol concentrations[121–123,125,126] as a result of resistance exercise training. However, serious design flaws or inadequate control for variables known to affect lipoprotein metabolism in many of these studies make the results difficult to interpret. Others reported no changes in total cholesterol, LDL-cholesterol, and HDL-cholesterol levels.[126–129]

One of the hypotheses proposed by some authors was that changes in lipids and lipo-proteins can be induced by high-repetition–low-intensity resistance training performed with little rest between sets or stations (circuit weight training), designed to maintain a high heart rate throughout the exercise session. This hypothesis was based mainly on the assumption that this type of resistance training (a predominantly anaerobic activity) contains enough of an aerobic component to activate the aerobic pathways. Because aerobic exercise was shown to favorably change lipids and lipoproteins, the assumption was that such resistance training will accomplish similar results.

Researchers put this hypothesis to the test by designing a weight training study. Volunteers were randomly assigned to one of three groups: a high-repetition–low-resistance group; a high-resistance–low repetition group, or the control group. When several of the confounding factors were controlled, they observed no changes in any lipoprotein levels in middle-aged individuals at low and high risk for heart disease after 20 weeks of strength training.[128,129] Researchers thus concluded that resistance exercise training does not change lipid and lipoproteins concentrations in the blood. This is now the prevailing consensus among experts in the field.

Finally, increased physical activity or regimented exercises are likely to favorably change the lipoprotein–lipid profile of the participant. In addition to the lipids and lipoproteins, there are a number of enzymatic changes, lipoprotein sub-fractions, and apolipoproteins that have not been discussed in this chapter. For those who are interested, an extensive and highly recommended review that goes beyond this chapter is written by Durstine and Haskell.[130]

> Most study findings support that strength or resistance training has an insignificant effect on lipid and lipoprotein metabolism.

■ SUMMARY

- A direct, continuous, and graded relationship exists between cholesterol and heart disease. Based on the results of these studies, the expert panel of the NCEP set the standards for desirable blood cholesterol at < 200 mg/dl.
- High blood concentrations of LDL-cholesterol are directly related to CHD. Conversely, high HDL-cholesterol concentrations are inversely related to CHD.
- Recent data support that high blood triglyceride concentrations are directly and independently related to CHD. Their prognostic value for predicting CHD is strengthened when used in combination with HDL-cholesterol and LDL-cholesterol.
- Aerobic exercise training or habitual physical activity of adequate duration, intensity, and volume favorably changes lipid and lipoprotein blood concentrations.
- Most of the increases in HDL-cholesterol occur at the weekly distance of 7 to 14 miles at moderate exercise intensities of approximately 12 minutes per mile. This exercise level is equivalent to approximately 1,200 to 1,600 kcal/week. Additional changes can be realized with greater weekly distances.
- It is reasonable to assume that any aerobic activity that meets or exceeds these levels of caloric expenditure and physical demand will result in similar increases in HDL-cholesterol levels.

- Exercise-induced favorable changes in HDL-cholesterol metabolism are the result of the interaction between the exercise components of intensity, frequency, duration of each exercise session, and length of the exercise training period. This interaction between these components comprises an exercise volume threshold. It is likely that changes in HDL-cholesterol are realized when this exercise volume threshold is achieved or surpassed.
- Resistance exercise training or weight training does not change lipid and lipoproteins concentrations in the blood.

■ REFERENCES

1. The Pooling Project Research Group. Relationship of blood pressure, serum cholesterol, smoking habit, relative weight and ECG abnormalities to incidence of major coronary events: final report of the pooling project. *J Chronic Dis* 1978;31(4):201–306.
2. Kannel WB, Castelli WP, Gordon T, McNamara PM. Serum cholesterol, lipoproteins, and the risk of coronary heart disease. The Framingham study. *Ann Intern Med* 1971; 74(1):1–12.
3. Chapman JM, Goerke LS, Dixon W, et al. Measuring the risk of coronary heart disease in adult population groups. The clinical status of a population group in Los Angeles under observation for two to three years. *Am J Public Health Nations Health* 1957; 47(4 Pt 2):33-42.
4. Keys A, Kimura N, Kusukawa, et al. Lessons from serum cholesterol studies in Japan, Hawaii and Los Angeles. *Ann Intern Med* 1958;48(1):83–94.
5. Keys A, Taylor HL, Blackburn H, et al. Coronary heart disease among Minnesota business and professional men followed fifteen years. *Circulation* 1963;28:381–395.
6. Paul O, Lepper MH, Phelae WH, et al. A longitudinal study of coronary heart disease. *Circulation* 1963;28:20–31.
7. Morris JN, Heady JA, Raffle PAB, et al. Coronary heart disease and physical activity of work. *Lancet* 1953;265(6796):1111–1120.
8. Goldbourt U, Holtzman E, Neufeld HN. Total and high density lipoprotein cholesterol in the serum and risk of mortality: evidence of a threshold effect. *Br Med J (Clin Res Ed)* 1985;290(6477):1239–1243.
9. Stamler J, Wentworth D, Neaton JD. The Multiple Risk Factor Intervention Trial (MRFIT)—important then and now. *JAMA* 2008;300(11):1343–1345.
10. Stamler J, Wentworth D, Neaton JD. Is the relationship between serum cholesterol and risk of premature death from coronary heart disease continuous and graded? Findings in 356,222 primary screenees of the Multiple Risk Factor Intervention Trial (MRFIT). *JAMA* 1986;256(20):2823–2828.
11. Executive Summary of the Third Report of the National Cholesterol Education Program (NCEP) Expert Panel on Detection, Evaluation, and Treatment of High Blood Cholesterol in Adults (Adult Treatment Panel III). *JAMA* 2001;285(19):2486–2497.
12. Brown MS, Goldstein JL. Receptor-mediated control of cholesterol metabolism. *Science* 1976;191(4223):150–154.
13. Brown MS, Goldstein JL. How LDL receptors influence cholesterol and atherosclerosis. *Sci Am* 1984;251(5):58–66.
14. Goldstein JL, Brown MS. Atherosclerosis: the low-density lipoprotein receptor hypothesis. *Metabolism* 1977;26(11):1257–1275.
15. Goldstein JL, Brown MS. The low-density lipoprotein pathway and its relation to atherosclerosis. *Annu Rev Biochem* 1977;46: 897–930.
16. Goldstein JL, Kita T, Brown MS. Defective lipoprotein receptors and atherosclerosis. Lessons from an animal counterpart of familial hypercholesterolemia. *N Engl J Med* 1983;309(5):288–296.
17. The Lipid Research Clinics Coronary Primary Prevention Trial results. I. Reduction

in incidence of coronary heart disease. *JAMA* 1984;251(3):351–364.

18. The Lipid Research Clinics Coronary Primary Prevention Trial results. II. The relationship of reduction in incidence of coronary heart disease to cholesterol lowering. *JAMA* 1984;251(3):365–374.

19. Manninen V, Tenkanen L, Koskinen P, et al. Joint effects of serum triglyceride and LDL cholesterol and HDL cholesterol concentrations on coronary heart disease risk in the Helsinki Heart Study. Implications for treatment. *Circulation* 1992;85:37–45.

20. Glynn RJ, Rosner B, Silbert JE. Changes in cholesterol and triglyceride as predictors of ischemic heart disease in men. *Circulation* 1982;66:724–731.

21. Austin MA. Plasma triglyceride as a risk factor for coronary heart disease. The epidemiologic evidence and beyond. *Am J Epidemiol* 1989;129(2):249–259.

22. Hokanson JE, Austin MA. Plasma triglyceride level is a risk factor for cardiovascular disease independent of high-density lipoprotein cholesterol level: a meta-analysis of population-based prospective studies. *J Cardiovas Risk* 1996;3:213–219.

23. Salonen T, Puska P. Relation of serum cholesterol and triglycerides to the risk of acute myocardial infarction, cerebral stroke and death in eastern Finnish male population. *Int J Epidemiol* 1983;12:26–31.

24. Cambien F, Jacqueson A, Richard JL, et al. Is the level of serum triglyceride a significant predictor of coronary death in "normocholesterolemic" subjects? The Paris Prospective Study. *Am J Epidemiol* 1986;124:624–632.

25. Pocock SJ, Shaper AG, Phillips AN. Concentration of high density lipoprotein cholesterol, triglycerides and total cholesterol in ischemic heart disease. *BMJ* 1989;298:988–1002.

26. Criqui MH, Heiss G, Cohn R, et al. Plasma triglyceride level and mortality from coronary heart disease. *N Engl J Med* 1993;328:1220–1225.

27. Assmann G, Schulte H. Relation of high-density lipoprotein cholesterol and triglycerides to incidence of atherosclerotic coronary artery disease (the PROCAM experience). *Am J Cardiol* 1992;70:733–737.

28. Wilson PWF, Larson MG, Castelli WP. Triglycerides, HDL cholesterol and coronary heart disease: a Framingham update on their interrelations. *Can J Cardiol* 1994;10(Suppl B): 5B–9B.

29. Barr DP, Russ EM, Eder HA. Protein-lipid relationships in human plasma. II. In atherosclerosis and related conditions. *Am J Med* 1951;11(4):480–493.

30. Miller GJ, Miller NE. Plasma-high-density-lipoprotein concentration and development of ischaemic heart-disease. *Lancet* 1975; 1(7897):16–19.

31. Glomset JA. Physiological role of lecithin-cholesterol acyltransferase. *Am J Clin Nutr* 1970;23(8):1129–1136.

32. Castelli WP, Doyle JT, Gordon T, et al. HDL cholesterol and other lipids in coronary heart disease. The cooperative lipoprotein phenotyping study. *Circulation* 1977;55(5): 767–772.

33. Gordon T, Castelli WP, Hjortland MC, et al. High density lipoprotein as a protective factor against coronary heart disease. The Framingham Study. *Am J Med* 1977;62(5): 707–714.

34. Kannel WB. High-density lipoproteins: epidemiologic profile and risks of coronary artery disease. *Am J Cardiol* 1983;52(4): 9B–12B.

35. Frick MH, Elo O, Haapa K, et al. Helsinki Heart Study: primary-prevention trial with gemfibrozil in middle-aged men with dyslipidemia. Safety of treatment, changes in risk factors, and incidence of coronary heart disease. *N Engl J Med* 1987;317(20): 1237–1245.

36. Castelli WP, Garrison RJ, Wilson PW, et al. Incidence of coronary heart disease and lipoprotein cholesterol levels. The Framingham Study. *JAMA* 1986;256(20):2835–2838.

37. Ehnholm C, Huttunen JK, Pietinen P, et al. Effect of a diet low in saturated fatty acids on plasma lipids, lipoproteins, and HDL subfractions. *Arteriosclerosis* 1984;4(3):265–269.

38. Ehnholm C, Huttunen JK, Pietinen P, et al. Effect of diet on serum lipoproteins in a population with a high risk of coronary heart disease. *N Engl J Med* 1982;307(14):850–855.

39. Jenkins DJ, Wolever TM, Rao AV, et al. Effect on blood lipids of very high intakes of fiber in diets low in saturated fat and cholesterol. *N Engl J Med* 1993;329(1):21–26.

40. Mensink RP, Katan MB. Effect of monounsaturated fatty acids versus complex carbohydrates on high-density lipoproteins in healthy men and women. *Lancet* 1987;1 (8525):122–125.

41. Mattson FH, Grundy SM. Comparison of effects of dietary saturated, monounsaturated, and polyunsaturated fatty acids on plasma lipids and lipoproteins in man. *J Lipid Res* 1985;26(2):194–202.

42. Grundy SM. Comparison of monounsaturated fatty acids and carbohydrates for lowering plasma cholesterol. *N Engl J Med* 1986; 314(12):745–748.

43. Schaefer EJ, Levy RI, Ernst ND, et al. The effects of low cholesterol, high polyunsaturated fat, and low fat diets on plasma lipid and lipoprotein cholesterol levels in normal and hypercholesterolemic subjects. *Am J Clin Nutr* 1981;34(9):1758–1763.

44. Paffenbarger RS, Hale WE. Work activity and coronary heart mortality. *N Engl J Med* 1975;292(11):545–550.

45. Paffenbarger RS Jr, Hale WE. Work activity of longshoremen as related to death from coronary heart disease and stroke. *N Engl J Med* 1970;282(20):1109–1114.

46. Cooper KH, Pollock ML, Martin RP, et al. Physical fitness levels vs. selected coronary risk factors. A cross-sectional study. *JAMA* 1976;236(2):166–169.

47. Hartung GH, Foreyt JP, Mitchell RE, et al. Relation of diet to high-density-lipoprotein cholesterol in middle-aged marathon runners, joggers, and inactive men. *N Engl J Med* 1980;302(7):357–361.

48. Malaspina JP, Bussiere H, Le Calve G. The total cholesterol/HDL cholesterol ratio: a suitable atherogenesis index. *Atherosclerosis* 1981;40(3-4):373–375.

49. Wood PD, Haskell W, Klein H, et al. The distribution of plasma lipoproteins in middle-aged male runners. *Metabolism* 1976;25(11): 1249–1257.

50. Adner MM, Castelli WP. Elevated high-density lipoprotein levels in marathon runners. *JAMA* 1980;243(6):534–536.

51. Tsopanakis C, Kotsarellis D, Tsopanakis AD. Lipoprotein and lipid profiles of elite athletes in Olympic sports. *Int J Sports Med* 1986;7(6):316–321.

52. Durstine JL, et al. Lipid, lipoprotein, and iron status of elite women distance runners. *Int J Sports Med* 1987;8(Suppl 2):119–123.

53. Enger SC, Stromme SB, Refsum HE. High density lipoprotein cholesterol, total cholesterol and triglycerides in serum after a single exposure to prolonged heavy exercise. *Scand J Clin Lab Invest* 1980;40(4): 341–345.

54. Hagan RD, Smith MG, Gettman LR. High density lipoprotein cholesterol in relation to food consumption and running distance. *Prev Med* 1983;12(2):287–295.

55. Hurter R, Peyman MA, Swale J, et al. Some immediate and long-term effects of exercise on the plasma-lipids. *Lancet* 1972;2(7779): 671–674.

56. Lehtonen A, Viikari V. The effect of vigorous physical activity at work on serum lipids with a special reference to serum high-density lipoprotein cholesterol. *Acta Physiol Scand* 1978;104(1):117–121.

57. Lehtonen A, Viikari J. Serum triglycerides and cholesterol and serum high-density lipoprotein cholesterol in highly physically active men. *Acta Med Scand* 1978;204(1–2): 111–114.

58. Martin RP, Haskell WL, Wood PD. Blood chemistry and lipid profiles of elite distance runners. *Ann NY Acad Sci* 1977;301: 346–360.

59. Thompson PD, Cullinane EM, Sady SP, et al. High density lipoprotein metabolism in endurance athletes and sedentary men. *Circulation* 1991;84(1):140–152.

60. Vodak PA, Wood PD, Haskell WL, Williams PT. HDL-cholesterol and other plasma lipid

and lipoprotein concentrations in middle-aged male and female tennis players. *Metabolism* 1980;29(8):745–752.

61. Huttunen JK, Laslinies E, Voutilainen E, et al. Effect of moderate physical exercise on serum lipoproteins. A controlled clinical trial with special reference to serum high-density lipoproteins. *Circulation* 1979;60(6):1220–1229.

62. Lopez A, Vial R, Balart L, Arroyave G. Effect of exercise and physical fitness on serum lipids and lipoproteins. *Atherosclerosis* 1974;20(1):1–9.

63. Thompson PD, Cullinane EM, Spady SP, et al. Modest changes in high-density lipoprotein concentration and metabolism with prolonged exercise training. *Circulation* 1988;78(1):25–34.

64. Wood PD, Stefanick ML, Williams PT, Haskell WL. The effects on plasma lipoproteins of a prudent weight-reducing diet, with or without exercise, in overweight men and women. *N Engl J Med* 1991;325(7):461–466.

65. LaRosa JC, Cleary P, Muesing RA, et al. Effect of long-term moderate physical exercise on plasma lipoproteins. The National Exercise and Heart Disease Project. *Arch Intern Med* 1982;142(13):2269–2274.

66. Gyntelberg F, Brennan R, Holloszy JO, et al. Plasma triglyceride lowering by exercise despite increased food intake in patients with type IV hyperlipoproteinemia. *Am J Clin Nutr* 1977;30(5):716–720.

67. Moore RA, Penfold WA, Simpson RD, et al. High-density lipoprotein, lipid, and carbohydrate metabolism during increasing fitness. *Ann Clin Biochem* 1979;16(2):76–80.

68. Sutherland WH, Woodhouse SP. Physical activity and plasma lipoprotein lipid concentrations in men. *Atherosclerosis* 1980;37(2):285–292.

69. Williams PT, Krauss RM, Wood PD, et al. Lipoprotein subfractions of runners and sedentary men. *Metabolism* 1986;35(1):45–52.

70. Haskell WL, Taylor HL, Wood PD, et al. Strenuous physical activity, treadmill exercise test performance and plasma high-density lipoprotein cholesterol. The Lipid Research Clinics Program Prevalence Study. *Circulation* 1980;62(4 Pt 2):IV53–IV61.

71. Brownell KD, Bachorik PS, Ayerle PS. Changes in plasma lipid and lipoprotein levels in men and women after a program of moderate exercise. *Circulation* 1982;65(3):477–484.

72. Desprès JP, Moorjani S, Tremblay A, et al. Heredity and changes in plasma lipids and lipoproteins after short-term exercise training in men. *Arteriosclerosis* 1988;8(4):402–409.

73. Wood PD, Stefanick ML, Dreon DM, et al. Changes in plasma lipids and lipoproteins in overweight men during weight loss through dieting as compared with exercise. *N Engl J Med* 1988;319(18):1173–1179.

74. Wood PD, Haskell WL, Blair SN, et al. Increased exercise level and plasma lipoprotein concentrations: a one-year, randomized, controlled study in sedentary, middle-aged men. *Metabolism* 1983;32(1):31–39.

75. Sopko G, Leon AS, Jacobs DR Jr, et al. The effects of exercise and weight loss on plasma lipids in young obese men. *Metabolism* 1985;34(3):227–236.

76. Stein RA, Michielli DW, Glantz MD, et al. Effects of different exercise training intensities on lipoprotein cholesterol fractions in healthy middle-aged men. *Am Heart J* 1990;119(2 Pt 1):277–283.

77. Altekruse EB, Wilmore JH. Changes in blood chemistries following a controlled exercise program. *J Occup Med* 1973;15(2):110–113.

78. Tran ZV, Weltman A, Glass GV, Mood DP. The effects of exercise on blood lipids and lipoproteins: a meta-analysis of studies. *Med Sci Sports Exerc* 1983;15(5):393–402.

79. Brunner D, Weisbort J, Meshulam N, et al. Relation of serum total cholesterol and high-density lipoprotein cholesterol percentage to the incidence of definite coronary events: twenty-year follow-up of the Donolo-Tel Aviv Prospective Coronary Artery Disease Study. *Am J Cardiol* 1987;59(15):1271–1276.

80. Gordon DJ, Probstfield JL, Garrison RJ, et al. High-density lipoprotein cholesterol and

cardiovascular disease. Four prospective American studies. *Circulation* 1989;79(1): 8–15.

81. Kokkinos PF, Holland JC, Narayan P, et al. Miles run per week and high-density lipoprotein cholesterol levels in healthy, middle-aged men. A dose-response relationship. *Arch Intern Med* 1995;155(4):415–420.

82. Lakka TA, Salonen JT. Physical activity and serum lipids: a cross-sectional population study in eastern Finnish men. *Am J Epidemiol* 1992;136(7):806–818.

83. LaPorte RE, Brenes G, Dearwater S, et al. HDL cholesterol across a spectrum of physical activity from quadriplegia to marathon running. *Lancet* 1983;1(8335):1212–1213.

84. Farrell PA, Barboriak J. The time course of alterations in plasma lipid and lipoprotein concentrations during eight weeks of endurance training. *Atherosclerosis* 1980; 37(2):231–238.

85. Kavanagh T, Shephard RJ, Lindley W, Pieper M. Influence of exercise and lifestyle variables upon high density lipoprotein cholesterol after myocardial infarction. *Arteriosclerosis* 1983;3(3):249–259.

86. Kokkinos PF, Fernhall B. Physical activity and high density lipoprotein cholesterol levels: what is the relationship? *Sports Med* 1999;28(5):307–314.

87. Drygas W, Jegler A, Kunski H. Study on threshold dose of physical activity in coronary heart disease prevention. Part I. Relationship between leisure time physical activity and coronary risk factors. *Int J Sports Med* 1988;9(4):275–278.

88. Williams PT, Wood PD, Haskell WL, Vranizan K. The effects of running mileage and duration on plasma lipoprotein levels. *JAMA* 1982;247(19):2674–2679.

89. Kraus WE, Houmard JA, Duscha BD, et al. Effects of the amount and intensity of exercise on plasma lipoproteins. *N Engl J Med* 2002;347(19):1483–1492.

90. Kokkinos PF, Holland JC, Pittaras AE, et al. Cardiorespiratory fitness and coronary heart disease risk factor association in women. *J Am Coll Cardiol* 1995;26(2):358–364.

91. Eaton CB, Lapane KL, Garber CE, et al. Physical activity, physical fitness, and coronary heart disease risk factors. *Med Sci Sports Exerc* 1995;27(3):340–346.

92. Gibbons LW, Blair SN, Cooper KH, Smith M. Association between coronary heart disease risk factors and physical fitness in healthy adult women. *Circulation* 1983;67(5):9 77–983.

93. Hartung GH, Reeves RJ, Foreyt JP, et al. Effect of alcohol intake and exercise on plasma high-density lipoprotein cholesterol subfractions and apolipoprotein A-I in women. *Am J Cardiol* 1986;58(1):148–151.

94. Upton SJ, Hagan RD, Lease P, et al. Comparative physiological profiles among young and middle-aged female distance runners. *Med Sci Sports Exerc* 1984;16(1):67–71.

95. Frey MA, Doerr BM, Laubach CL, et al. Exercise does not change high-density lipoprotein cholesterol in women after ten weeks of training. *Metabolism* 1982;31(11):1142–1146.

96. Moll ME, Williams RS, Lester RM, et al. Cholesterol metabolism in non-obese women: failure of physical conditioning to alter levels of high density lipoprotein cholesterol. *Atherosclerosis* 1979;34(2):159–166.

97. Shephard RJ, Youldon PE, Cox M, West C. Effects of a 6-month industrial fitness program on serum lipid concentrations. *Atherosclerosis* 1980;35(3):277–286.

98. Cauley JA, Kriska AM, LaPorte RE, et al. A two year randomized exercise trial in older women: effects on HDL-cholesterol. *Atherosclerosis* 1987;66(3):247–258.

99. Klebanoff R, Miller VT, Fernhall B. Effects of exercise and estrogen therapy on lipid profiles of postmenopausal women. *Med Sci Sports Exerc* 1998;30(7):1028–1034.

100. Lindheim SR, Notelovitz M, Feldman EB, et al. The independent effects of exercise and estrogen on lipids and lipoproteins in postmenopausal women. *Obstet Gynecol* 1994; 83(2):167–172.

101. Binder EF, Birge SJ, Kohrt WM. Effects of endurance exercise and hormone replacement therapy on serum lipids in older women. *J Am Geriatr Soc* 1996;44(3):231–236.

102. Leclerc S, Allard C, Talbot J, et al. High density lipoprotein cholesterol, habitual physical activity and physical fitness. *Atherosclerosis* 1985;57(1):43–51.

103. Kokkinos PF, Narayan P, Colleran J, et al. Effects of moderate intensity exercise on serum lipids in African-American men with severe systemic hypertension. *Am J Cardiol* 1998;81(6):732–735.

104. Myhre K, Mjøs OD, Bjørsvik G, Strømme SB. Relationship of high density lipoprotein cholesterol concentration to the duration and intensity of endurance training. *Scand J Clin Lab Invest* 1981;41(3):303–309.

105. Duncan JJ, Gordon NF, Scott CB. Women walking for health and fitness. How much is enough? *JAMA* 1991;266(23):3295–3299.

106. Santiago MC, Leon AS, Serfass RC. Failure of 40 weeks of brisk walking to alter blood lipids in normolipemic women. *Can J Appl Physiol* 1995;20(4):417–428.

107. King AC, Haskell WL, Young DR, et al. Long-term effects of varying intensities and formats of physical activity on participation rates, fitness, and lipoproteins in men and women aged 50 to 65 years. *Circulation* 1995;91(10):2596–2604.

108. Williams PT. Relationships of heart disease risk factors to exercise quantity and intensity. *Arch Intern Med* 1998;158(3):237–245.

109. Williams PT. High-density lipoprotein cholesterol and other risk factors for coronary heart disease in female runners. *N Engl J Med* 1996;334(20):1298–1303.

110. Kokkinos PF, Hurley BF. Strength training and lipoprotein-lipid profiles. A critical analysis and recommendations for further study. *Sports Med* 1990;9(5):266–272.

111. Paffenbarger RS, Hale WE. Work activity and coronary heart mortality. *N Engl J Med* 1975;292(11):545–550.

112. Paffenbarger RS Jr, Laughlin ME, Gima AS, Black RA. Work activity of longshoremen as related to death from coronary heart disease and stroke. *N Engl J Med* 1970;282(20):1109–114.

113. Clarkson PM, Hintermister R, Fillyaw M, Stylos L. High density lipoprotein cholesterol in young adult weight lifters, runners and untrained subjects. *Hum Biol* 1981;53(2):251–257.

114. Farrell PA, Maksud MG, Pollock ML, et al. A comparison of plasma cholesterol, triglycerides, and high density lipoprotein-cholesterol in speed skaters, weightlifters and non-athletes. *Eur J Appl Physiol Occup Physiol* 1982;48(1):77–82.

115. Cuppers HJ, Erdmann D, Schubert H, et al. Glucose tolerance, serum insulin, and serum lipids in athletes. *Curr Probl Clin Biochem* 1982;11:155–165.

116. Berg A, Ringwald G, Deus B, et al. Physical performance and serum cholesterol fractions in healthy young men. *Clin Chim Acta* 1980;106(3):325–330.

117. Hurley BF, Seals DR, Hagberg JM, et al. High-density-lipoprotein cholesterol in body-builders vs. powerlifters. Negative effects of androgen use. *JAMA* 1984;252(4):507–513.

118. Yki-Jarvinen H, Koivisto VA, Taskinen MR, Nikkila E. Glucose tolerance, plasma lipoproteins and tissue lipoprotein lipase activities in body builders. *Eur J Appl Physiol Occup Physiol* 1984;53(3):253–259.

119. Stone MH, Wilson GD. Resistive training and selected effects. *Med Clin N Am* 1985;69(1):109–122.

120. Fang CL, Sherman WM, Crouse SF, Tolson H. Exercise modality and selected coronary risk factors: a multivariate approach. *Med Sci Sports Exerc* 1988;20(5):455–462.

121. Johnson CC, Stone MH, Lopez SA, et al. Diet and exercise in middle-aged men. *J Am Diet Assoc* 1982;81(6):695–701.

122. Weltman A, Janny C, Rians CB, et al. The effects of hydraulic-resistance strength training on serum lipid levels in prepubertal boys. *Am J Dis Child* 1987;141(7):777–780.

123. Fripp RR, Hodgson JL. Effect of resistive training on plasma lipid and lipoprotein levels in male adolescents. *J Pediatr* 1987;111(6 Pt 1):926–931.

124. Goldberg L, Elliot DL, Schutz RW, et al. Changes in lipid and lipoprotein levels after weight training. *JAMA* 1984;252(4):504–506.

125. Ullrich IH, Reid CM, Yeater RA. Increased HDL-cholesterol levels with a weight lifting program. *South Med J* 1987;80(3):328–331.

126. Hurley BF, et al. Resistive training can reduce coronary risk factors without altering $\dot{V}O_2$max or percent body fat. *Med Sci Sports Exerc* 1988;20(2):150–154.

127. Campbell DE. Influence of several physical activities on serum cholesterol concentrations in young men. *J Lipid Res* 1965;6(4): 478–480.

128. Kokkinos PF, Hurley BF, Vacaro P, et al. Effects of low- and high-repetition resistive training on lipoprotein-lipid profiles. *Med Sci Sports Exerc* 1988;20(1):50–54.

129. Kokkinos PF, Hurley BF, Smutok MA, et al. Strength training does not improve lipoprotein-lipid profiles in men at risk for CHD. *Med Sci Sports Exerc* 1991;23(10): 1134–1139.

130. Durstine JL, Haskell WL. Effects of exercise training on plasma lipids and lipoproteins. In JO Holloszy, ed. *Exercise and Sports Science Reviews*. Baltimore: Williams & Wilkins; 1994;22:477–521.

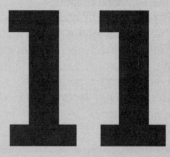
Diabetes Mellitus and Physical Activity

D iabetes mellitus is defined by the Expert Committee on the Diagnosis and Classification of Diabetes Mellitus as a group of metabolic diseases characterized by hyperglycemia (high concentrations of blood glucose) resulting from defects in insulin production, insulin action, or both.[1]

■ TYPES OF DIABETES

Two broad categories characterize diabetes: type 1 and type 2 diabetes.

Type 1 diabetes, formerly referred to as *insulin-dependent diabetes mellitus*, accounts for 5% to 10% of all diagnosed cases. Because type 1 diabetes typically occurs in children and adolescents, it also used to be termed *juvenile diabetes*. This autoimmune disease most often results from irreparable damage to the insulin-producing cells (beta cells) of the pancreas after antibody attacks.[2] It is characterized by an absolute deficiency of *insulin*, the hormone that regulates blood glucose.

Type 2 diabetes, formerly referred to as *non-insulin–dependent diabetes mellitus*, accounts

for about 90% to 95% of diagnosed diabetes cases. It usually appears in adults after the age of 40. The progression from a non-diabetic state to type 2 diabetes is likely the result of the complex interaction between genetic predisposition and environmental, dietary, and social influences.

In the pre-diabetic state, which is characterized by insulin resistance, the insulin signaling that leads to efficient transport of glucose across the cell membrane is diminished. Consequently, the amount of insulin required to transport a certain amount of glucose into the cells is increased, so the insulin levels in these individuals are elevated (**Figure 11.1**). As the degree of insulin resistance increases, the need for insulin also rises. Eventually, insulin secretion becomes defective and no longer adequate to compensate for the increased insulin resistance.[3]

■ PRE-DIABETES

Prior to the abnormally elevated fasting blood glucose levels that leads to the diagnosis of type 2 diabetes, most individuals exhibit subtle abnormalities in blood glucose and insulin concentrations, a condition known as the **pre-diabetes**.

These abnormalities include:

• Insulin resistance and elevated insulin levels known as *hyperinsulinemia*
• Impaired fasting glucose (IFG) or impaired glucose tolerance (IGT). Both IFG and IGT may coexist in some individuals.

Insulin Resistance

Insulin resistance is defined as a state in which insulin requirements for the efficient transport of a set amount of glucose across the

Figure 11.1 Insulin requirements for normal, pre-diabetic, and diabetic conditions. Note the gradual increase in insulin secretion in pre-diabetic states. This is a response by the system to compensate for the increased insulin resistance and maintain a constant amount of glucose uptake by the cells. In the diabetic state, beta cell exhaustion leads to reduced insulin secretion.

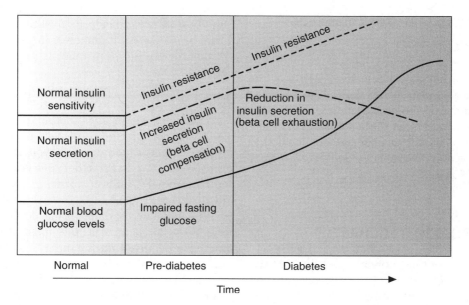

cell membrane are increased. To maintain a normal rate of blood glucose transport into the cell, higher levels of insulin are secreted, a condition known as **hyperinsulinemia**.

As stated previously, in the pre-diabetic state, insulin signaling leading to efficient glucose transport across the cell membrane (insulin sensitivity) is diminished. Stating it another way, insulin resistance increases. Consequently, the amount of insulin required to transport a certain amount of glucose into the cells is increased. To compensate for this, insulin secretion by the beta cells increases and insulin levels in these individuals are elevated (see Figure 11.1).

With the higher blood glucose levels observed in type 2 diabetes, intuitively you would think that insulin concentrations should also be higher. However, by the time a person develops type 2 diabetes, his or her insulin secretion has become inadequate. Approximately 50% of the beta cells lose their ability to produce insulin and this is enough to compensate for the insulin resistance.[3] With time, the progressive increase of resistance leads to a greater need for insulin. Gradually, the pancreas loses its ability to produce it and blood levels of insulin decline. Most of the individuals with type 2 diabetes are obese and obesity, at least in part, is responsible for some degree of insulin resistance.[4,5]

Impaired Fasting Glucose

Impaired Fasting Glucose is a condition in which the fasting blood glucose level is 100 to

125 milligrams per deciliter (mg/dl) after an overnight fast. The level is higher than the normal blood glucose levels of 70 to 99 mg/dl, but not high enough to be classified as diabetes.

Impaired Glucose Tolerance

Impaired Glucose Tolerance is a condition in which the blood glucose level is 140 to 199 mg/dl after a 2-hour oral glucose tolerance test. This level is also higher than normal but not high enough to be classified as diabetes. The risk for progression to diabetes among those with pre-diabetes is high but not inevitable. Diabetes and pre-diabetic conditions are summarized in **Table 11.1**.

■ EPIDEMIOLOGY

According to the National Institute of Diabetes and Digestive and Kidney Diseases approximately 20.8 million Americans have diabetes and about 30% are unaware of their diagnosis.[6] It is estimated that the total prevalence of diabetes in the United States will be double in 2050 when compared to the prevalence in 2005.[7] The increase in the prevalence among the youth is also alarming. In the last 10 years, the prevalence of type 2 diabetes has more than tripled in children as young as 10 years of age. Physical inactivity, improper diet habits, and obesity are the culprits for this increase.[8] The prevalence of diabetes in the United States for the different races is presented in **Figure 11.2**.

Similar trends are also observed worldwide. The prevalence of diabetes for all age groups worldwide was estimated to be 2.8% in 2000 and is projected to be 4.4% in 2030. The total number of people with type 2 diabetes for the next two to three decades is projected to rise from 171 million in 2000 to 366 million in 2030 (**Table 11.2**).[9]

The incidence of diabetes has doubled over the past 30 years but the most dramatic increase occurred during the 1990s. Most of the increase in absolute incidence of diabetes occurred in individuals with BMI $\geq$ 30 kg/m^2.[10] One and a half million new cases of diabetes were diagnosed in people age 20 or older in 2005,[6] most of them between the ages 40–59 years (**Figure 11.3**).

Table 11.1 Classification of Diabetes and Pre-Diabetic Conditions Based on Blood Glucose Levels

	Blood Glucose Levels
Normal	70–99 (mg/dl)
Pre-diabetes	
–Impaired fasting glucose (IFG)	100–125 mg/dl
–Impaired glucose tolerance (IGT)	140–199 mg/dl
Diabetes	> 125 mg/dl

Source: Report of the Expert Committee on the Diagnosis and Classification of Diabetes Mellitus. *Diabetes Care* 1998;21(7):S5–S19.

Figure 11.2 Prevalence of physician-diagnosed diabetes in adults aged 20 and older by race/ethnicity and sex.

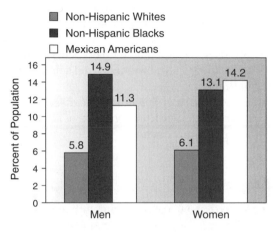

Source: NHANES: 2005–2006; NCHS and NHLBI; Lloyd–Jones, et al. *Circulation* 2009;119;e11–e161.

Figure 11.3 Estimated number of new cases of diagnosed diabetes in U.S. adults aged 20 years or older, by age group (2005).

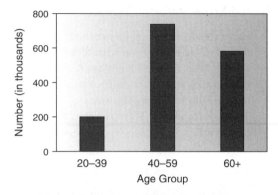

Source: From 2001–2003 National Health Interview Survey estimates projected to year 2005.

Diabetes was the sixth leading cause of death in 2002. According to U.S. death certificate reports, diabetes contributed to a total of 224,092 deaths. Overall, the risk for death among people with diabetes is about twice that of people without diabetes of similar age.

In 2007, the direct medical cost attributable to diabetes was $116 billion and indirect cost (disability, work loss, premature mortality) was $58 billion, for a total cost of $174 billion.[11]

■ COMPLICATIONS OF DIABETES IN THE UNITED STATES

The National Institute of Diabetes and Digestive and Kidney Diseases lists a number of co-morbidities attributed to diabetes that include but are not limited to heart disease and stroke, high blood pressure, blindness, kidney disease,

Table 11.2 Estimated Prevalence of Type 2 Diabetes

Year	Estimated Number of Cases in the United States	Estimated Number of Cases Worldwide
2,000	17.7 million	171 million
2,030	33.3 million	336 million

Source: Wild S, et al., Global prevalence of diabetes: estimates for the year 2000 and projections for 2030. *Diabetes Care* 2004;27(5):1047–1053.

nervous system disease, amputations, dental disease, and complications of pregnancy.[6]

Heart Disease and Stroke

- Heart disease and stroke account for about 65% of deaths in people with diabetes.
- Adults with diabetes have heart disease death rates about two to four times higher than adults without diabetes.
- The risk for stroke is two to four times higher among people with diabetes.

High Blood Pressure

- About 73% of adults with diabetes have blood pressure greater than or equal to 130/80 mm Hg or use prescription medications for hypertension.

Blindness

- Diabetes is the leading cause of new cases of blindness among adults aged 20 to 74 years.
- Diabetic retinopathy causes 12,000 to 24,000 new cases of blindness each year.

Kidney Disease

- Diabetes is the leading cause of kidney failure, accounting for 44% of new cases in 2002. During the same year, 44,400 people with diabetes began treatment for end-stage kidney disease and 153,730 people with end-stage kidney disease due to diabetes were living on chronic dialysis or with a kidney transplant.

Nervous System Disease

- About 60% to 70% of people with diabetes have mild to severe forms of nervous system damage. The results of such damage include impaired sensation or pain in the feet or hands, slowed digestion of food in the stomach, carpal tunnel syndrome, and other nerve problems.
- Almost 30% of people with diabetes aged 40 years or older have impaired sensation in the feet.
- Severe forms of diabetic nerve disease are a major contributing cause of lower-extremity amputations.

Amputations

- More than 60% of non-traumatic lower-limb amputations occur among people with diabetes.
- In 2002, about 82,000 non-traumatic lower-limb amputations were performed in people with diabetes.

Dental Disease

- Periodontal (gum) disease is more common in people with diabetes. Among young adults, those with diabetes have about twice the risk of those without diabetes.
- Almost one third of people with diabetes have severe periodontal diseases with loss of attachment of the gums to the teeth measuring 5 millimeters or more.

Complications of Pregnancy

- Poorly controlled diabetes before conception and during the first trimester of pregnancy can cause major birth defects in 5% to 10% of pregnancies and spontaneous abortions in 15% to 20%.

- Poorly controlled diabetes during the second and third trimesters of pregnancy can result in excessively large babies, posing a risk to both mother and child.

Other Complications

- Uncontrolled diabetes often leads to biochemical imbalances that can cause acute life-threatening events, such as diabetic ketoacidosis and coma.
- People with diabetes are more susceptible to many other illnesses and, once they acquire these illnesses, often have worse prognoses. For example, they are more likely to die with pneumonia or influenza than people who do not have diabetes.

■ PHYSIOLOGY AND PATHOPHYSIOLOGY OF DIABETES

Diabetes is characterized by the inadequacy or inability of the cells to utilize carbohydrates for their energy needs. More specifically, in diabetics, blood glucose cannot enter the cells to be used for their energy needs.

As mentioned in Chapter 4, once consumed, all carbohydrates are degraded to glucose, the simplest form of sugar. Glucose is an important source of energy for humans. This is especially true for certain tissues such as the brain that depend almost exclusively on glucose for energy requirements. Low blood glucose concentrations can cause serious complications and even death. Blood glucose concentrations thus are tightly controlled by the hormonal regulation of glucose uptake by the cells and glucose production by the liver.[12]

Muscle cells are the principal sites for glucose uptake. For glucose to be used by the cells, it must enter the cells. However, glucose cannot pass through the cell membrane; it must be "carried" into the cell by specific proteins known as **glucose-transporters**. For this to occur, insulin must be available. Insulin is required to activate the transporter GLUT-4, the primary transporter involved in the transport of glucose within muscle cells. In this process, insulin binds to the insulin receptors located on the cell membrane. In turn, GLUT-4 receptors, located within the cell, are sequestered to the membrane of the cell. Glucose binds with the receptors and transport into the cell increases (**Figure 11.4**).

Figure 11.4 Metabolic pathways for intramuscular glucose metabolism.

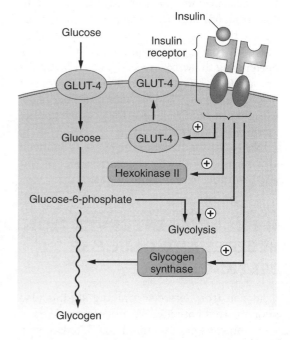

Source: From Perseghin G, et al. *N Engl J Med* 1996;1357–1356.

■ MECHANISM OF EXERCISE-INDUCED GLUCOSE UPTAKE

Exercise is a natural stimulus for increased glucose uptake by the working muscle cells via the **GLUT-4 transporter**. The mechanism that increases the translocation of the GLUT-4 receptors to the membrane does not depend on insulin (insulin-independent). Rather, GLUT-4 receptor translocation is activated by muscular contractions,[13] hypoxia,[14,15] nitric oxide,[16–18] bradykinin,[19,20] and increased concentrations of calcium.[21–23] Consequently, glucose transport into the cell increases several-fold (**Figure 11.5**).

This is in accord with the increased energy demand during physical activity or exercise. To meet the increased energy demand, glucose transport into the muscle cells increases. Nature thus has provided an ingenious way to make sure energy requirements of the muscles performing the work are met, even if insulin is not available (insulin secretion is suppressed during exercise). The activity itself becomes the stimulus and regulator for glucose uptake by the working cells.

Naturally, for diabetics the exercise-induced glucose uptake by the cell carries significant and favorable health implications.

■ EXERCISE INTERVENTION STUDIES AND GLUCOSE METABOLISM

Evidence from exercise training studies also supports that both aerobic and anaerobic exercises improve glucose uptake and insulin sensitivity after only a few weeks of training. Smutok et al.[24,25] randomly assigned middle-aged individuals with impaired glucose tolerance to 16 weeks of aerobic or anaerobic

Figure 11.5　Insulin and exercise signaling pathways that regulate glucose metabolism in muscle and fat cells. The exercise-induced translocation of GLUT-4 to the plasma membrane is independent of that for insulin.

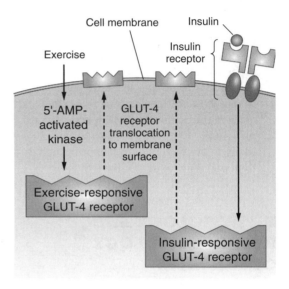

Source: From Shepherd PR, Kahn BB. Glucose transporters and insulin action—implications for insulin resistance and diabetes mellitus. *N Engl J Med* 1999;341(4):248–257.

(strength) exercise training. Baseline blood glucose and insulin levels were compared to those at the end of the exercise training period (16 weeks) following glucose ingestion during an oral glucose tolerance test. Individuals in the aerobic exercise group had significantly lower blood glucose and insulin concentrations at 90 and 120 minutes. The findings were even more impressive in the strength training group where blood glucose concentrations were significantly lower 30 minutes after glucose ingestion (**Figures 11.6** and **11.7**). In a similar study, Miller et al. reported strikingly similar and even more impressive findings after 16 weeks of

Figure 11.6 Blood glucose levels before and after 16 weeks of either aerobic or strength training following a glucose challenge.

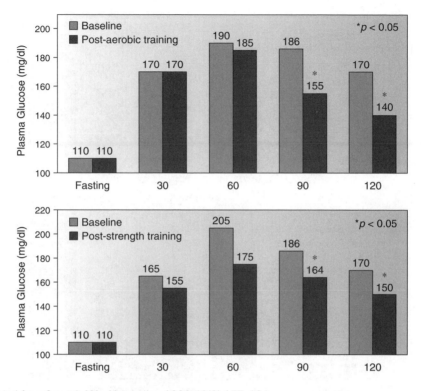

Source: Adapted from Smutok MA. *Metabolism* 1993;42(2):177–184.

strength training in older, healthy individuals. Blood glucose and insulin concentrations in this study were significantly lower following strength training at 30 minutes post glucose ingestion (**Figure 11.8**).[26] Others have reported significant reductions in both glucose and insulin concentrations after aerobic and strength exercise training.[27,28] Collectively, the findings of these studies support that, after exercise training, less insulin is required to dispose the same and even more blood glucose. In other words, both aerobic and strength training improve insulin sensitivity.

The findings that strength training improves glucose uptake suggest that exercise-induced changes in carbohydrate metabolism are independent of improvements in oxygen uptake.[26] These findings are in accord with the physiologic demands of the muscle performing an anaerobic task (weight training). During such tasks, the anaerobic pathways are challenged to meet the increased in energy demand of the working muscles. Accordingly, the body responds to improve anaerobic formation of ATP.

Both aerobic and strength training improve insulin sensitivity. Consequently, glucose uptake by the cells increases at lower insulin level.

Figure 11.7 Blood insulin levels before and after 16 weeks of aerobic or strength training following a glucose challenge.

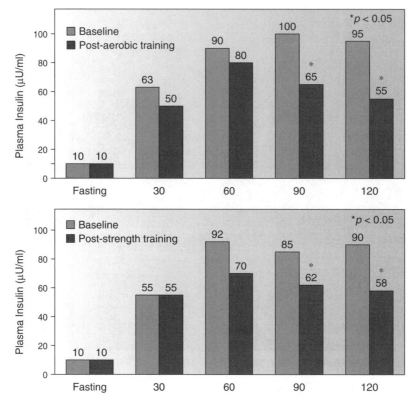

Source: Adapted from Smutok MA. *Metabolism* 1993;42(2):177–184.

Figure 11.8 Strength training and glucose metabolism.

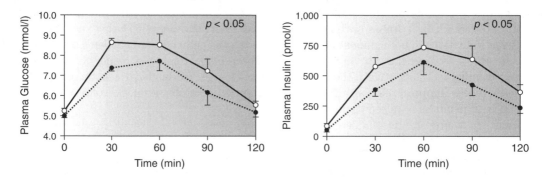

Source: Adapted from Miller JP, et al. *J Appl. Physiol* 1994;77(3):1122–1227.

■ EXERCISE AND DIABETES PREVENTION

In addition to its therapeutic effects, exercise has a more profound effect in the prevention of the disease. Strong evidence from large cohort studies supports the assertion that exercise and physical activity in general provide a highly effective way to delay or avert the development of type 2 diabetes. In addition, physical activity has been shown to reduce the risk of mortality in diabetics.

Leisure time physical activity expressed in kilocalories expended per week was associated with the development of type 2 diabetes in 5,990 men.[29] The main findings of the study as reported by the investigators are:

1. The incidence of diabetes was inversely related to weekly caloric expenditure.
2. The incidence rate declined as energy expenditure increased from less than 500 to 3,500 kcal.
3. There was a 6% reduction in the adjusted risk for developing diabetes for each 500-kcal increment in energy expenditure per week.

Similar findings were reported in 8,633 non-diabetic men during an average follow-up of 6 years. The low-fit group had a 1.9-fold increase in the risk for impaired fasting glucose and 3.7-fold increase in the risk for developing diabetes.[30,31] In the Physicians' Health Study, 21,271 male physicians age 40 to 84 years and free of diabetes, cardiovascular disease, and cancer at baseline were followed for an average of 5 years. The age-adjusted risk for developing diabetes was inversely related with increasing frequency of exercise per week. Those who exercised as little as one time per week had a 23% reduction in risk. The risk was 38% lower in those who exercised two to four times per week and 42% lower in those exercising five or more times per week. Controlling for additional coronary risk factors did not alter the findings substantially.[32]

To date, the largest study to assess the association between physical activity and the risk of diabetes is the Nurse's Health Study.[33] A total of 70,102 female nurses ages 40 to 65 years who did not have diabetes, heart disease, or cancer at baseline (1986) were followed for 8 years. Fitness categories were established based on the physical activity expressed as MET-hours per week. After adjusting for confounding factors, the investigators observed the following:

- An inverse and significant relationship between fitness and the relative risk for developing diabetes. The risk was significantly lower across all fitness categories.
- A dose-response relationship with greater volume of physical activity yielding more favorable (lower) risk for diabetes. The relative risk for diabetes was 23% lower for women with the physical activity score of 2.1 to 4.6 MET-hours per week (the category next to the lowest level of physical activity), when compared to the lowest category (**Table 11.3**).
- A dose-response relationship between the walking pace and the risk for diabetes. Faster pace yielded lower risk (**Table 11.4**).
- The intensity of the activity (walking pace of 20–30 minutes/mile) required to elicit health benefits is relatively low and attainable by most individuals. Even the higher pace of < 20 minutes per mile is attainable by most individuals.
- Equivalent energy expenditures from different activities and intensities confer similar health benefits.

Table 11.3 Percent Reduction in Relative Risk According to MET-Hours per Week

	MET-Hours per Week				
	0–2	2.1–4.6	4.7–10.4	10.5–21.7	≥ 21.8
Relative risk reduction as compared to group with 2 or less MET-Hours		23%	25%	38%	46%

Source: Hu FB, Sigal RJ, Rich-Edwards JW, et al. Walking compared with vigorous physical activity and risk of type 2 diabetes in women: a prospective study. *JAMA* 1999;282:1433–1439.

This is a unique study for two reasons. First, it provided much needed information on the association between diabetes and physical activity on women. Second, the large number of participants allowed the investigators to examine the association between exercise intensity (walking vs. more vigorous activities) and the risk for developing diabetes.

■ INTERVENTIONAL STUDIES

The epidemiologic findings of the aforementioned studies are supported by two interventional studies.[34,35] Tuomilehto and co-investigators randomly assigned 522 middle-aged, overweight men ($n = 172$) and women ($n = 350$) with impaired glucose tolerance to either the intervention group or control group. The intervention group was instructed to follow a healthy diet, reduce weight, and increase physical activity. They were followed for a mean period of 3.2 years.

At the end of the follow-up period, the cumulative incidence of diabetes was 11% for the intervention group and 23% in the control group. The risk for diabetes was reduced by 58% in the intervention group (**Figure 11.9**). The investigators concluded that the observed changes in the incidence of diabetes were the direct result of the implemented lifestyle modifications.[35]

In the Diabetes Prevention Program Research Group, the investigators randomly assigned 3,234 non-diabetic individuals with elevated fasting blood glucose levels to one of

Table 11.4 Percent Reduction in Relative Risk According to Walking Pace

	Walking Pace		
	> 30 min/mile	20–30 min/mile	< 20 min/mile
Relative risk reduction as compared to group walking at the pace of > 30 min/mile		28%	59%

Source: Hu FB, Sigal RJ, Rich-Edwards JW, et al. Walking compared with vigorous physical activity and risk of type 2 diabetes in women: a prospective study. *JAMA* 1999;282:1433–1439.

Figure 11.9   Incidence of diabetes during the follow-up period.

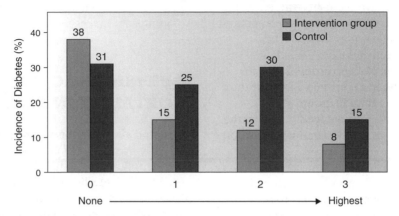

Source: Adapted from The Finnish Diabetes Prevention Study Group. *N Engl J Med* 2001;344(18): 1343–1350.

three groups: lifestyle-modification, metformin (one of the newest and most effective medications available to treat diabetes), and placebo. The lifestyle modification group included weight reduction of at least 7% of their initial body weight through a heart-healthy diet and engaging in moderate intensity physical activity (brisk walking) for at least 150 minutes per week. At the end of the follow-up period (2.8 years), investigators reported the following:

- Both the medication (metformin) and lifestyle interventions were equally effective in lowering blood glucose concentrations when compared to the placebo group (**Figure 11.10**).

Figure 11.10   Fasting blood glucose concentrations for the three groups in the Diabetes Prevention Program Research Group study.

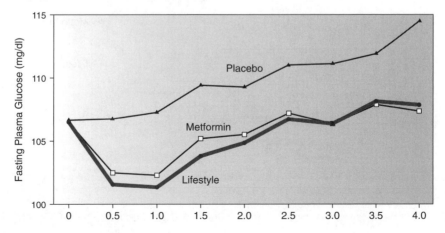

Source: Adapted from Diabetes Prevention Program Research Group. *N Engl J Med* 2002;346(6): 393–403.

- Both the medication and lifestyle interventions were effective in reducing the incidence of diabetes when compared to the placebo group (**Figure 11.11**).
- The estimated cumulative incidence was 28.9% for the placebo group, 21.7% for the medication group, and 14.4% for the lifestyle-intervention group.
- The incidence was reduced by 58% in the lifestyle group and 31% in the medication group.
- The lifestyle intervention was significantly more effective in preventing the incidence of diabetes than medication. To prevent one case of diabetes, the investigators calculated that 6.9 persons have to participate in the lifestyle-intervention group and 13.9 would have to receive medication.
- Finally, lifestyle intervention resulted in more participants maintaining normal blood glucose values over a period of 4 years than the medication or placebo groups.[34]

■ PHYSICAL ACTIVITY AND MORTALITY IN DIABETICS

The association of fitness and risk of all-cause mortality was assessed in 1,263 diabetic men in a 2-year follow-up study. After adjustment for age, baseline cardiovascular disease, fasting plasma glucose level, high cholesterol level, overweight, current smoking, high blood pressure, and parental history of cardiovascular disease, the mortality risk in physically unfit men was 2.1 times higher compared to their physically fit counterparts.[30]

In a similar study, physical activity was assessed every 2 years for a follow-up period of

Figure 11.11   Cumulative incidence of diabetes in the Diabetes Prevention Program Research Group study.

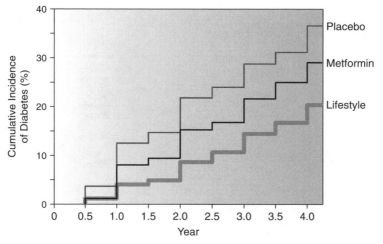

Source: Data from Diabetes Prevention Program Research Group. *N Engl J Med* 2002;346(6):393–403.

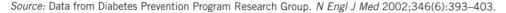

14 years in over 2,800 diabetic men. Physical activity quintiles were formed based on MET-hours per week, and the association of physical activity and mortality was assessed. The investigators reported an inverse association between physical activity and cardiovascular risk and mortality. Walking also was associated with decreased mortality. Walking pace predicted the risk of mortality independent from duration of walking. The maximum risk reduction for both cardiovascular risk and mortality was evident at the physical activity level of 12 to 21.7 MET-hours per week. This level of work is achievable by either 3 to 5 hours per week of brisk walking, 2 to 3 hours of jogging or 1 to 2 hours of running.

Similar findings were reported in a study of 5,125 diabetic women in the Nurses' Health Study.[36] Physically active women had significantly lower risk for cardiovascular events compared to physically inactive. A faster pace was independently associated with lower risk also.

Collectively, the findings of the two studies regarding walking pace strengthen the previous finding[33] that exercise intensity has an independent effect and perhaps confers additional health benefits.

The prevalence of diabetes is three- to four-fold higher in obese individuals compared to those of normal weight.[7] The association between cardiovascular mortality and fitness in obese diabetics is not well-defined. A recent study by Church et al. examined the association of exercise capacity (aerobic fitness) and cardiovascular mortality in diabetics with different body weight (normal, overweight and obese) in 2,316 diabetic men.[37]

The investigators concluded that low fitness was associated with increased risk for cardiovascular mortality in individuals with normal body weight as well as those characterized as overweight and obese. Considering the increased prevalence of obesity worldwide, this finding

has significant public health implications. It suggests that increased physical activity can yield health benefits for the diabetic individual regardless of body composition status.

■ EXERCISE GUIDELINES FOR THE DIABETIC PATIENT

Exercise for the diabetic patient must be carefully monitored. Exercise, diet, and insulin (if the patient is taking insulin) must interact precisely to bring the desired outcome. Because exercise has an insulin-like effect, hypoglycemia during and after exercise is the most common problem in diabetics who engage in physical activity. The problem is more common in diabetics who take insulin and less common in those on oral hypoglycemic agents. Excessive insulin or accelerated absorption of insulin from the ejection site both may cause hypoglycemia. It is also important to realize that hypoglycemia occurs not only during exercise, but also 4 to 6 hours following exercise.

Exercise and Type 1 Diabetes

As previously mentioned, exercise promotes glucose uptake by the working cells. Theoretically, patients with type 1 diabetes will require relatively less insulin to transport the same amount of glucose from the blood into the cells. Regular exercise therefore is likely to reduce the insulin requirements of patients with type 1 diabetes.

In addition to the reduction in insulin requirements for the exercising diabetic individual, regular exercise also leads to improved physical fitness of the individual. Consequently, the patient's sense of well-being and ability to cope with physical and psychological stresses that associated with the disease can be enhanced.

However, it is very important to understand that there is a strong interaction between exercise, diet, and insulin. When an optimum balance among these three factors is achieved, the diabetic patient can achieve optimum benefits. Of course, this is not easy. Each patient is different and each may have a different diet. Therefore, exercise must be tailored specifically for the individual patient. Furthermore, in certain conditions, exercise can be harmful and therefore should not be recommended. Because of the personalized exercise program that is required for such patients, only general guidelines for exercise can be addressed here. It also must be emphasized that the diabetic patient will be best served if he or she seeks professional help in developing a personalized program that will specifically meet their needs. Such programs must take into consideration the following:

1. Amount of insulin the individual is using
2. Individual's diet before and after exercise
3. Musculoskeletal and body weight limitations
4. Time of day the individual exercises
5. The type, intensity, and duration of exercise
6. Weather conditions during exercise
7. Access to exercise facilities
8. Co-morbidities

Weight Training Exercises and Diabetes

In addition to the aerobic exercises, diabetic patients can derive similar benefits in blood sugar control with weight training. It has been known for some time that any type of muscular work promotes glucose entry into the muscle cells.[22] All muscular contractions therefore will yield similar benefits when workloads are similar. This is especially good news for patients who cannot walk or jog. For these patients, weight training exercises are a viable alternative.

For patients who have little time to exercise or, for whatever reasons, cannot participate in a weight training program, push-ups, sit-ups, and hand grip exercises may be beneficial, especially when they are performed several times during the day. Putting it simply, any exercise is better than no exercise.

Although without a doubt exercise has many benefits to offer the type 1 diabetic individual, it is strongly recommended that these individuals work closely with their physician.

Exercise and Type 2 Diabetes

Type 2 diabetic patients who are not taking insulin can exercise without the concerns that type 1 diabetics must face. Exercise recommendations for the patient with type 2 diabetes are similar to those presented for patients with type 1 diabetes.

It should be kept in mind that the effects of exercise on glucose metabolism diminish after 24 to 48 hours. For this reason, it is advisable that diabetic patients perform some form of physical activity almost every day. However, sedentary individuals should not begin exercising 5 to 6 days a week initially. Instead, the duration, frequency, and intensity of the program should progress slowly and carefully until the individual can be physically active on most days of the week.

A good program will be one that challenges the leg muscles (walk or jog) and upper body (weight training) five to six times per week. Refraining from intense exercise training 1 to 2 days per week is recommended. However, it is also recommended that the diabetic patient engages in some physical activity on all days of the week.

One approach will be to engage in moderate intensity exercise 3 to 5 days a week and slow walk or gardening the other days. Another approach will be mixing the activities. One can engage in weight training for the upper body twice a week and aerobic activity involving the legs three times week. This is possible because weight training is equally beneficial. As mentioned before, in studies comparing the benefits of weight training and jogging, patients with abnormally high blood sugar levels benefited similarly from weight training and jogging.[25,26,38]

■ THE METABOLIC SYNDROME

The **metabolic syndrome** refers to a cluster of specific cardiovascular disease risk factors that include high blood pressure, elevated triglycerides, low levels of high-density lipoprotein (HDL), impaired fasting glucose, and excess abdominal fat. Insulin resistance is thought to be the underlying pathophysiology.[39] The metabolic syndrome thus is also called the *insulin resistance syndrome*.

The biologic mechanisms at the molecular level between insulin resistance and metabolic risk factors are not yet fully understood and appear to be complex. However, it is known that some of the underlying causes of this syndrome are overweight or obesity, physical inactivity, and genetic factors. In addition, most people with insulin resistance have central obesity (excess accumulation of fat around the abdomen region versus the hips).

Epidemiology

The metabolic syndrome has become increasingly common in the United States. An estimated 47 million U.S. adults currently fall within the criteria of the metabolic syndrome.[40]

Clustering of these metabolic risk factors has been noted in the pediatric population in the last decade.[41–43]

Diagnoses

The criteria for diagnosing the metabolic syndrome have not been standardized. The Third Report of the National Cholesterol Education Program (NCEP) Expert Panel on Detection, Evaluation, and Treatment of High Blood Cholesterol in Adults (Adult Treatment Panel III) proposed that the metabolic syndrome is identified by the presence of three or more of the following components:

Central obesity (waist circumference)	
Men	> 40 inches
Women	> 35 inches
Fasting blood triglycerides	≥ 150 mg/dl
Blood HDL cholesterol	Men < 40 mg/dl
	Women < 50 mg/dl
Blood pressure	≥ 130/85 mm Hg
Fasting glucose	≥ 110 mg/dl

Exercise

Exercise has a favorable effect on all the cardiac risk factors that comprise the metabolic syndrome. Current recommendations for the management of the metabolic syndrome encourage lifestyle modifications that include increased physical activity.

Findings from several studies support that exercise is likely to positively affect individuals with the metabolic syndrome. The HERITAGE Family Study, a relatively large study of 621 men and women, was designed to investigate the contribution of regular exercise to modifications of cardiovascular risk factors in type 2 diabetes.[44] Participants followed a standardized exercise training program for 20 weeks. One hundred and five individuals in the study were classified at baseline as having the metabolic syndrome but over 30% of those were no longer classified as having the metabolic syndrome after 20 weeks of exercise training. This study provides strong evidence that regular exercise is effective in treating individuals with the metabolic syndrome or multiple cardiovascular risk factors.

A similar study of 874 healthy participants found a strong and inverse association between physical activity and the metabolic syndrome. A significant reduction in the risk for developing the metabolic syndrome was observed with a moderate change in activity levels, suggesting that low-fit individuals can significantly reduce their risk by modest increases in their physical activity level.[45]

The associations between leisure-time physical activity and cardiovascular and metabolic risk factors were also assessed in a population-based cohort of 612 middle-aged men without the metabolic syndrome. At the 4-year follow-up, and after adjustment for age, BMI, smoking, alcohol, and socioeconomic status or potentially mediating factors (insulin, glucose, lipids, and blood pressure), the investigators reported that men engaging in more than 3 hours per week of moderate or vigorous physical activity were half as likely as sedentary men to have the metabolic syndrome. The association was even stronger for those engaging in more vigorous activities. Men in the upper third of fitness level of the cohort were 75% less likely than unfit men to develop the metabolic syndrome had even.[46]

In children, the findings are similar. The clustering of metabolic risk factors was inversely related to physical activity in 589 pre- or early pubertal Danish children. The investigators concluded that potential beneficial effect of activity may be greatest in children with lower cardiorespiratory fitness. Accordingly, the investigators suggested that children, particularly those who are less fit, should be encouraged to engage in physical activity to improve their metabolic health and to establish healthy habits.[47]

Although studies examining the association between exercise and the metabolic syndrome are relatively few, the findings support that even moderate increases in physical activity can offer substantial protection from the risk of developing the metabolic syndrome. Moderate increases in exercise or physical activity thus are likely beneficial and are recommended for the prevention and management of the metabolic syndrome.

■ SUMMARY

- Diabetes mellitus is defined as a metabolic disease characterized by hyperglycemia (high concentrations of blood glucose) resulting from defects in insulin production, insulin action, or both. It is characterized by the inadequacy or inability of the cells to utilize carbohydrates for their energy needs.

- Type 1 diabetes is characterized by an absolute deficiency of insulin, most often the result of irreparable damage to the insulin-producing cells of the pancreas from antibody attacks. It typically occurs in children and adolescents.

- Type 2 diabetes is characterized by insulin resistance that leads to a diminished glucose transport across the cell membrane. To compensate for the decreased transport, insulin secretion for a given blood glucose concentration increases. Gradually, the pancreas loses its ability to produce insulin.

- Obesity, at least in part, is responsible for some degree of insulin resistance.

- Pre-diabetes is a condition characterized by blood glucose levels that are higher than normal but not high enough to be classified as diabetes.

- Exercise is a natural stimulus for increased glucose uptake by the working muscle cells via the GLUT-4 transporter. The exercise-induced translocation of the GLUT-4 receptors to the membrane of the cell is insulin-independent.
- The findings from interventional studies support that insulin resistance and glucose disposal are improved following aerobic or resistance exercises.
- Exercise and physical activity in general are a highly effective way to delay or avert the development of type 2 diabetes and to reduce the risk of mortality in diabetics.
- In at least one interventional study, exercise and other lifestyle interventions were two times more effective in preventing the incidence of type 2 diabetes than the diabetic medication, metformin.
- Exercise for the diabetic individual is highly recommended but must be carefully monitored. Exercise, diet, and insulin (if the patient is taking insulin) must interact precisely to bring the desired outcome. This is especially important for individuals with type 1 diabetes.
- The metabolic syndrome refers to a cluster of specific cardiovascular disease risk factors. Insulin resistance is thought to be the underlining pathophysiology. For this, the metabolic syndrome is also called the insulin resistance syndrome.
- The underlying causes of this syndrome are overweight/obesity, physical inactivity, and genetic factors. In addition, most people with insulin resistance have central obesity.
- Exercise has a favorable effect on all the cardiac risk factors that comprise the metabolic syndrome. Relatively moderate increases in physical activity can offer substantial protection from the risk of

developing the metabolic syndrome. Moderate increases in exercise or physical activity thus are likely to be beneficial and is recommended for the prevention and management of the metabolic syndrome.

■ REFERENCES

1. Report of the Expert Committee on the Diagnosis and Classification of Diabetes Mellitus. *Diabetes Care* 1998;21(7):S5–S19.
2. Atkinson MA, MacLaren NK. The pathogenesis of insulin-dependent diabetes mellitus. *N Engl J Med* 1994;331(21):1428–1436.
3. Polonsky KS, Sturis J, Bell GI. Seminars in Medicine of the Beth Israel Hospital, Boston. Non-insulin-dependent diabetes mellitus—a genetically programmed failure of the beta cell to compensate for insulin resistance. *N Engl J Med* 1996;334(12):777–783.
4. Bogardus C, Lillioja S, Mott DM, et al. Relationship between degree of obesity and in vivo insulin action in man. *Am J Physiol* 1985;248(3 Pt 1):E286–E291.
5. Kolterman OG, Gray RS, Griffin J, et al. Receptor and postreceptor defects contribute to the insulin resistance in noninsulin-dependent diabetes mellitus. *J Clin Invest* 1981;68(4):957–969.
6. National Institute of Diabetes and Digestive and Kidney Diseases. National Diabetes Statistics fact sheet: general information and national estimates on diabetes in the United States, 2005. Bethesda, MD: U.S. Department of Health and Human Services, National Institute of Health; 2005.
7. Mokdad AH, Ford ES, Bowman BA, et al. Prevalence of obesity, diabetes, and obesity-related health risk factors, 2001. *JAMA* 2003;289(1):76–79.
8. Lloyd-Jones D, Adams R, Cartyhenon M, et al. Heart disease and stroke statistics, 2009 update: a report from the American Heart Association Statistics Committee and Stroke

Statistics Subcommittee. *Circulation* 2009; 119:480–486.

9. Wild S, Roglic G, Green A, et al. Global prevalence of diabetes: estimates for the year 2000 and projections for 2030. *Diabetes Care* 2004;27(5):1047–1053.

10. Fox CS, Penicina MJ, Meigs JB, et al. Trends in the incidence of type 2 diabetes mellitus from the 1970s to the 1990s: the Framingham Heart Study. *Circulation* 2006;113(25):2914–2918.

11. National Diabetes Statistics, 2007 fact sheet. Bethesda, MD: U.S. Department of Health and Human Services, National Institutes of Health; 2008.

12. Shepherd PR, Kahn BB. Glucose transporters and insulin action—implications for insulin resistance and diabetes mellitus. *N Engl J Med* 1999;341(4):248–257.

13. Nesher R, Karl IE, Kipnis DM. Dissociation of effects of insulin and contraction on glucose transport in rat epitrochlearis muscle. *Am J Physiol* 1985;249(3 Pt 1):C226–C232.

14. Azevedo JL Jr, Carey JO, Pories WJ, et al. Hypoxia stimulates glucose transport in insulin-resistant human skeletal muscle. *Diabetes* 1995;44(6):695–698.

15. Cartee GD, Douen AG, Rambal T, et al. Stimulation of glucose transport in skeletal muscle by hypoxia. *J Appl Physiol* 1991;70(4): 1593–1600.

16. Balon TW, Nadler JL. Evidence that nitric oxide increases glucose transport in skeletal muscle. *J Appl Physiol* 1997;82(1):359–363.

17. Etgen GJ Jr, Fryburg DA, Gibbs EM. Nitric oxide stimulates skeletal muscle glucose transport through a calcium/contraction- and phosphatidylinositol-3-kinase-independent pathway. *Diabetes* 1997;46(11):1915–1919.

18. Roberts CK, Barnard RJ, Scheck SH, Balon TW. Exercise-stimulated glucose transport in skeletal muscle is nitric oxide dependent. *Am J Physiol* 1997;273(1 Pt 1):E220–E225.

19. Asahi Y, Hayashi H, Wang L, Ebina Y. Fluoro-microscopic detection of myc-tagged GLUT4 on the cell surface. Co-localization of the translocated GLUT4 with rearranged actin by insulin treatment in CHO cells and L6 myotubes. *J Med Invest* 1999;46(3-4):192–199.

20. Taguchi T, Kishikawa H, Motoshima H, et al. Involvement of bradykinin in acute exercise-induced increase of glucose uptake and GLUT-4 translocation in skeletal muscle: studies in normal and diabetic humans and rats. *Metabolism* 2000;49(7):920–930.

21. Goodyear LJ, Giorgino F, Sherman LA, et al. Insulin receptor phosphorylation, insulin receptor substrate-1 phosphorylation, and phosphatidylinositol 3-kinase activity are decreased in intact skeletal muscle strips from obese subjects. *J Clin Invest* 1995; 95(5):2195–2204.

22. Holloszy JO, Hansen PA. Regulation of glucose transport into skeletal muscle. *Rev Physiol Biochem Pharmacol* 1996;128:99–193.

23. Ryder JW, Chibalin AV, Zierath JR. Intracellular mechanisms underlying increases in glucose uptake in response to insulin or exercise in skeletal muscle. *Acta Physiol Scand* 2001;171(3):249–257.

24. Smutok MA, Reece C, Kokkinos PF, et al. Aerobic versus strength training for risk factor intervention in middle-aged men at high risk for coronary heart disease. *Metabolism* 1993; 42(2):177–184.

25. Smutok MA, Reece CE, Kokkinos PF, et al. Effects of exercise training modality on glucose tolerance in men with abnormal glucose regulation. *Int J Sports Med* 1994;15(6): 283–289.

26. Miller JP, Pratley RE, Goldberg AP, et al. Strength training increases insulin action in healthy 50- to 65-yr-old men. *J Appl Physiol* 1994;77(3):1122–1127.

27. Reitman JS, Vasquez B, Klimes I, Nagulesparan M. Improvement of glucose homeostasis after exercise training in non–insulin-dependent diabetes. *Diabetes Care* 1984;7(5):434–441.

28. Craig BW, Everhart J, Brown R. The influence of high-resistance training on glucose tolerance in young and elderly subjects. *Mech Ageing Dev* 1989;49(2):147–157. (see comments)

29. Helmrich SP, Ragland DR, Leung RW, Paffenbarger RS Jr. Physical activity and reduced occurrence of non–insulin-dependent diabetes mellitus. *N Engl J Med* 1991;325(3):147–152. (see comments)

30. Wei M, Gibbons LW, Kampert JB, et al. Low cardiorespiratory fitness and physical inactivity as predictors of mortality in men with type 2 diabetes. *Ann Intern Med* 2000;132(8):605–611. (see comment)

31. Wei M, Gibbons LW, Mitchell TL, et al. The association between cardiorespiratory fitness and impaired fasting glucose and type 2 diabetes mellitus in men. *Ann Intern Med* 1999;130(2):89–96. Erratum, 1999:131(5):394.

32. Manson JE, Nathan DM, Drolewski AS, et al. A prospective study of exercise and incidence of diabetes among U.S. male physicians. *JAMA* 1992;268(1):63–67.

33. Hu FB, Sigal RJ, Rich-Edwards JW, et al. Walking compared with vigorous physical activity and risk of type 2 diabetes in women: a prospective study. *JAMA* 1999;282(15):1433–1439.

34. Knowler WC, Barrett-Connor E, Fowler SE, et al. Reduction in the incidence of type 2 diabetes with lifestyle intervention or metformin. *N Engl J Med* 2002;346(6):393–403. (see comments)

35. Tuomilehto J, Lindström J, Eriksson JG, et al. Prevention of type 2 diabetes mellitus by changes in lifestyle among subjects with impaired glucose tolerance. *N Engl J Med* 2001;344(18):1343–1350. (see comments)

36. Hu FB, Stampfer MJ, Solomon C, et al. Physical activity and risk for cardiovascular events in diabetic women. *Ann Intern Med* 2001; 134(2):96–105. (see comment)

37. Church TS, La Monte MJ, Barlow CE, Blair SN. Cardiorespiratory fitness and body mass index as predictors of cardiovascular disease mortality among men with diabetes. *Arch Intern Med* 2005;165(18):2114–2120.

38. Ryan AS, Hurlbut DE, Lott ME, et al. Insulin action after resistive training in insulin resistant older men and women. *J Am Geriatr Soc* 2001;49(3):247–253.

39. Kahn R, Buse J, Ferrannini E, et al. The metabolic syndrome: time for a critical appraisal: joint statement from the American Diabetes Association and the European Association for the Study of Diabetes. *Diabetes Care* 2005; 28(9):2289–2304. (see comments)

40. Executive Summary of the Third Report of the National Cholesterol Education Program (NCEP) Expert Panel on Detection, Evaluation, and Treatment of High Blood Cholesterol in Adults (Adult Treatment Panel III). *JAMA* 2001;285(19):2486–2497.

41. Sinaiko AR, Steinberger J, Moran A, et al. Relation of insulin resistance to blood pressure in childhood. *J Hypertens* 2002;20:509–517.

42. Steinberger J. Insulin resistance and cardiovascular risk in the pediatric patient. *Prog Pediatr Cardiol* 2001;12:169–175.

43. Bao W, Srinivasan SR, Wattigney WA, Berenson GS. Persistence of multiple cardiovascular risk clustering related to syndrome X from childhood to young adulthood: the Bogalusa Heart Study. *Arch Intern Med* 1994;154:1842–1847.

44. Katzmarzyk PT, Leon AS, Willmore JH, et al. Targeting the metabolic syndrome with exercise: evidence from the HERITAGE Family Study. *Med Sci Sports Exerc* 2003;35(10):1703–1709.

45. Franks PW, Ekelund U, Brage S, et al. Does the association of habitual physical activity with the metabolic syndrome differ by level of cardiorespiratory fitness? *Diabetes Care* 2004; 27(5):1187–1193.

46. Laaksonen DE, Lakka HM, Salonen JT, et al. Low levels of leisure-time physical activity and cardiorespiratory fitness predict development of the metabolic syndrome. *Diabetes Care* 2002;25:1612–1618.

47. Brage S, Wedderkopp N, Ekelund U, et al. Features of the metabolic syndrome are associated with objectively measured physical activity and fitness in Danish children: the European Youth Heart Study (EYHS). *Diabetes Care* 2004;27(9):2141–2148.

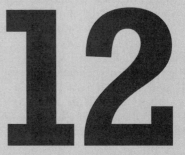

CHAPTER

12

High Blood Pressure and Physical Activity

A s discussed in Chapter 7, the pressure generated by the left ventricle during systole is known as the systolic blood pressure (SBP). The pressure that the blood exerts on the blood vessels during diastole (the relaxing phase of the heart beat) is known as the diastolic blood pressure (DBP). Hypertension (high blood pressure) is considered a chronic elevation in either SBP ($\geq$ 140 mm Hg) or DBP ($\geq$ 90 mm Hg) at rest.

Hypertension was not recognized as a menace of health until the latter part of the twentieth century. In fact, even up until the 1960s some experts in the field believed that arterial disease was the cause of hypertension and not the result.[1] Use of drugs to lower blood pressure was scoffed as "treatment of the manometer rather than of the patient." The prevailing belief among physicians was that the rise in blood pressure was an essential compensatory mechanism (and, thus, essential blood pressure) to maintain adequate perfusion as the individual advanced in age. Attempts to lower blood pressure were therefore discouraged.[1]

Pioneering research by Dr. Edward Freis in the 1940s to the 1970s, however, challenged the prevailing opinion among the medical community that reduction in elevated blood pressure per se was not beneficial. Freis and the Veterans Administration study group in the mid 1960s to early 1970s proved conclusively that treatment of hypertension reduces strokes and cardiovascular complications.[2–9] Since then, several large scale trials have been implemented that have significantly enhanced our knowledge of the diagnosis and treatment of hypertension.

Chronic hypertension is now recognized as a major and the most common risk factor for developing cardiovascular disease.[10–13] This relationship is direct, strong, continuous, graded, consistent, predictive, and independent.[14] The risk of cardiovascular morbidity and mortality increases progressively and linearly as blood pressure rises with no evidence of a plateau.[10,13,15] The mortality risk doubles for every 20 mm Hg increase in SBP above the threshold of 115 mm Hg and for every 10 mm Hg increase in the DBP threshold of 75 mm Hg (**Figure 12.1**).[16]

The World Health Organization reported in 2002 that the number of people with hypertension worldwide is estimated as much as 1 billion, with 7.1 million deaths per year attributable to hypertension.[17] Over 58 million Americans are diagnosed with hypertension.[12,13] The prevalence of hypertension increases with age (**Figure 12.2**), and a higher percentage of men have high blood pressure up to age 45, while women surpass men after 54 years of age.[18] For a 55-year-old individual with normal blood pressure, the risk of

Figure 12.1 CVD risk and blood pressure. Note that the risk for CVD doubles with each 20 mm Hg increase in SBP beyond 115 mm Hg and each 10 mm Hg in DBP beyond 75 mm Hg.

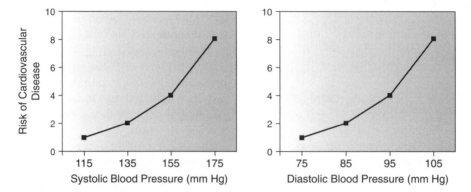

Source: Modified from NHLBI. The seventh report of the Joint National Committee on Prevention, Detection, Evaluation, and Treatment of High Blood Pressure (JNC 7). *Hypertension* 2003;42:1206.

developing hypertension during the remaining of his or her life is estimated to be 90%.[19] The prevalence of hypertension is higher in African-American men and women than Caucasians. African Americans also develop hypertension at an earlier age and the average blood pressures are much higher than those of Caucasians. The estimated direct and indirect cost for high blood pressure for 2009 is 73.4 billion (**Table 12.1**).[18]

Figure 12.2 Prevalence of high blood pressure according to age and gender.

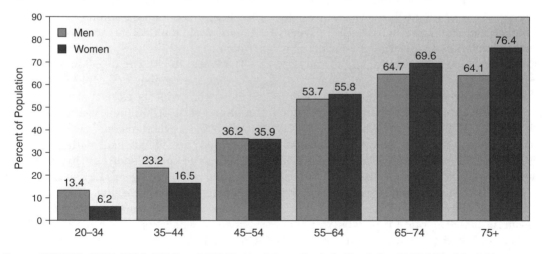

Source: NHANES: 2005–2006; NCHS and NHLBI; Lloyd-Jones D, et al. *Circulation* 2009;119:e11–e161.

Table 12.1 High Blood Pressure

Population Group	Prevalence in 2006 Age 20+	Mortality in 2006 (All Ages)	Estimated Cost in 2009
Both genders	73,600,000	57,356	73.4 billion
Men	35,300,000	24,046	
Women	38,300,000	33,310	
White men	34.1%	17,312	
White women	30.3%	25,814	
Black men	44.4%	6,746	
Black women	43.9%	6,592	

Source: Lloyd-Jones D, Adams R, Carnethon M, et al. Heart disease and stroke statistics—2009 update: a report from the American Heart Association Statistics Committee and Stroke Statistics Subcommittee. *Circulation* 2009;119: e1–e161.

■ METHODS OF ASSESSING BLOOD PRESSURE

Blood pressure (BP) can be assessed directly and indirectly. **Direct assessment of BP** requires the insertion of a catheter into an artery that is connected to a calibrated pressure transducer. This allows the continuous beat-by-beat measure of arterial blood pressure. Obviously, this method is highly impractical for everyday use and is only used in some research.

Indirect assessment of BP is done by the use of the sphygmomanometer and stethoscope (**Figure 12.3**). This method of measuring blood pressure is based on the work by Riva-Rocci (1896), Hill and Bernard (1897), and Korotkoff (1905). The indirect method is based on the occlusion of blood flow through the brachial artery by a cuff wrapped around the upper arm. Occlusion of the artery is accomplished by the cuff inflated above the systolic blood pressure (SBP; about 180–200 mm Hg). Then, the cuff is deflated slowly.

As the pressure within cuff is gradually falls to the level of the peak pressure generated by the left ventricle during contraction, blood begins to flow through the brachial artery, producing a sharp rhythmic sound with each heart beat. The sound changes in quality and intensity as the pressure within the cuff decreases progressively, and finally disappears. These sounds are known as the *Korotkoff sounds* and are described as phases:

- **Phase I:** The pressure level at which the first faint but clear tapping sounds are heard.
- **Phase II:** The period during which a murmur or swishing sounds are heard.
- **Phase III:** The period during which the sounds are crisper and increase in intensity.
- **Phase IV:** The time when a distinct, abrupt, muffling sound (usually of a soft blowing quality) is heard.
- **Phase V:** The pressure level when the last sound is heard and after which all sound disappears.

Figure 12.3 BP assessment using sphygmomanometer and stethoscope.

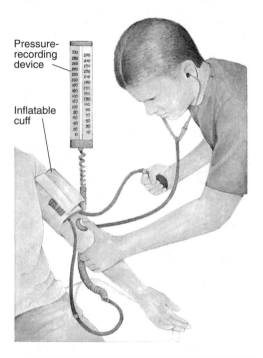

- Pressure-recording device
- Inflatable cuff

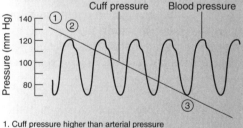

Cuff pressure   Blood pressure

Pressure (mm Hg)

1. Cuff pressure higher than arterial pressure
2. Arterial pressure and cuff pressure equal; sounds can now be heard
3. Cuff pressure falls below arterial pressure; sounds no longer audible

---

Systolic blood pressure is the pressure at which the first audible sound is heard (Phase I).

Diastolic blood pressure in adults is the pressure that corresponds with the last sound (Phase V) and Phase IV in children.

Recording BP by the indirect method appears relatively easy. However, it is perhaps the simplicity of the method that creates an environment of carelessness that may lead to erroneous results. For this reason, a detailed explanation of BP, based on the recommendations of the American Heart Association is presented below.

- The individual should be seated in a quiet, comfortable environment with the arm resting at heart level. Allow 5 minutes of rest in this position.
- Chose the right size cuff. The use of a narrow cuff overestimates blood pressure. Proper bladder width should be 40% to 50% of the upper arm circumference and a bladder length at least 80% of arm circumference.
- Wrap the cuff around the upper arm snugly but not too tight. The center of the bladder should be placed directly over the brachial artery.
- Locate the brachial artery along the inner arm by palpitation.
- Position the stethoscope below the cuff and directly over the palpable brachial artery.
- Inflate the cuff to approximately 30 mm Hg above the cuff pressure to which the radial pulse is no longer palpable.
- Release the air in the cuff so that the pressure falls at the rate of 2- to 3-mm Hg per second.
- Note the systolic blood pressure at the onset of at least two consecutive beats (Phase I).
- Note the diastolic blood pressure at the cessation of sound (Phase V) for adults. Listen for about 10 to 20 mm Hg below this sound to confirm disappearance of sound and then deflate rapidly.
- Record pressure and wait 1 to 2 minutes before repeating the procedure in the same arm.

In some patients, the Korotkoff sounds do not disappear. In such cases, Phase IV (the change of the sounds) should be recorded as the diastolic blood pressure.

■ DETERMINANTS OF HYPERTENSION

The primary determinants of BP are cardiac output and peripheral resistance. A chronic increase in cardiac output, peripheral resistance, or both will result in hypertension. Numerous hemodynamic, metabolic, and humoral factors are known to affect cardiac output and peripheral resistance. Many of these factors have been investigated as culprits of essential hypertension and several leading theories have been advanced. However, a unifying concept of the pathogenesis of hypertension has not been established. Clearly, the processes leading to essential hypertension are complex and multi-factorial.

■ STRUCTURAL ARTERIAL CHANGES IN HYPERTENSION

It is well accepted that essential hypertension is associated with increased peripheral resistance. Structural changes in the resistance vessels have been suspected as the cause for the increased peripheral resistance. Several studies confirmed that the diameter of resistance vessels in hypertensive patients is structurally narrower than in individuals with normal BP and that the lumina and wall/lumen ratios of small resistance arteries are structurally altered.[20,21]

The morphologic alterations of the vessels are in response to increased tension within the vessel wall. The significance of these structural changes of the resistance arteries and the rela-

tionship of cardiovascular design and function can be fully realized when one considers the laws of Laplace and Poiseuille. According to the Laplace relationship, wall stress is directly proportional to the pressure within the cavity (vessel) and the radius of the vessel and inversely proportional to the wall thickness.

Laplace's Law: $T = P \times r/w$

where:

T = tension per unit wall layer (wall stress)

P = transmural pressure (pressure within the artery)

r = radius of the artery

w = wall thickness

To maintain constant wall stress (T), an increase in transmural pressure (P) must be accompanied by an increase in relative wall thickness (W) and/or a decrease in the radius. The relative wall thickness is achieved through medial and smooth muscle cell hypertrophy and hyperplasia, and by increased interstitial matrix.

Structural changes in the vessels ultimately results in significant changes in the rate of blood flow. This is explained by Poiseullie's Law, which states that blood flow is directly proportional to the fourth power of the inner radius of the vessel while resistance is inversely related to the fourth power of the radius. Thus, small changes in the radius of the arteries lead to large changes in blood flow and peripheral resistance.

A small reduction in the diameter of blood vessels will lead to a large increase in peripheral resistance and a large reduction in blood flow, ultimately resulting in relatively higher blood pressures.

■ NORMAL BLOOD PRESSURE VALUES

Traditionally, normal BP values were considered an SBP < 140 mm Hg and a DBP < 90 mm Hg. However, recent findings support that the risk of cardiovascular disease begins to rise at a much lower blood pressure values. Data from over 1 million individuals support that death from cardiovascular disease increases progressively and linearly from blood pressure levels starting at 115/75 mm Hg. The risk for cardiovascular death doubles for every 20 mm Hg increase in SBP beyond this level or 10 mm Hg increase in DBP.[22] In addition, longitudinal data from the Framingham Heart Study indicated that the relative risk for cardiovascular disease is more than twofold higher in those with SBP of 130 to 139 mm Hg and DBP of 85 to 89 mm Hg as compared to those with blood pressure below 120/80 mm Hg.[23] Collectively, these findings support that the association between blood pressure and cardiovascular risk should be re-evaluated.

■ PRE-HYPERTENSION

Based on the aforementioned information,[22,23] in 2003 the Seventh Report of the Joint National Committee on Prevention, Detection, Evaluation, and Treatment of High Blood Pressure (JNC 7) revised the criteria of normal blood pressure values by introducing a new category referred to as **pre-hypertension** (Table 12.2).[12]

Pre-hypertensive individuals are at one and a half- to twofold higher risk for developing hypertension and major cardiovascular disease compared to those with normal BP. An estimated 37.4% Americans have pre-hypertension, which translates to 41,900,000 million men and 27,800,000 women.[16,24,25]

The JNC 7 Committee emphasized that pre-hypertension is not a disease category. Rather, it is a designation intended to identify individuals with elevated risk of developing hypertension. Pre-hypertensive individuals are not candidates for antihypertensive therapy unless they have co-morbidities such as diabetes or kidney disease. The emphasis for these individuals should be lifestyle changes to reduce the risk for developing hypertension.

Pre-hypertension refers to a new category of blood pressure that includes individuals with systolic blood pressure between 120 to 139 mm Hg and/or diastolic blood pressure between 80 to 89 mm Hg.

Table 12.2 Classification of Blood Pressure for Adults Age 18 and Older According to JNC 7

Category	Systolic		Diastolic
Normal	< 120	and	< 80
Pre-hypertension	120–139	or	80–89
Stage 1 hypertension	140–159	or	90–99
Stage 2 hypertension	≥ 160	or	≥ 100

Source: Chobanian AV, et al. The Seventh Report of the Joint National Committee on Prevention, Detection, Evaluation, and Treatment of High Blood Pressure: the JNC 7 report. *JAMA* 2003;289(19):2560–2572.

■ PERILS OF HIGH BLOOD PRESSURE

Chronic hypertension is a major and the most common risk factor for developing cardiovascular disease including left ventricular hypertrophy, heart failure, and stroke.[10–14] The relationship between elevated blood pressure and cardiovascular disease is direct, strong, continuous, graded, consistent, predictive, and independent of other risk factors. The risk of cardiovascular morbidity and mortality increases in a curvilinear fashion as blood pressure rises with no evidence of a plateau.[11,14] For example, in patients with blood pressure > 180/110 mm Hg, the risk of developing coronary heart disease is about five times higher than those with blood pressure < 120/80 mm Hg.[11]

It is also important to emphasize that the risk increases when SBP, DBP, or both are elevated. The association of increased DBP with cardiovascular disease risk and perhaps the existence of a threshold beyond which the risk is elevated significantly was demonstrated in a large study of approximately 420,000 individuals with a mean follow-up time of over 11 years. The findings of this study support that DBP

threshold for increased risk was 70 mm Hg. Beyond this threshold of 70 mm Hg and up to 110 mm Hg, the risk increased linearly.[10]

The significance of increased risk when both SBP and DBP are elevated was described in another large study (MRFIT), where approximately 350,000 individuals were followed for a mean of over 10 years (**Table 12.3**).[11] Based on information given in Table 12.3, the following points can be emphasized:

1. The risk of death from heart disease increases steadily as SBP or DBP increases. For example, if we concentrate on just the first column, it becomes evident that as the SBP increases from less than 120 mm Hg to 160 mm Hg or greater, the risk also increases progressively from 1.0 to 4.19. That is, the risk of CHD is over four times higher in those with SBP that is 160 mm Hg or more. This is despite a DBP value below 80 mm Hg.

2. Similarly, if one maintains a SBP below 120, but the DBP rises progressively, the rise in risk is also progressive, reaching 3.23 times at a DBP value of 100 mm Hg or greater (first horizontal block).

Table 12.3 Risk for Coronary Heart Disease Mortality Based on Systolic and Diastolic Blood Pressures at Rest

Systolic Blood Pressure (mm Hg)	Diastolic Blood Pressure (mm Hg)				
	< 80	80–84	85–89	90–99	100
< 120	1.00	1.35	1.36	0.98	3.23
120–129	1.19	1.30	1.49	1.49	1.84
130–139	1.67	1.61	1.67	1.91	2.64
140–159	2.57	2.22	2.67	2.56	2.99
≥ 160	4.19	3.20	3.41	3.41	4.57

Source: Stamler J, Stamler R, Neaton JD. Blood pressure, systolic and diastolic, and cardiovascular risks. US population data. *Arch Intern Med* 1993;153(5):598–615.

3. The risk is even higher when both SBP and DBP are elevated. At a SBP of 160 mm Hg or higher and DBP of 100 mm Hg or higher, the risk is 4.57 times that of someone with BP less than 120/80 mm Hg.

■ BENEFITS OF LOWERING BLOOD PRESSURE

Lowering elevated blood pressure results in a reduction in the rates of death from heart disease and stroke. Interestingly, the decrease in BP does not have to be drastic for substantial health benefits. Reductions in DBP of 5 mm Hg over a period of 5 years was associated with at least 34% less stroke and at least 21% less CHD. Reductions of 7.5 mm Hg and 10 mm Hg are associated with 46% and 56% less in stroke and 29%, and 37% less CHD, respectively.[10]

Reduction in DBP	Reduction in Stroke	Reduction in CHD
7.5	46%	29%
10	56%	37%

Relatively small reductions in blood pressure lead to significant and large reductions in both stroke and coronary heart disease.

■ EXERCISE AS THERAPY FOR HYPERTENSION

The potential of increased physical activity to lower elevated blood pressure or to prevent/attenuate the development of hypertension was suggested by several epidemiologic studies. After allowing for the traditional confounding factors, the findings of these studies suggest that habitual physical activity as reported by the participants is associated with lower blood pressure.[26-29] These findings are supported by other studies where physical activity was assessed more objectively by an exercise treadmill test.[26,30] For example, in one study of middle-aged women who were classified as high-fit based on their peak exercise time during an treadmill test, significantly lower DBP values (5 and 7 mm Hg) were found when compared to women of low and moderate fitness levels, respectively.[30] In addition, cross-sectional and large-scale longitudinal population studies reported that the relative risks for developing hypertension in sedentary men and women with normal blood pressure at rest were approximately 35% to 70% higher, respectively, when compared to their physically active peers.[31-33]

Exercise Interventional Studies

Based on the aforementioned epidemiologic evidence, the natural next question for investigators was to assess the potential of structured exercise program to lower BP in hypertensive individuals or those with elevated BP. In addition to whether or not exercise lowers BP values, these studies addressed several other questions such as the mode, amount, and intensity of exercise required for changes.

Initial studies showed significant reductions in blood pressure. However, several deficiencies in their design such as lack of a control group, small number of participants in each study, and poorly controlled exercise programs made their findings questionable and subject to criticism. After these initial reports, an overwhelming number of well-controlled studies that followed have consistently shown that regularly performed aerobic exercise of mild to moderate intensity lowers BP in patients with essential hypertension.[34-52]

Most of these exercise intervention studies have assessed the efficacy of aerobic exercise to lower BP in hypertensive patients. An overwhelming number of these studies reported that regularly performed aerobic exercise lowers BP in patients with mild to moderate essential hypertension when compared to non-exercising controls. Although some variability exists among the several reviews and meta-analyses, the general conclusion is that aerobic exercise training is effective in lowering BP in hypertensive individuals.[53–57] As suggested

by at least one study,[36] the magnitude of the exercise-induced BP reduction is related to the initial BP level.

In 2001, researchers analyzed the findings of 21 well-controlled exercise intervention studies for blood pressure control.[54] The average exercise-related BP reduction in these studies was 10.5 mm Hg for SBP and 7.6 mm Hg for DBP. In the control group, the average reduction was only 3.8 mm Hg and 1.3 mm Hg for SBP and DBP, respectively (**Table 12.4**). These findings are supported by a recent meta-analysis of

Table 12.4 Summary of Findings from Exercise Studies in Hypertensive Individuals

Study Investigators	Reference no.	Mean Age of Participants	Exercise Intensity (% of MHR)	SBP Reduction	DBP Reduction
Akinpelu et al.	34	58	60–70	8.5	0
Baglivo et al.	35	59	–	19	15
Cononie et al.	36	70–79	50–85	10	9
Dengel et al.	37	50-70	60–70	10	10
Gordon	38	12–65	60–85	8	6
Higashi et al.	39	52	Low	13	4
Ishikawa et al.	40	30–39	60	13	9
Keleman et al.	41	47	–	13	12
Koga et al.	42	49	50	7	6
Kokkinos et al.	43	57	60–80	7	5
Martin et al.	44	44	60–80	7	10
Matsusaki et al.	45	47	60 & 85	9	6
Motoyama et al.	46	68–84	Low	15	9
Rogers et al.	47	40	50–60	15	6
Seals et al.	48	> 49	50	10	7
Seals and Reiling	49	50–74	50	10	8
Somers et al.	50	–	–	9.7	6.8
Tanaka et al.	51	70	70	6	2
Zanettini et al.	52	70–85	70–85	15	11.5

Source: Kokkinos PF, Narayan P, Papademetriou V. Exercise as hypertension therapy. *Cardiol Clin* 2001;19(3): 507–516.

randomized controlled trials involving 72 trials, 105 study groups, and 3,936 participants. Cornelissen and Fagard[53] concluded that exercise training lowers resting SBP values by 6.9 mm Hg and DBP by 4.9 in hypertensive individuals.

Consequently, the American College of Sports Medicine and other authorities endorsed the concept that a sedentary lifestyle increases the risk for hypertension, whereas increased occupational or leisure time physical activity is associated with lower levels of blood pressure.[14,56,58] Increased physical activity is now strongly recommended as part of the lifestyle modification as adjunct to pharmacologic therapy proposed by the Joint National Committee.[12,13,59]

Gender and Exercise-Induced Reduction in Blood Pressure

Participants in most exercise studies on blood pressure are men, so relatively little information exists on the effects of exercise training on hypertensive women. The question of whether exercise is as effective in lowering blood pressure in women as it is in men cannot be answered definitively. However, the average blood pressure reduction reported by the three studies of women was 10 mm Hg for SPB and 7.7 mm Hg for DBP after exercise training.[40,42,47] These changes are comparable to the exercise-induced blood pressure reductions reported for hypertensive men. There is also some evidence derived from a meta-analysis suggesting that exercise-induced BP reduction may be greater in women than men.[60] Based on the available evidence, it appears that exercise is at least equally effective in lowering blood pressure in women as it is in men.

Age, Exercise, and Blood Pressure Reduction

Regardless of the antihypertensive properties of physical activity or exercise, its efficacy as a therapy (as with any other therapy) depends greatly on its implementation. It is less likely that people will subscribe to exercise if it is too painful or, even worse, cause injury or death.

This is especially relevant for the aging population for two main reasons. First, the prevalence of hypertension increases with advancing age. More than half of the people aged 60 to 69 years of age and approximately 75% of those 70 years of age or older are affected by hypertension.[12,61] Second, older individuals are more likely to have health issues that compromise their ability to exercise. Physical activity or exercise in these individuals thus presents challenges not encountered in younger groups.

The question of whether exercise reduces blood pressure in older individuals has been addressed in several studies,[40,62] and it appears that changes in blood pressure may be somewhat related to age. According to a meta-analysis, exercise-induced blood pressure reduction appears to be greater in middle-aged hypertensive patients than in both younger and older patients.[62] The reasons for this are not clear. Similarly, in the multi-center trial, the magnitude of blood pressure reduction was greater in younger (age range 30–49 years) than older (age range 50–69 years) hypertensive men and women.[40]

Although the findings linking the influence of age to the magnitude of blood pressure reduction are somewhat conflicting, it is clear that hypertensive patients of advanced age can tolerate exercise well and benefit from a properly designed exercise program. In a group of 70- to 79-year-old hypertensive patients, Cononie et al.[36] reported reductions of 8, 9, and 8 mm Hg in systolic, diastolic, and mean blood pressure values, respectively, after 6 months of aerobic exercise. In a similar study, the investigators noted 15, 9, and 11 mm Hg reductions in systolic, diastolic, and mean blood pressure, respectively, in 68- to 84-year-old hypertensive patients.[36,46]

Exercise Intensity Influences

Exercise intensity is important to consider, especially when physical activity is implemented in an aging population. The intensity of exercise is the most difficult to quantify and perhaps carries a greater potential for injury. The challenge over the years thus has been to determine the exercise intensity that will maximize health benefits at a relatively low risk for injury. Stating it in another way, how intense does exercise need to be and still maintain a low risk/benefit ratio? Early exercise interventional studies implemented relatively high intensities to train their young participants. Because high-intensity exercise carries a high risk for cardiac complications and other injuries,[63] health professions were reluctant to prescribe exercise to older or high-risk patients. The challenge was to identify the exercise intensity with the lowest risk/benefit ratio.

Several studies now support that low-to-moderate intensity exercise (35% to 79% of age-predicted maximum heart rate) is effective in lowering blood pressure.[28,45–47,64,65] Furthermore, in studies designed to compare the effects of different exercise intensities, low intensity exercise was more effective in lowering blood pressure than high intensity.[45,46,64,65] For example, Hagberg et al.[64] compared blood pressure changes in two groups; one group exercised at 53% of maximum oxygen uptake (low-intensity) and the other group exercised at 73% of maximum oxygen uptake (high-intensity). Significant reductions in DBP were observed in both groups following training. However, SBP was only reduced in the low-intensity group. In another study of similar design, both SBP and DBP were reduced significantly in hypertensive individuals exercising at 50% of their maximum oxygen uptake (low-intensity), but not in those exercising at 75% of their maximum oxygen uptake (high-intensity).[45] The findings of the Trial of Hypertension Prevention[66] also support that moderate intensity physical activity (3.0–6.0 MET) for at least 2 to 3 days a week is an appropriate recommendation for the general public for the prevention of primary hypertension.

The reduction of blood pressure by moderate-to-low exercise intensities is particularly important for the hypertensive patient. When compared to high intensity, low intensity exercise carries a lower risk for cardiac complications.[63] Physicians may be more comfortable advising patients, especially older patients, to pursue a low-intensity versus a high-intensity exercise program. Patients are also more inclined to participate and sustain a lower rather than a higher intensity exercise program. These factors, along with the low cost, lack of pharmacological side-effects, and additional cardiovascular benefits associated with exercise[67] are likely to increase patient participation in exercise programs and lead to a better control of hypertension.

Exercise Implementation in Patients with Stage 2 Hypertension

Individuals with stage 2 hypertension (SBP ≥ 160 mm Hg or DBP 100 mm Hg), are difficult to manage and are at an increased risk for CHD.[11] They often receive more than one antihypertensive medication and are likely to have multiple co-morbidities. They also have low exercise tolerance and are more likely to raise their BP values to relatively high and certainly unsafe levels during exercise. Needless to say, exercise in such patients is difficult to implement and certainly more risky. Naturally, low-intensity exercise training in this subgroup of patients is preferred.

Researchers examined the efficacy of exercise to lower blood pressure in individuals with stage 2 hypertension. Participants were middle-aged and older and had left ventricular hypertrophy (enlarged heart). All patients were treated with the maximum dose tolerated of antihypertensive medications to control BP. They were randomly assigned to either a control group (medication only) or intervention (exercise plus medication) group. Those in the exercise intervention group participated in a low-to-moderate intensity aerobic exercise (treadmill or stationary bike) program for 32 weeks.

At 16 weeks, a significant reduction in BP and left ventricular mass regression in these patients was noted. In some patients, the BP reduction was so substantial that it warranted a reduction in the antihypertensive medication the patient was receiving prior to the exercise program. At 32 weeks, BP in the exercise group was still significantly lower from baseline even after a 33% reduction in antihypertensive medication was achieved.[43] In addition, the patients reported substantial improvements in their quality of life. These findings support the following:

- Carefully designed exercise is safe and can be tolerated well by patients with stage 2 hypertension.
- Exercise is efficacious in reducing blood pressure even in individuals with stage 2 hypertension.
- Exercise works well with antihypertensive medications and has an additive effect in lowering blood pressure, reducing left ventricular mass, and improving cardiac function.
- Exercise training may lead to a reduction in the amount of antihypertensive medication necessary to control blood pressure for some patients.

Most studies support that regularly performed aerobic activities of moderate intensity can significantly lower blood pressure in hypertensive individuals of all ages and both genders.

Resistance Training and Hypertension

Most interventional studies have examined the efficacy of aerobic exercise in lowering BP. Resistance exercise or strength training and their potential health benefits have been ignored for several decades. In particular, strength training as a way to lower BP was discouraged by physicians and other health professionals largely because several investigators reported extremely high elevations in BP during weight lifting exercises at 80% to 100% of repetition maximum (1-RM).[68,69]

For example, in two studies the mean peak pressure during the double-leg press for the group reached 320/250 mm Hg in individuals with normal blood pressure at rest with pressures in one subject exceeding 480/350 mm Hg.[68] Peak pressures with the single-arm curl exercise reached a mean group value of 255/190 mm Hg when repetitions were continued to failure. In mildly hypertensive individuals, BP reached 345/245 mm Hg during squatting.[69] It was concluded that the intra-abdominal and intra-thoracic (Valsalva response) pressure increases during the lift combined with the mechanical compression of blood vessels were the reasons for the extreme elevations in BP.[68,69]

Two important points need to be emphasized. First, the BP response was during the lifting of a heavy weight to exhaustion. Lifting lower weight does not have nearly such profound effect on BP. Second, breath holding during the lift (known as Valsalva maneuver), increases intra-thoracic pressure and consequently BP. Normal breathing during the lift (not holding the breath) virtually eliminates the large BP rise.

In recent years, strength training has become popular among older men and women. This is the result of several reports that strength training may be a promising intervention to reduce the risk of falls by reversing or attenuating the age-related decline in bone mineral density, muscle mass, and power.[70] These reports sparked interest in re-examining the safety of resistance exercises for hypertensive patients and the possible antihypertensive effects.

The available information on the effects of strength training on resting BP is limited and conflicting. For example, a possible antihypertensive effect of strength training has been suggested by some[71–73] but not all studies.[36,74] In two of these studies, a small (5 mm Hg), but significant reduction was observed in DBP.[71,72] In the third study,[73] the reduction of 7 mm Hg for SBP and 6 mm Hg for DBP was comparable to the reduction in BP observed in the control group. In contrast, others found no changes in BP following 6 months of strength training in a group of 70- to 79-year-old men and women.[36] Similarly, researchers found no significant changes in BP in previously sedentary middle-aged men after 20 weeks of strength training.[74] In a more recent meta-analysis, Kelly and Kelly concluded that the reduction in blood pressure as a result of resistance training was approximately 3 mm Hg.[75]

Consequently, the American College of Sports Medicine concluded that strength training has not been consistent in lowering BP in hypertensive patients. They recommended that the efficacy of resistance training in lowering BP be investigated further. In general, resistance training is not recommended as the only form of exercise to lower BP in hypertensive individuals.[56,76]

> The efficacy of strength or resistance training to lower blood pressure has not yet been determined and resistance training as a means of lowering blood pressure should not be recommended.

Ambulatory Blood Pressure and Exercise

Traditional BP assessment represents only a snapshot of an individual's BP values. The need to assess BP during the course of 24 hours or longer (ambulatory blood pressure, ABP) was recognized early on and led to the development of devices to accomplish such a task. Early ABP devices were cumbersome, expensive, and relatively inaccurate. As technology improved, however, ABP monitoring became more and more accessible and accurate. Today's ABP devices consist of a digital recorder (approximately the size of a MP3 player) that is connected to a regular BP cuff. The cuff is worn around the arm and can be programmed to inflate at various time intervals (usually every 20–30 minutes). The BP value is recorded and stored in the digital recorder to be downloaded later to a computer.

Ambulatory blood pressure provides a more comprehensive assessment of BP and is a good predictor of cardiovascular events and a better predictor of target organ damage than resting BP values.[77,78] Information on BP assessments over a 24-hour period in exercise studies is limited and findings inconclusive. Only a relatively small number of studies have used ambulatory device[49,50,52,73,79–82] and one large trial (HARVEST Trial).[27]

Several problems with these studies make interpretation of the findings difficult. For example, some studies report average 24-hour BP, others report daytime BP, and some report only nighttime BP values. A small number of participants were used in some studies and other studies did not use a control group.

Overall, changes in BP over a 24-hour period are not as optimistic as the results reported by the traditional auscultatory method.

Due to its relatively large population, the HARVEST trial, provided more reliable information on the exercise-related 24-hour BP changes. Oakatubu and colleagues reported that young hypertensive individuals who engaged in physical activity for at least once a week during the previous two months exhibited significantly lower 24-hour and daytime DBP than the inactive group.[27] Based on the limited data, the American College of Sports Medicine concluded that the average reduction in daytime blood pressure was about 3/3.2 mm Hg.[56]

In a recent study, researchers provided evidence to support that fit individuals have lower BP values during a 24-hour period. In a group of over 600 men and women, they noted significantly lower BP during the day, night, and over 24 hours for the high- and moderate-fit groups when compared to those of low fitness group.[83] The differences in BP values between the low- and high-fit individuals were similar in magnitude with the changes reported by interventional studies,[54,55] These findings support the notion that physical activity and fitness results in lower BP throughout routine daily activities. The clinical significance of this is discussed later in this chapter.

> Overall, changes in blood pressure over a 24-hour period are not as optimistic as the results reported by the traditional auscultatory method.

Left Ventricular Hypertrophy and Exercise

Left ventricular hypertrophy (LVH) is considered an independent risk factor for cardiovascular disease.[84] The risk of cardiovascular morbid events, including sudden cardiac death, increases threefold in patients with LVH when compared to those without it.[84] LVH is more prevalent in individuals with hypertension than in those with normal BP. Naturally, it is desirable to attenuate the development of LVH or reverse the process and consequently reduce the risk of mortality associated with it.

Exercise training studies addressing the efficacy of exercise in lowering the risk of mortality in individuals with LVH have not been conducted. However, evidence from epidemiologic studies supports that physical activity and fitness do provide protection against cardiovascular events. In a 2002 study, the investigators examined if physical activity can attenuate the elevated risk of stroke associated with increased left ventricular mass (LVM; **Figure 12.4**).[85] The risk of stroke in sedentary individuals with elevated LVM was 3.5 times greater when compared to sedentary individuals with normal LVM. Among physically fit individuals with elevated LVM, the investigators concluded that the risk of stroke was similar to that observed in individuals with normal LVM. This is an important observation because it suggests

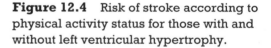

Figure 12.4 Risk of stroke according to physical activity status for those with and without left ventricular hypertrophy.

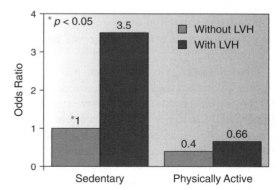

Source: Data from Rodriguez CJ, et al. *JACC* 2002; 39(2):1462–1488.

that even in the presence of elevated LVM, exercise attenuates its deleterious effects.

Researchers examined the efficacy of exercise to reduce LVM in hypertensive patients with LVH. A reduction in the thickness of the posterior and septal walls were noted with a significant reduction (12%) in LVM index after only 16 weeks of moderate intensity exercise[43] (**Figures 12.5** and **12.6**). Interestingly, the 12% reduction in LVM index is similar to the reduction achieved by medication therapy.[86] Other investigators also reported similar reduction in LVM index[52] or a trend towards a lower LVM index[35] with aerobic training. One study that reported an increase in LVM index used weight training.[41] More favorable changes and improvement in cardiac function may be possible with longer periods of exercise training.

■ Exaggerated Blood Pressure Response to Exercise

In apparently healthy individuals, SBP increases as exercise intensity increases in a

Figure 12.5 Cardiac wall thickness at baseline and after 16 weeks of exercise training in hypertensive individuals.

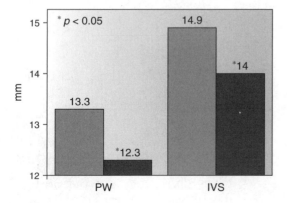

Source: Data from Kokkinos P, et al. *New Engl J Med* 1995;333:1462–1467.

Figure 12.6 LVMI at baseline and after 16 weeks of exercise training in hypertensive individuals.

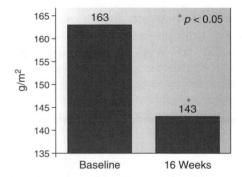

Source: Data from Kokkinos P, et al. *New Engl J Med* 1995;333:1462–1467.

dose-response fashion and reaches a plateau at approximately 180 to 200 mm Hg. DBP remains very close and even below resting levels. However, in some individuals, there is a disproportional increase in the BP response during exercise. In other words, SBP can rise substantially higher than 200 mm Hg and, similarly, DBP can rise to undesirably higher levels than resting values. Although a definitive abnormal rise threshold has not yet been established, most studies support that a SBP > 200 mm Hg or DBP > 110 mm Hg at peak or near peak exercise is considered an exaggerated BP response to exercise.

A systolic blood pressure > 200 mm Hg or diastolic blood pressure > 110 mm Hg at peak or near peak exercise is considered an exaggerated blood pressure response to exercise.

Some studies suggest that such a rise in exercise blood pressure is associated with future development of hypertension,[87,88] heart disease, and cardiovascular mortality;[89–91] however, others found no relationship.[92,93]

Evidence supports that fitness levels may play a significant role in the exercise blood pressure response. More specifically, moderate aerobic exercise training may attenuate the excessive elevations of BP during physical activity. Researchers found that higher fitness levels, as indicated by peak exercise time, were inversely associated with BP values at 6 minutes of exercise. In addition, peak exercise time was the strongest predictor of SBP response at 6 minutes of exercise in normotensive and hypertensive middle-aged women.[30] In other words, those with a low exercise capacity were more likely to have an exaggerated BP response during exercise. In another study, researchers reported significantly lower SBP and DBP levels at submaximal and maximal workloads in hypertensive patients following 16 weeks of aerobic training.[94] Significantly lower exercise SBP at a submaximal exercise workload was also reported in postmenopausal women after 8 weeks of aerobic training.[48]

■ Exaggerated Blood Pressure Response to Submaximal Exercise and Left Ventricular Hypertrophy

There is evidence that an abnormal rise in SBP during submaximal levels of exercise is associated with LVH. In fact, blood pressure at submaximal workloads may be a better predictor of LVH than peak exercise blood pressure.[31,35,75] In a recent study,[95] researchers demonstrated that men and women with normal BP values at rest but an abnormal rise in SBP during exercise equivalent to a brisk walk, had a significantly higher LVM and were more likely to have LVH. The exercise SBP at 5 METs and the change in BP from rest to the workload of 5 METs were the strongest predictors of LVH. Because 5 METs are equivalent to the metabolic demand of most daily activities, this finding suggests that the SBP at 5 METs reflects the SBP during the entire day. Furthermore, the daily exposure of the cardiovascular system to an increased hemodynamic load (high levels of SBP) presents the impetus for LVM increases observed in these patients.

Blood pressure at workloads that approximate the metabolic demand of daily activities (about 4–5 METs) appears to be the stimulus for LVM increases and is a better predictor of LVH than peak exercise BP levels.

Furthermore, researchers identified that the SBP of 150 mm Hg at the exercise levels of 5 METs was the threshold for LVH. Those beyond this BP threshold had a significantly higher LVM index when compared to individuals with an exercise BP below the 150 mm Hg threshold (**Figure 12.7**). The likelihood for LVH increased fourfold for every 10 mm Hg increment in SBP beyond this threshold. There was also a 42% reduction in the risk for LVH for every 1-MET increase in the workload.

Figure 12.7 LVMI and exercise SBP at 5 METs in individuals with normal BP levels at rest.

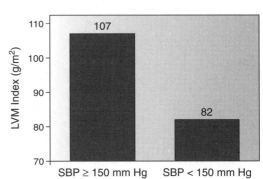

Source: Data from Kokkinos P, et al. *Hypertension* 2007;49:1–7.

Table 12.5 Resting and Exercise BP for Individuals with Optimal BP and Pre-Hypertension

	Resting BP	Exercise BP at 5 METs	Change
Optimal BP (<120/80 mm Hg)	110±5	129±10	19
Pre-hypertension (120–139/80–89 mm Hg)	131±6	148±10	17

Source: Kokkinos P, Pittaris A, Narayan P, et al. Exercise capacity and blood pressure associations with left ventricular mass in prehypertensive individuals. *Hypertension* 2007;49(1):55–61.

Interestingly, when the change in BP from rest to the exercise level of 5 METs was compared in the pre-hypertensive group and those with a BP < 120/80 mm Hg (normotensive), we noted that the change was similar (19 mm Hg vs. 17 mm Hg) for the normotensive and pre-hypertensive groups, respectively, yet the resting BP was significantly higher in the pre-hypertensive group (**Table 12.5**). Because the change in BP value was similar between the two groups and the resting BP was higher, the simplest and most likely explanation would be that it is the resting BP that provided the stimulus for the change in LVM and not the exercise BP, yet, the statistical procedures applied to determine the predictors of LVH revealed the opposite. This suggested the possibility that other factors were involved and should be considered.

■ Fitness, Exercise BP, and LVH

As the data were probed further, it became apparent that the peak exercise time was inversely related to the exercise BP. In other words, the higher the fitness level of the individual, the lower the BP value during exercise or work. This led to the hypothesis that the fitness level of the individual played a role in the BP response during exercise or physical exertion. Consequently, researchers categorized the individuals into three groups (low-fit, moderate-fit, and high-fit) based on the peak exercise time. When the change in BP from rest to exercise at 5 METs was examined, a much different picture emerged. The change in BP was 10 mm Hg higher in the low-fit group compared to the moderate and high-fit groups (**Table 12.6**).

Table 12.6 Blood Pressure Changes from Rest to Exercise and Left Ventricular Mass Index According to Fitness Levels

Group	Resting BP (mm Hg)	Exercise BP (mm Hg)	Change	LVMI (m/kg$^{2.7}$)	Prevalence of LVH (%)
Low-Fit	131	155 ± 14	24	48 ± 12	48.3
Moderate-Fit	132	146 ± 10	14	41 ± 9	18.7
High-Fit	130	144 ± 10	14	41 ± 9	21.6

In summary, researchers found that when compared to the low-fit group, moderate- and high-fit individuals exhibited significantly lower SBP at an exercise workload of 5 METs, a lower LVM index, and a lower prevalence of LVH (**Figure 12.8**). This suggests that moderate improvements in cardiorespiratory fitness achieved by moderate intensity physical activity can lead to lower hemodynamic loads during routine daily activities. Consequently, the workload of the left ventricle is reduced as is cardiac performance, ultimately resulting in lower LVM.

Support for improved hemodynamics and cardiac performance as a result of improved cardiorespiratory fitness was evident when researchers compared the daytime SBP of men and women. As depicted in **Figure 12.9**, moderate- and high-fit men and women had significantly lower daily SBP.[83]

> Fitness is associated with significantly lower systolic blood pressure at an exercise workload of 5 METs, lower left ventricular mass index, and lower prevalence of left ventricular hypertrophy.

Figure 12.9   Daytime ABP for men and women according to fitness levels.

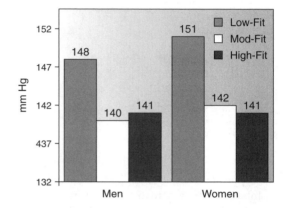

Source: Data from Kokkinos P, et al. *Journal of Hypertension* 2006;19:251–258.

■ Lowering Exercise BP with Exercise

The association between fitness and lower BP values supported by epidemiologic evidence is further substantiated by an interventional study conducted in 1997.[94] In that study, hypertensive patients underwent exercise training for 16

Figure 12.8   LVMI and exercise BP in individuals with normal BP levels at rest.

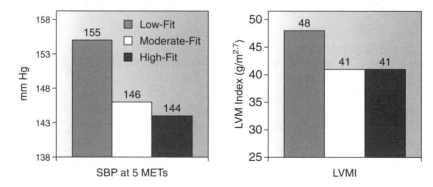

Source: Data from Kokkinos P, et al. *Hypertension* 2007;49:55–61.

weeks, three times per week. Blood pressure values during a standardized exercise test were recorded at baseline and again after 16 weeks. Changes in BP values after the 16 weeks of training were significantly lower at all submaximal workloads. Furthermore, blood pressure was lower by 20 mm Hg at maximal workload (**Figure 12.10**). This is clinically significant because it showed that BP during physical work can be attenuated with moderate levels of exercise training. This was evident even at the higher peak exercise workloads that were achieved (they did more work) after 16 weeks of training. Interestingly, the peak exercise heart rate was the same for pre- (153 ± 14 bpm) and post- (153 ± 11 bpm) exercise training, suggesting that the lower BP value during exercise was the result of lower peripheral resistance.

■ Pre-Hypertension, LVH, and Physical Activity

As discussed earlier in this chapter, pre-hypertension is a designation chosen by the JNC 7 Committee to identify individuals with an elevated risk for developing hypertension. Indeed, pre-hypertensive individuals have a significantly higher risk for developing hypertension and cardiovascular disease compared to those with normal BP.[16,24]

The factors involved in the increased risk are not well defined. Pre-hypertension may mark the beginning of a progressive increase in left ventricular mass (LVM) and a decline in cardiac function. Such changes are not accompanied by symptoms until later stages and therefore may go unnoticed for years. Because increased LVM is an independent predictor of cardiovascular disease and mortality,[84,96,97] researchers[95] investigated the potential that early changes in left ventricular structure may occur in pre-hypertensive individuals. Such changes may explain part of the increased risk. In a group of 790 men and women with pre-hypertension, we sought to determine the following:

1. The prevalence of left ventricular hypertrophy in pre-hypertensive individuals.

Figure 12.10 SBP at different workloads at baseline and after 16 weeks of aerobic training in hypertensive men.

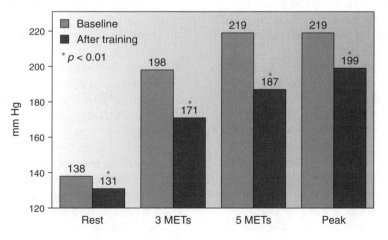

Source: Data from Kokkinos P, et al. *Am J Cardiology* 1997;79(10):1424–1426.

2. The association between LVM and blood pressure.
3. The association between fitness level, blood pressure, and LVM.

Summary of Findings and Clinical Significance

These findings support the following:

- LVH is prevalent in pre-hypertensive individuals. Over 26% of the pre-hypertensive individuals had LVH and only 3% in those with blood pressure of less than 120/80 mm Hg, considered as the optimal BP. In a similar study, the prevalence of LVH in pre-hypertensive individuals was 11.4%. However, the average age in this population was about half of the average age of the population (26.8 vs. 52 years). Collectively, these findings suggest that age also may play a role in the development of LVH.
- Improved physical fitness appears to prevent or at least attenuate the development of LVH. The likelihood of LVH was reduced by 42% for every 1-MET increase in exercise capacity.
- The presence of LVH can be predicted by the systolic BP at exercise level of 5 METs or the change in SBP from rest to the exercise levels of 5 METs.
- The likelihood of having LVH increased by fourfold for every 10 mm Hg increments above the exercise SBP threshold of 150 mm Hg. Over 86% of the individuals with LVH who achieved or exceeded the SBP threshold of 150 mm Hg were correctly identified as having LVH (sensitivity of test). Approximately 94% of those who achieved SBP levels below this threshold were identified as not having LVH (negative predictive value). The sensitivity

of 86% is substantially higher than the 6% to 53% range offered by standard electrocardiogram (ECG) criteria.[98,99]
- The prevalence of LVH was significantly higher in the low-fit individuals compared to moderate- and high-fit individuals (48.3% vs. 18.7% vs. 21.6%, respectively).
- Collectively, these findings have significant clinical value.
- Structural and functional changes in the heart occur much earlier than first thought. LVH can occur in younger pre-hypertensive individuals.
- Normal resting BP, or more accurately stated, what was considered normal resting blood pressure (< 140/90 mm Hg), does not indicate the absence of LVH. Keep in mind that 26% of middle-aged pre-hypertensive individuals in the study had LVH.
- Because the metabolic demand of most routine daily activities is approximately 3 to 5 METs, these findings suggest that the BP at the exercise level of 5 METs represents the BP during routine daily activities. This was further substantiated by findings that the 24-hour ABP was lower in fit compared to unfit individuals,[83] as discussed previously. The stimulus for the changes in the left ventricle (LVH) thus is not the resting BP, but the pressure during the entire day.
- This further suggests that moderate physical activity consisting of daily brisk walks of 30 to 40 minutes in duration can lower BP and prevent the development of LVH.
- Finally, exercise BP may be used by physicians to screen individuals who are likely to have LVH for further evaluation or to be more aggressive in treating such individuals. However, more studies are needed to support these findings.

Antihypertensive Mechanisms of Exercise

The underlying mechanisms responsible for the reduction in BP elicited by exercise training remain elusive and controversial. Current opinion prevails that exercise training must act upon a number of mechanisms. Ultimately, the effects of that action result in the reduction of total peripheral resistance, cardiac output, or both. It is generally agreed that the changes in BP are independent of changes in body weight, body composition,[76] and dietary influences. In addition, diet and exercise-induced reductions in blood pressure do not appear to be additive in this study.[38] However, it is likely that a combination of diet and exercise will be more beneficial for the hypertensive individual. Further studies regarding this issue are needed.

Reductions in cardiac output, sympathetic nerve activity, plasma norepinephrine levels, and total peripheral resistance have been reported.[48,100,101] In a meta-analysis involving 72 trials, 105 study groups, and 3,936 participants, Cornelissen and Fagard reported reductions in systemic vascular resistance, plasma norepinephrine, and plasma renin activity as the main reasons for the decrease in BP following exercise.[53] A reduction in total peripheral resistance is suggested also by changes observed in a group of hypertensive patients. Peak exercise blood pressure was significantly lower (219 ± 24 mm Hg vs. 199 ± 34 for SBP and 108 ± 10 mm Hg vs. 98 ± 13 mm Hg for DBP) at a similar maximal heart rate (153 ± 15 vs. 153 ± 11 bpm) at higher workloads, after aerobic exercise training.[94] Improved endothelial function is another possible mediator of the hypotensive response observed with exercise training. Improvement in reactive hyperemia following exercise has been demonstrated in hypertensive patients.[39]

Endothelial Function and Exercise in Hypertensive Patients

In the past two decades, several studies have shown that endothelial function is impaired in hypertensive patients.[102,103] Endothelial function has been shown to improve in healthy men following exercise training. In other studies, the effects of exercise on endothelial function were assessed in hypertensive and older individuals with normal BP values. Both studies showed that after 12 weeks of moderate intensity exercise, endothelial function improved in both hypertensive and normotensive subjects.[104,105]

Exercise Recommendations

The predicted reductions in mortality from stroke, coronary heart disease, and all causes are substantial even with modest reductions in SBP in the entire hypertensive population.[14] As stated earlier, the expected reduction in stroke and coronary heart disease with a 7.5 mm Hg reduction in DBP through antihypertensive medication is at least 46% and 29%, respectively.[10] The average reduction of 10.5 mm Hg for SBP and 7.6 mm Hg for DBP reported in the exercise studies reviewed is likely to yield similar benefits for the hypertensive patient.

Increased physical activity is also associated with reduced incidence of hypertension.[31,33] An appropriate recommendation for a public health policy on primary prevention of hypertension thus should include the implementation of a low-to-moderate intensity exercise program for most, and preferably all, days of the week, as stated by the American College of Sports Medicine (**Table 12.7**).[56] In patients with borderline BP values, increased physical activity may prevent the progression to hypertension. This is in line with the goals of Joint National Committee for Hypertension to not

Table 12.7 American College of Sports Medicine Exercise Guidelines for Lowering Blood Pressure

Exercise Type	Primarily endurance physical activity, supplemented by resistance exercise
Frequency	Most, and preferable all, days of the week
Duration	30 or more minutes of continuous or accumulated activity per day
Intensity	Moderate intensity activity (40% to < 60% of $\dot{V}O_2max$ [brisk walk]).

only treat hypertension but prevent it[12,13] and the Position Stand of the American College of Sports Medicine.[56]

As the U.S. population ages, hypertension becomes more prevalent and increasingly more difficult to treat. As more pharmacologic agents are used to control the rise in BP, the incidence of side effects increases and compliance is likely to decrease. Implementation of a regular exercise regimen alone or as an adjunct to medical therapy in hypertensive patients can improve BP control at relatively lower doses of antihypertensive pharmacologic agents and reduce adverse events.

The need for the implementation of physical activity as part of a therapeutic regimen becomes more apparent in patients with more severe stages of hypertension. These patients usually require more medication for BP control, experience more side-effects, and have a higher rate of non-compliance. Lower BP levels achieved by the implementation of an exercise program can lead to substantial reductions in the amount of medication without compromising BP control. This is likely to reduce the financial burden and improve quality of life for these patients.

Quality of life is also an important factor to consider. Once antihypertensive treatment is initiated, it is likely to continue for a lifetime unless patients make drastic lifestyle changes.[106] This raises a serious concern as to

the effect of antihypertensive medication will have on the general well-being of the patient and quality of life. The Treatment of Mild Hypertension Study (TOMHS) reported that in addition to the contribution in BP control, increased physical activity improved quality of life and had positive effects on the general well-being of the hypertensive patients.[106] Men and women also reported significant improvement in the quality of sleep with exercise.[107]

■ Exercise Programs for the Obese Hypertensive Patient

The hypertensive obese patient presents a special challenge. These patients are likely to have other cardiovascular risk factors and health-related conditions, including type 2 diabetes mellitus, dyslipidemia, and even sub-clinical CHD. When designing an exercise program for the hypertensive obese patient, these factors should be considered. It is strongly recommended that these patients undergo a detailed medical evaluation before engaging in any exercise. An exercise tolerance test to rule out CHD is also recommended especially for patients over the age of 40, a family history of CHD, or multiple risk factors. Obese patients may have concomitant musculoskeletal problems, heat intolerance, difficulty breathing, and movement restrictions, feel uncomfortable exercising due to their weight, and lack motivation.

When exercise programs are designed for these patients, exercise intensity and duration should be manipulated to promote a safe and effective antihypertensive and weight loss program. Exercise intensity should be tailored to meet individual patient needs and abilities. For the moderate-to-severely obese patient (BMI ≥ 35), the program should emphasize brisk walking and non-weight-bearing activities such as stationary biking, swimming, and other water exercises. The exercise intensity should be low and progressively increase to moderate. Patients of relatively poor fitness levels who are over the age of 50 should be advised to begin exercising at low intensities (heart rate of approximately 95 bpm to 100 bpm). As their fitness level improves, the exercise intensity can be increased progressively. Initially, the exercise duration should be 10 minutes per day, two 5-minute sessions per day (morning and evening), three days per week. As fitness levels increases, the exercise duration can progressively increase to 40 to 60 minutes per day, 5 days per week. In general, the exercise program should aim to promote a caloric expenditure of 300 to 500 kcal per day and 1,000 to 2,000 kcal per week. Such an approach in combination with a prudent diet is likely to reduce body weight. Manipulation of the exercise components (duration, frequency, and intensity) may be necessary to achieve this goal. The kcal energy expenditure for an activity that is specific to a person's weight can be estimated by multiplying the body weight in kg by the MET value and duration of the activity. For example, walking at the intensity of 4 METs (15 min/mile) expends 4 kcal/kg of body weight per hour. A 100-kg person walking for 30 minutes expends the following formula: (4 METs × 100 kg body weight) × (30 min/60 min) = 200 kcal. To expend 300 kcal,

the same individual would have to walk for 45 minutes. If walking at a pace of 3 miles per hour (i.e., a 3 MET level), he or she would have to walk for 60 minutes to expend 300 kcal. The MET equivalent for select activities is presented on **Table 12.8**.

For patients under the age of 50 or for those who are in a relatively good physical condition and not restricted by body weight (overweight to obese; BMI between 25 and 34.9), exercising at a low intensity may not present a challenge and patients may discontinue the program. Such patients may be better served if the exercise intensity is moderate (approximately 110 to 130 bpm). Periodic and progressive adjustments in the exercise intensity should be made when necessary. Exercise intensity should rise progressively every 2 to 4 weeks of regular exercise. Some recommend that increases are in the increments of approximately five heartbeats per minute, but not to exceed the upper limits of safe exercise (< 80% of PMHR). For example, a patient whose lower limit of the exercise heart rate is 100 bpm can increase it to 105 bpm.

Obese individuals are likely to have additional cardiovascular risk factors and health-related conditions, including sub-clinical CHD. When designing an exercise program for the hypertensive, obese patient these factors should be considered. Exercise should be tailored to meet individual patient needs and abilities. Exercise intensity and duration should be manipulated to promote a safe and effective antihypertensive and weight-loss program.

■ Exercise Guidelines for the Hypertensive Patient on Beta-Blockers

Certain medications used to control hypertension deserve special attention. Medications

Table 12.8 Approximate MET Levels for Select Physical Activities

Physical Activities	Mean MET Level
Volleyball	3
Water aerobics/calisthenics	4
Walking:	
4.0 mph (15 min/mile)	5
4.5 mph (~13 min/mile)	6
5.0 mph (12 min/mile)	8
Stair climbing	5
Conditioning exercise (health club exercises)	5
Dancing (aerobic)	5
Tennis	6.5
Dancing (social, square, tap)	7
Cycling (10 mph)	7
Circuit weight training	8
Running	
12 min/mile	8.7
10 min per mile	10
8 min per mile	12.5

known as beta-blockers are effective in controlling BP and offer cardioprotection for individuals with heart disease. A list of the most commonly used beta-blockers available is provided in **Table 12.9**.

A specific characteristic of beta-blockers is that they attenuate an increase in the exercise heart rate by partially blocking the beta-receptors in the heart (thus the name beta-blockers). As a result, the heart is protected against likely damage that may occur with higher heart rates. However, for those taking beta-blockers and exercising, using the maximum HR method (220 – age) to determine the intensity of exercise is no longer valid because a maximum heart rate cannot be achieved.

When one is treated with beta-blockers for high blood pressure or any other reason, the exercise heart rate can only be determined after the individual has undergone a graded exercise test.

A specific characteristic of the antihypertensive medications known as beta-blockers is that they attenuate an increase in the exercise heart rate, so the maximum heart rate during exercise is rarely achieved. The maximum HR method (220 – age) for determining exercise intensity is no longer valid. For these individuals, the exercise heart rate can only be determined by a graded exercise test.

Table 12.9 Common Beta-Blocker Medications

Generic Name	Brand Name
Acebutolol	Sectral
Atenolol	Tenormin
Bisopropolol	Zebeta
Metoprolol	Lopressor, Toprol
Nadolol	Corgard
Pindolol	Visken
Propranolol	Inderal
Satalol	Betapace
Timolol	Blocarden
Betaxolol	Kerlone
Bisoprolol	Zebeta
Penbutolol	Levatol
Carvedilol (alpha and beta-blocker)	Coreg
Labetalol (alpha and beta-blocker)	Trandate, Normodyne

■ SUMMARY

- Systolic blood pressure < 140 mm Hg and diastolic blood pressure < 90 mm Hg are considered to be normal blood pressure values. A chronic increase beyond these values in either SBP or DBP is considered hypertension.
- Blood pressure can be assessed directly and indirectly. The indirect method is by using a sphygmomanometer; a stethoscope is the most commonly used tool.
- The primary determinants of BP are cardiac output and peripheral resistance.
- Chronic elevations in BP result in structural changes of the heart and blood vessels.
- The risk of death from heart disease increases steadily as the SBP or DBP value increases. Conversely, even small reductions in elevated BP result in a reduction of death from heart disease and stroke.
- Pre-hypertension is a new classification for individuals with SBP values between 120 and 139 mm Hg and DBP values between 80 and 89 mm Hg.
- The relative risk for cardiovascular disease in these individuals is twice as likely when compared to those with normal BP. The emphasis on these individuals should be lifestyle changes to reduce the risk for developing hypertension.
- Mild- to moderate-intensity aerobic exercise is effective in lowering BP in those with all stages of hypertension.
- Left ventricular hypertrophy (LVH) is an independent risk factor for cardio-vascular disease and is prevalent in pre-hypertensive and hypertensive individuals.

- Pre-hypertensive individuals who exhibit an abnormal BP response (≥ 150 mm Hg) during exercise at workloads equivalent to routine daily (3–5 METs) are likely to have higher left ventricular mass (LVM).
- The likelihood for LVH increases fourfold for every 10 mm Hg increment in systolic blood pressure beyond this threshold.
- Exercise capacity or increased fitness attenuates the BP rise during exercise and during daily activities. In turn, fit individuals exhibit lower BP during the day (24-hour BP) and at absolute submaximal exercise workloads. These individuals also have lower LVM.
- The risk of stroke increases in individuals with increased LVM. Available data suggest this increased risk of stroke is attenuated by increased physical activity.
- In general, the available data support that the implementation of regular exercise alone or as an adjunct to medical therapy in hypertensive patients can improve BP control at relatively lower doses of antihypertensive pharmacologic agents, and reduces adverse events.

■ REFERENCES

1. Freis ED. Hypertension: pathophysiology, diagnosis, and management. In: *Historical Development of Antihypertensive Treatment*, 2nd ed. JHL Brenner, ed. New York: Raven Press; 1995:2741–2751.
2. Freis ED. Treatment of hypertension with chlorothiazide. *JAMA* 1959;169(2):105–108.
3. Freis ED. Essential hypertension. *Heart Bull* 1959;8(3):52–54.
4. Freis ED. The value of antihypertensive therapy. *Bull N Y Acad Med* 1969;45(9):951–962.
5. Freis ED. The Veterans Administration cooperative study on antihypertensive agents: implications for stroke prevention. *Stroke* 1974;5(1):76–77.
6. Freis ED, Wanko A, Wilson IM, et al. Treatment of essential hypertension with chlorothiazide (diuril); its use alone and combined with other antihypertensive agents. *JAMA* 1958;166(2):137–140.
7. Poblete PF, Kyle MC, Pipberger AV, Freis ED. Effect of treatment on morbidity in hypertension. Veterans Administration Cooperative Study on Antihypertensive Agents. Effect on the electrocardiogram. *Circulation* 1973;48(3):481–490.
8. Effects of treatment on morbidity in hypertension. Results in patients with diastolic blood pressures averaging 115 through 129 mm Hg. *JAMA* 1967;202(11):1028–1034.
9. Effects of treatment on morbidity in hypertension. II. Results in patients with diastolic blood pressure averaging 90 through 114 mm Hg. *JAMA* 1970;213(7):1143–1152.
10. MacMahon S, Peto R, Cutler J, et al. Blood pressure, stroke, and coronary heart disease. Part 1, Prolonged differences in blood pressure: prospective observational studies corrected for the regression dilution bias. *Lancet* 1990;335(8692):765–774.
11. Stamler J, Stamler R, Neaton JD. Blood pressure, systolic and diastolic, and cardiovascular risks. US population data. *Arch Intern Med* 1993;153(5):598–615.
12. Chobanian AV, Bakris GL, Black HR, et al. The seventh report of the Joint National Committee on Prevention, Detection, Evaluation, and Treatment of High Blood Pressure: the JNC 7 report. *JAMA* 2003;289(19):2560–2572. Erratum 2003;289(19):2573–2575 (see comments).
13. The sixth report of the Joint National Committee on prevention, detection, evaluation, and treatment of high blood pressure. *Arch Intern Med* 1997;157(21):2413–2446.
14. National High Blood Pressure Education Program Working Group report on primary prevention of hypertension. 1993. *Arch Intern Med* 1993;153(2):186–208.
15. Collins R, Peto R, MacMahon S, et al. Blood pressure, stroke, and coronary heart disease.

Part 2, Short-term reductions in blood pressure: overview of randomised drug trials in their epidemiological context. *Lancet* 1990; 335(8693):827–838.

16. Vasan RS, Larson MG, Leip EP, et al. Assessment of frequency of progression to hypertension in non-hypertensive participants in the Framingham Heart Study: a cohort study. *Lancet* 2001;358(9294):1682–1686.

17. World Health Organization. *World Health Report 2002: Reducing Risks to Health, Promoting Healthy Life*. Geneva: WHO;2002.

18. Lloyd-Jones D, Adams R, Carnethon M, et al. Heart disease and stroke statistics—2009 update: a report from the American Heart Association Statistics Committee and Stroke Statistics Subcommittee. *Circulation* 2009; 119:480–486.

19. Vasan RS, Beiser A, Seshandri S, et al. Residual lifetime risk for developing hypertension in middle-aged women and men: The Framingham Heart Study. *JAMA* 2002;287(8): 1003–1010.

20. Conway J. A vascular abnormality in hypertension. A study of blood flow in the forearm. *Circulation* 1963;27(4 Pt 1):520–529.

21. Folkow B, Grimby G, Thulesius O. Adaptive structural changes of the vascular walls in hypertension and their relation to the control of the peripheral resistance. *Acta Physiol Scand* 1958;44(3–4):255–272.

22. Lewington S, Clarke R, Oizilbash N, et al. Age-specific relevance of usual blood pressure to vascular mortality: a meta-analysis of individual data for one million adults in 61 prospective studies. *Lancet* 2002;360(9349): 1903–1913. Erratum 2002;261(9362):1060 (see comments).

23. Vasan RS, Larson MG, Leip EP, et al. Impact of high-normal blood pressure on the risk of cardiovascular disease. *N Engl J Med* 2001; 345(18):1291–1297. (see comments).

24. Liszka HA, Mainous AG 3rd, King DE, et al. Prehypertension and cardiovascular morbidity. *Ann Fam Med* 2005;3(4):294–299.

25. Qureshi AI, Suri MF, Kirmani JF, Divani AA. Prevalence and trends of prehypertension and hypertension in United States: National Health and Nutrition Examination Surveys 1976 to 2000. *Med Sci Monit* 2005;11(9): CR403–CR409.

26. Gibbons LW, Blair SN, Cooper KH, Smith M. Association between coronary heart disease risk factors and physical fitness in healthy adult women. *Circulation* 1983;67(5): 977–983.

27. Palatini P, Graniero GR, Mormino P, et al. Relation between physical training and ambulatory blood pressure in stage I hypertensive subjects. Results of the HARVEST Trial. Hypertension and Ambulatory Recording Venetia Study. *Circulation* 1994;90(6): 2870–2876.

28. Reaven PD, Barrett-Connor E, Edelstein S. Relation between leisure-time physical activity and blood pressure in older women. *Circulation* 1991;83(2):559–565.

29. Staessen JA, Fagard R, Amery A. Life style as a determinant of blood pressure in the general population. *Am J Hypertens* 1994;7(8): 685–694.

30. Kokkinos PF, Holland JC, Pittaras AE, et al. Cardiorespiratory fitness and coronary heart disease risk factor association in women. *J Am Coll Cardiol* 1995;26(2):358–364.

31. Blair SN, Goodyear NW, Gibbons LW, Goper KH. Physical fitness and incidence of hypertension in healthy normotensive men and women. *JAMA* 1984;252(4):487–490.

32. Haapanen N, Miilunpalo S, Vuori I, et al. Association of leisure time physical activity with the risk of coronary heart disease, hypertension and diabetes in middle-aged men and women. *Int J Epidemiol* 1997; 26(4):739–747. (see comment)

33. Paffenbarger RS Jr, Wing AL, Hyde RT, Jung DL. Physical activity and incidence of hypertension in college alumni. *Am J Epidemiol* 1983;117(3):245–257.

34. Akinpelu AO. Responses of the African hypertensive to exercise training: preliminary observations. *J Hum Hypertens* 1990; 4(2):74–76.

35. Baglivo HP, Fabriques G, Burrieza H, et al. Effect of moderate physical training on left ventricular mass in mild hypertensive

persons. *Hypertension* 1990;15(2 Suppl): I153–I156.

36. Cononie CC, Graves JE, Pollock ML, et al. Effect of exercise training on blood pressure in 70- to 79-yr-old men and women. *Med Sci Sports Exerc* 1991;23(4):505–511.

37. Dengel DR, Galecki AT, Hagberg JM, Pratley RE. The independent and combined effects of weight loss and aerobic exercise on blood pressure and oral glucose tolerance in older men. *Am J Hypertens* 1998;11(12): 1405–1412.

38. Gordon NF, Scott CB, Levine BD. Comparison of single versus multiple lifestyle interventions: are the antihypertensive effects of exercise training and diet-induced weight loss additive? *Am J Cardiol* 1997;79(6): 763–767.

39. Higashi Y, Sasaki S, Sasaki N, et al. Daily aerobic exercise improves reactive hyperemia in patients with essential hypertension. *Hypertension* 1999;33(1 Pt 2):591–597.

40. Ishikawa K, Ohta T, Zhang J, et al. Influence of age and gender on exercise training-induced blood pressure reduction in systemic hypertension. *Am J Cardiol* 1999;84(2): 192–196.

41. Kelemen MH, Effron MB, Valenti SA, Stewart KJ. Exercise training combined with antihypertensive drug therapy. Effects on lipids, blood pressure, and left ventricular mass. *JAMA* 1990;263(20):2766–2771.

42. Koga M, Ideshi M, Matsusaki M, et al. Mild exercise decreases plasma endogenous digitalislike substance in hypertensive individuals. *Hypertension* 1992;19(2 Suppl): II231–I1236.

43. Kokkinos PF, Naryan P, Colleran JA, et al. Effects of regular exercise on blood pressure and left ventricular hypertrophy in African-American men with severe hypertension. *N Engl J Med* 1995;333(22): 1462–1467.

44. Martin JE, Dubbert PM, Cushman WC. Controlled trial of aerobic exercise in hypertension. *Circulation* 1990;81(5):1560–1567.

45. Matsusaki M, Ideda M, Tashiro E, et al. Influence of workload on the antihypertensive

effect of exercise. *Clin Exp Pharmacol Physiol* 1992;19(7):471–479.

46. Motoyama M, Sunami Y, Kinoshita F, et al. Blood pressure lowering effect of low intensity aerobic training in elderly hypertensive patients. *Med Sci Sports Exerc* 1998;30(6): 818–823.

47. Rogers MW, Probst MM, Gruber JJ, et al. Differential effects of exercise training intensity on blood pressure and cardiovascular responses to stress in borderline hypertensive humans. *J Hypertens* 1996;14(11): 1369–1375.

48. Seals DR, Reiling MJ. Effect of regular exercise on 24-hour arterial pressure in older hypertensive humans. *Hypertension* 1991; 18(5):583–592.

49. Seals DR, Silverman HG, Reiling MJ, Davy KP. Effect of regular aerobic exercise on elevated blood pressure in postmenopausal women. *Am J Cardiol* 1997;80(1):49–55.

50. Somers VK, Conway J, Johnston J, Sleight P. Effects of endurance training on baroreflex sensitivity and blood pressure in borderline hypertension. *Lancet* 1991;337(8754):1363–1368. (see comment).

51. Tanaka H, Bassett DR Jr, Howley ET, et al. Swimming training lowers the resting blood pressure in individuals with hypertension. *J Hypertens* 1997;15(6):651–657.

52. Zanettini R, Bettega D, Agostoni O, et al. Exercise training in mild hypertension: effects on blood pressure, left ventricular mass and coagulation factor VII and fibrinogen. *Cardiology* 1997;88(5):468–473.

53. Cornelissen VA, Fagard RH. Effects of endurance training on blood pressure, blood pressure-regulating mechanisms, and cardiovascular risk factors. *Hypertension* 2005;46(4):667–675.

54. Kokkinos PF, Narayan P, Papademetriou V. Exercise as hypertension therapy. *Cardiol Clin* 2001;19(3):507–516.

55. Kokkinos PF, Papademetriou V. Exercise and hypertension. *Coron Artery Dis* 2000; 11(2):99–102.

56. Pescatello LS, Franklin B, Fagard R, et al. American College of Sports Medicine posi-

tion stand. Exercise and hypertension. *Med Sci Sports Exerc* 2004;36(3):533–553.

57. Kelley GA, Kelley KA, Tran ZV. Aerobic exercise and resting blood pressure: a meta-analytic review of randomized, controlled trials. *Prev Cardiol* 2001;4(2):73–80.

58. Physical exercise in the management of hypertension: a consensus statement by the World Hypertension League. *J Hypertens* 1991;9(3):283–287.

59. The fifth report of the Joint National Committee on Detection, Evaluation, and Treatment of High Blood Pressure (JNC V). *Arch Intern Med* 1993;153(2):154–183.

60. Halbert JA, Silgay CA, Finucane P, et al. The effectiveness of exercise training in lowering blood pressure: a meta-analysis of randomised controlled trials of 4 weeks or longer. *J Hum Hypertens* 1997;11(10):641–649.

61. Burt VL, Welton P, Roccella EJ, et al. Prevalence of hypertension in the US adult population. Results from the Third National Health and Nutrition Examination Survey, 1988–1991. *Hypertension* 1995;25(3):305–313. (see comment).

62. Hagberg JM, Brown MD. Does exercise training play a role in the treatment of essential hypertension? *J Cardiovasc Risk* 1995;2(4):296–302.

63. Friedewald VE Jr, Spence DW. Sudden cardiac death associated with exercise: the risk-benefit issue. *Am J Cardiol* 1990;66(2):183–188.

64. Hagberg JM, Montain SJ, Martin WH 3rd, Ehsani AA. Effect of exercise training in 60- to 69-year-old persons with essential hypertension. *Am J Cardiol* 1989;64(5):348–353.

65. Pescatello LS, Fargo AE, Leach CN Jr, Scherzer HH. Short-term effect of dynamic exercise on arterial blood pressure. *Circulation* 1991;83(5):1557–1561.

66. Borhani NO. Significance of physical activity for prevention and control of hypertension. *J Hum Hypertens* 1996;10(Suppl 2):S7–S11.

67. Fletcher GF, Blair SN, Blumenthal J, et al. Statement on exercise. Benefits and recommendations for physical activity programs for all Americans. A statement for health professionals by the Committee on Exercise and Cardiac Rehabilitation of the Council on Clinical Cardiology, American Heart Association. *Circulation* 1992;86(1):340–344.

68. MacDougall JD, Tuxen D, Sale DG, et al. Arterial blood pressure response to heavy resistance exercise. *J Appl Physiol* 1985;58(3):785–790.

69. Palatini P, Mos L, Munari L, et al. Blood pressure changes during heavy-resistance exercise. *J Hypertens Suppl* 1989;7(6):S72–S73.

70. Hurley BF, Roth SM. Strength training in the elderly: effects on risk factors for age-related diseases. *Sports Med* 2000;30(4):249–268.

71. Harris KA, Holly RG. Physiological response to circuit weight training in borderline hypertensive subjects. *Med Sci Sports Exerc* 1987;19(3):246–252.

72. Hurley BF, Hagberg JM, Goldberg AP, et al. Resistive training can reduce coronary risk factors without altering $\dot{V}O_2$max or percent body fat. *Med Sci Sports Exerc* 1988;20(2):150–154.

73. Blumenthal JA, Siegel WC, Appelbaum M. Failure of exercise to reduce blood pressure in patients with mild hypertension. Results of a randomized controlled trial. *JAMA* 1991;266(15):2098–2104.

74. Smutok MA, Reece C, Kokkinos PF, et al. Aerobic versus strength training for risk factor intervention in middle-aged men at high risk for coronary heart disease. *Metabolism* 1993;42(2):177–184.

75. Kelly GA, Kelly KS. Progressive resistance exercise and resting blood pressure: a meta-analysis of randomized controlled trials. *Hypertension* 2000;35:838–843.

76. American College of Sports Medicine. Physical activity, physical fitness and hypertension. Position stand. *Med Sci Sports Exerc* 1993;25:ix.

77. Polónia J, Martins L, Bravo-Faria D, et al. Higher left ventricle mass in normotensives with exaggerated blood pressure responses to exercise associated with higher ambulatory blood pressure load and sympathetic activity. *Eur Heart J* 1992;13(Suppl A):30–36.

78. Verdecchia P, Schillaci G, Reboldi G, et al. Different prognostic impact of 24-hour mean blood pressure and pulse pressure on stroke and coronary artery disease in essential hypertension. *Circulation* 2001;103(21): 2579–2584.

79. Cooper AR, Moore LA, McKenna J, Riddoch CJ. What is the magnitude of blood pressure response to a programme of moderate intensity exercise? Randomised controlled trial among sedentary adults with unmedicated hypertension. *Br J Gen Pract* 2000;50(461): 958–962.

80. Cox KL, Puddy IB, Morton AR, et al. Exercise and weight control in sedentary overweight men: effects on clinic and ambulatory blood pressure. *J Hypertens* 1996;14(6): 779–790.

81. Jessup JV, Lowenthal DT, Pollock ML, Turner T. The effects of endurance exercise training on ambulatory blood pressure in normotensive older adults. *Geriatr Nephrol Urol* 1998;8(2):103–109.

82. Marceau M, Kouamé N, Lacourcière Y, Cléroux J. Effects of different training intensities on 24-hour blood pressure in hypertensive subjects. *Circulation* 1993;88(6): 2803–2811.

83. Kokkinos P, Pittaras A, Manolis A, et al. Exercise capacity and 24-h blood pressure in prehypertensive men and women. *Am J Hypertens* 2006;19(3):251–258.

84. Levy D, Garrison RJ, Savage DD, et al. Prognostic implications of echocardiographically determined left ventricular mass in the Framingham Heart Study. *N Engl J Med* 1990;322(22):1561–1566.

85. Rodriguez CJ, Sacco RL, Sciacca RR, et al. Physical activity attenuates the effect of increased left ventricular mass on the risk of ischemic stroke: The Northern Manhattan Stroke Study. *J Am Coll Cardiol* 2002; 39(9):1482–1488.

86. Dahlof B, Pennert K, Hansson L. Reversal of left ventricular hypertrophy in hypertensive patients. A meta-analysis of 109 treatment studies. *Am J Hypertens* 1992;5(2):95–110.

87. Miyai N, Arita M, Miyashita K, et al. Blood pressure response to heart rate during exercise test and risk of future hypertension. *Hypertension* 2002;39(3):761–766.

88. Singh JP, Larson MG, Manolio TA, et al. Blood pressure response during treadmill testing as a risk factor for new-onset hypertension. The Framingham Heart Study. *Circulation* 1999;99(14):1831–1836.

89. Filipovsky J, Ducimetiere P, Safar ME. Prognostic significance of exercise blood pressure and heart rate in middle-aged men. *Hypertension* 1992;20(3):333–339.

90. Mundal R, Kjeldsen SE, Sandvik L, et al. Exercise blood pressure predicts cardiovascular mortality in middle-aged men. *Hypertension* 1994;24(1):56–62.

91. Mundal R, Kjeldsen SE, Sandvik L, et al. Exercise blood pressure predicts mortality from myocardial infarction. *Hypertension* 1996;27(3 Pt 1):324–329.

92. Fagard RH, Pardaens K, Staessen JA, Thijs L. Prognostic value of invasive hemodynamic measurements at rest and during exercise in hypertensive men. *Hypertension* 1996;28(1): 31–36.

93. Manolio TA, Burke GL, Savage PJ, et al. Exercise blood pressure response and 5-year risk of elevated blood pressure in a cohort of young adults: the CARDIA study. *Am J Hypertens* 1994;7(3):234–241.

94. Kokkinos PF, Pittaris A, Narayan P, et al. Effects of aerobic training on exaggerated blood pressure response to exercise in African-Americans with severe systemic hypertension treated with indapamide +/– verapamil +/– enalapril. *Am J Cardiol* 1997; 79(10):1424–1426.

95. Kokkinos P, Pittaris A, Narayan P, et al. Exercise capacity and blood pressure associations with left ventricular mass in prehypertensive individuals. *Hypertension* 2007;49(1):55–61.

96. Bikkina M, Levy D, Evans JC, et al. Left ventricular mass and risk of stroke in an elderly cohort. The Framingham Heart Study. *JAMA* 1994;272(1):33–36. (see comment)

97. Koren MJ, Devereaux RB, Casale PN, et al. Relation of left ventricular mass and geometry to morbidity and mortality in uncomplicated essential hypertension. *Ann Intern Med* 1991;114(5):345–352.

98. Devereux RB. Is the electrocardiogram still useful for detection of left ventricular hypertrophy? *Circulation* 1990;81(3):1144–1146.

99. Levy D, Labib SB, Anderson KM, et al. Determinants of sensitivity and specificity of electrocardiographic criteria for left ventricular hypertrophy. *Circulation* 1990;81(3): 815–820.

100. Cléroux J, Kouamé N, Nadeau A, et al. Aftereffects of exercise on regional and systemic hemodynamics in hypertension. *Hypertension* 1992;19(2):183–191. (see comment).

101. Floras JS, Sinkey CA, Aylward PF, et al. Postexercise hypotension and sympathoinhibition in borderline hypertensive men. *Hypertension* 1989;14(1):28–35.

102. Linder L, Kiowski W, Bühler FR, Lüscher TF. Indirect evidence for release of endothelium-derived relaxing factor in human forearm circulation in vivo. Blunted response in essential hypertension. *Circulation* 1990;81(6): 1762–1767.

103. Panza JA, Quyyumi AA, Bruch JE Jr, Epstein SE. Abnormal endothelium-dependent vascular relaxation in patients with essential hypertension. *N Engl J Med* 1990;323(1):22–27. (see comment).

104. DeSouza CA, Shapiro LF, Clevenger CM, et al. Regular aerobic exercise prevents and restores age-related declines in endothelium-dependent vasodilation in healthy men. *Circulation* 2000;102(12):1351–1357.

105. Higashi Y, Sasaki S, Kurisu S, et al. Regular aerobic exercise augments endothelium-dependent vascular relaxation in normotensive as well as hypertensive subjects: role of endothelium-derived nitric oxide. *Circulation* 1999;100(11):1194–1202. (see comments)

106. Grimm RH Jr, Grandits GA, Cutler JA, et al. Relationships of quality-of-life measures to long-term lifestyle and drug treatment in the Treatment of Mild Hypertension Study. *Arch Intern Med* 1997;157(6):638–648. (see comment)

107. King AC, Oman RF, Brassington GS, et al. Moderate-intensity exercise and self-rated quality of sleep in older adults. A randomized controlled trial. *JAMA* 1997;277(1):32–37. (see comments).

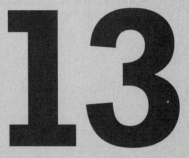
Obesity and Physical Activity

*Sudden death is more common in those
who are naturally fat than in the lean.*
Hippocrates (460–377 BC)

This quotation is evidence that obesity was a health problem even in ancient Athens, where the appreciation for beauty of the body and importance of health and fitness throughout society were held in such high regard.

In the United States and most of the industrialized world, obesity has reached epidemic proportions.[1] This chapter reviews the epidemiology, causes, and cardiovascular risks involved with obesity. The effects of physical activity, overweight/obesity, and cardiovascular risk are presented also.

■ CLASSIFICATION AND ASSESSMENT OF OVERWEIGHT AND OBESITY

Obesity is defined as the accumulation of excess body fat, usually $\geq 25\%$ of the total body weight for men and $\geq 33\%$ for women.[2]

Body composition is comprised of three major structural components: muscle, bone, and fat. Assessing body fat is not a simple task. Because direct assessment of body fat is not practical (see Chapter 2), several indirect techniques and technologies thus have been developed over the years to assess body composition. The most commonly used methods and techniques for estimating or assessing body composition and their advantages and disadvantages are described in **Table 13.1**.

Because direct body fat assessment is impractical for large populations, body mass index (BMI) was adopted by the American Heart Association (AHA) as a practical clinical indicator of adiposity.[3] BMI, calculated as weight (in kg) divided by height (in m) squared

(kg/m^2), has been shown in large epidemiologic studies to correlate well with total body fat and to be related to cardiovascular and all-cause mortality.[4–6] The estimated BMI for different weight and height is presented in **Table 13.2**.

The National Heart, Lung, and Blood Institute and World Health Organization have adapted a single set of cut-points at 5 BMI internals (**Table 13.3**) to classify overweight and obesity.[2] Based on this classification, men and women with a BMI ≥ 30 kg/m^2 are considered obese and at high risk for mortality. However, it is important to keep in mind that BMI may not accurately reflect true adiposity for some populations. For example, a relatively muscular male weighing 100 kg, 1.80 meters in height, and approximately 20% actual body fat has a BMI of 30.86 (BMI = $100/1.8^2$). According to the proposed classification system (Table 13.3), this individual is falsely classified as obese.

BMI has been shown in large epidemiologic studies to correlate well with total body fat and to be related to cardiovascular and all-cause mortality. However, it is important to keep in mind that BMI may not accurately reflect true adiposity for some populations. It also fails to take body fat distribution into account.

■ ABDOMINAL BODY FAT

Body mass index also fails to take body fat distribution into account. Fat cells in the abdominal area tend to be more metabolically active, taking up and releasing more fat than the fat cells of lower body areas (gluteal and femoral). Strong evidence supports that the excess accumulation of adipose tissue in the abdomen, characteristic of the type of fat distribution seen in men (android, abdominal, or central obesity) is associated with a higher risk for
(Continued on page 346)

Table 13.1 Various Methods of Assessing Body Composition

Method or Technique Name	Method of Assessment	Advantages	Disadvantages
Densitometry of Underwater Weighing	Subject exhales fully all air. Then he/she submerses in water for only a few seconds. Weight is assessed under water.	Considered the gold standard. It is based on the Archimedes Principle. This method computes percentage body fat from body density (body mass/body volume).	Expensive and time consuming. Requires a laboratory equipped with a water tank and trained personnel. Individuals must exhale forcefully to reduce all possible air from lungs. Then they are submersed in water for several trials, each lasting several seconds. This may not be tolerated well by some subjects, who will either not undergo the procedure or make it difficult to obtain an accurate reading.
Dual-Energy X-Ray Absorptiometry (DXA)	Uses two low-energy distinct x-ray beams that penetrate bone and soft tissue areas to the depth of 30 cm. Computer software reconstructs the attenuated beams and produces an image of the tissues to quantify muscle and fat mass.	Quick; takes approximately 12 minutes to complete and correlates very highly with densitometry. Total body mass or regional tissue mass can be assessed.	Expensive, requires trained personnel and proper equipment.
Bod-Pod	Relatively new procedure that uses an elliptically shaped box that the subject sits in. It is based on air displacement plethysmography.	Quick; takes approximately 3–5 minutes and has high reproducibility. Does not require any special skills by technician.	Expensive. Claustrophobia may be an issue with some participants.
Magnetic Resonance Imaging (MRI)		Can distinguish between changes in muscle mass and fat. Good for studies designed to assess changes in muscle mass (i.e., resistance [weight] training).	Highly expensive, requires highly trained technicians. Cost prohibitive for large cohort studies.

Method or Technique Name	Method of Assessment	Advantages	Disadvantages
Bioelectrical Impedance	A light current is introduced to the individual.	Quick, relatively inexpensive	Tends to over-predict body fat. Requires trained personnel and standardized conditions (hydration, environmental temperature) that may not be possible in all situations.
Skinfold Test	Requires a caliper that measures body fat at standardized anatomical body sites.	Relatively easy and inexpensive to perform (requires a caliper). No special laboratory required other than a room for some privacy. Time requirements are only a few minutes per subject, thus allowing large numbers of individuals to be processed.	Skilled and experienced personnel are required.
Body Mass Index	Weight and height are needed.	The simplest and least expensive method, requiring only the weight (kg) and height (m) data of the individual.	This is only an index of body composition. It does not measure body fat, but only assumes that higher BMI translates to higher body fat content. This may or may not be true and can vary greatly for different populations.
Waist Circumference and Waist:Hip Ratio	Measurements of waist and hip circumference.	Simple, inexpensive, and relatively quick to perform.	Both waist circumference and the waist-to-hip ratio are an index of body composition. They do not measure body fat. However, they both provide an index of fat distribution.

Table 13.2 Body Mass Index Based on Weight and Heigh

Height (inches)	Body Weight (lbs)													
	120	130	140	150	160	170	180	190	200	210	220	230	240	250
58	25	27	29	31	33	36	38	40	42	44	46	48	50	52
59	24	26	28	30	32	34	36	38	40	42	44	46	48	50
60	23	25	27	29	31	33	35	37	39	41	43	45	47	49
61	23	25	26	28	30	32	34	36	38	40	42	43	45	47
62	22	24	26	27	29	31	33	35	37	38	40	42	44	46
63	21	23	25	27	28	30	32	34	35	37	39	41	43	44
64	21	22	24	26	27	29	31	33	34	36	38	39	41	43
65	20	22	23	25	27	28	30	32	33	35	37	38	40	42
66	19	21	23	24	26	27	29	31	32	34	36	37	39	40
67	19	20	22	23	25	27	28	30	31	33	34	36	38	39
68	18	20	21	23	24	26	27	29	30	32	33	35	36	38
69	18	19	21	22	24	25	27	28	30	31	32	34	35	37
70		19	20	22	23	24	26	27	29	30	32	33	34	36
71		18	20	21	22	24	25	26	28	29	31	32	33	35
72		18	19	20	22	23	24	26	27	28	30	31	33	34
73			18	20	21	22	24	25	26	28	29	30	32	33
74			18	19	21	22	23	24	26	27	28	30	31	32
75				19	20	21	22	24	25	26	27	29	30	31
76				18	19	21	22	23	24	26	27	28	29	30
77				18	19	20	21	23	24	25	26	27	28	30

Body mass index < 18 is not recommended and therefore these values are not represented in this table.

Source: Jakicic JM, Clark K, Coleman E, et al. American College of Sports Medicine Position Stand on appropriate intervention strategies for weight loss and prevention of weight regain for adults. *Med Sci Sports Exerc* 2001;33(12):2401–2516.

cardiovascular morbidity and mortality than peripheral distribution of body fat.[7] Abdominal obesity is also an independent risk factor for ischemic stroke in all race and ethnic groups. The risk is about three times greater for those in the highest quartile of abdominal girth when compared to those in the lowest quartile.[8]

Cardiovascular risk may be overestimated for a woman with BMI of 30 or 32, if adiposity is distributed in the pelvic and not the abdomen area. If a direct body fat assessment is not available for these individuals, waist circumference measurement provides a practical method for assessing cardiovascular risk associated with central distribution of fat. Waist circumference correlates more strongly and directly with abdominal fat and cardiovascular risk than waist-to-hip ratio and BMI data. Waist

Table 13.3 Classification of Body Weight and Obesity Based on BMI and Waist Circumference

Body Weight	Obesity Class	BMI (kg/m²)	Waist Circumference	Associated Health Risk
Underweight		< 18.5		
Normal	–	18.5–24.9		Average
Overweight	–	25.0–29.9	Men: ≥ 94 cm Women: ≥ 80 cm	Increased
Obesity	I	30.0–34.9	Men: ≥ 102 cm Women: ≥ 102 cm	Moderate
Moderate Obesity	II	35.0–39.9		High
Severe Obesity	III	≥ 40		Very High

circumference >102 cm for men and > 88 cm for women is associated with increased cardiovascular risk.[9,10]

Excess accumulation of adipose tissue in the abdomen is associated with a higher risk for cardiovascular morbidity and mortality than peripheral distribution of body fat. Waist circumference correlates more strongly and directly with abdominal fat and cardiovascular risk than waist-to-hip ratio and BMI.

■ EPIDEMIOLOGY

Overweight and obesity are not simply cosmetic problems, but serious health conditions. They are both considered to be a leading risk factor a number of chronic health conditions such as diabetes, hypertension, coronary heart disease, and premature mortality in developed nations. The prevalence of obesity has risen significantly in both genders during the past 2 to 3 decades (**Figure 13.1**). Approximately 55% to 60% of U.S. adults are classified as over-

weight (BMI ≥ 25 kg/m²) and approximately 25% of these individuals are obese (BMI ≥ 30 kg/m²).[11,12] According to the National Health and Nutrition Examination Survey (NHANES), age-adjusted prevalence of overweight and obesity increased from 64.5% in 1999–2000 to 66.3% in 2003–2004. The prevalence of obesity alone (BMI ≥ 30 kg/m²) increased during this period from 30.5% to 34.2% and for extreme obesity from 4.7% to 5.9%.[13]

The estimated excess number of deaths annually in 2000 that were attributable to obesity among adults in the United States was nearly 112,000 relative to normal weight.[14] Some reports suggest that the number could be as high as 300,000.[15]

■ CHILDREN AND ADOLESCENTS

The statistics of obesity for children and adolescents during the past 2 decades are even more alarming than adults. The number of overweight children during this period has doubled.[16] As illustrated in **Figure 13.2**, the prevalence of

Figure 13.1 Age-adjusted prevalence of obesity in adults 20 to 74 years of age from 1974 to 2004.

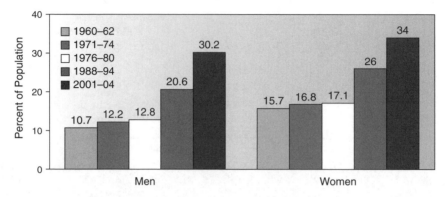

Source: From Lloyd-Jones D, et al. Heart disease and stroke statistics—2009 update. A report from the American Heart Association Statistics Committee and Stroke Statistics Subcommittee. *Circulation* 2009;119:e21–e181.

overweight children between the ages 6 to 11 years increased from 4% in 1971–1974 to 17.5% in the years 2001–2004. Similarly, the prevalence of obesity and overweight in adolescents (12–19 years of age) increased by almost three-fold, from 6.1% to 17%.[13] Based on the 2000 Centers for Disease Control and Prevention (CDC) growth chart for the United States, nearly 10 million children aged 6 to 9 and adolescents 6 to 19 years of age are considered obese. In 1999 to 2000, 10% of preschool children aged 2 to 5 were overweight. This rate increased to 14% during the 2003–2004 periods.[13] Obviously, children are becoming overweight and obese at progressively younger age.[17] Although these statistics are derived primarily from Americans, there is

Figure 13.2 Prevalence of overweight in U.S. children and adolescents by age from 1974 to 2004.

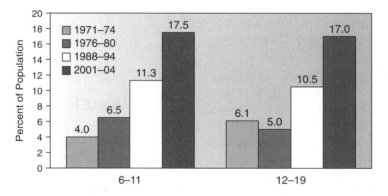

Source: From Lloyd-Jones D, et al. Heart disease and stroke statistics—2009 update. A report from the American Heart Association Statistics Committee and Stroke Statistics Subcommittee. *Circulation* 2009;119:e21–e181.

strong evidence that the incidence of obesity is increasing globally.[6]

This trend in childhood obesity raises concerns of an even greater preponderance of adult obesity in the future. Even more alarming, it raises concern that childhood obesity will lead to chronic health problems in adulthood. These trends were been substantiated recently by the findings of a large study of 10,235 men and 4,318 women born from 1930 through 1976. During a follow-up period of 46 years, investigators assessed the relationship between BMI in childhood (7 through 13 years of age) and coronary heart disease (CHD). The adjusted risk for CHD increased with higher BMI in both men and women. In addition, the association between BMI and CHD was stronger for boys than girls but increased with age for both sexes.[18] For each 1-unit increase in BMI at every age from 7 to 13 years, the risk for CHD increased significantly for both genders. Because children are becoming overweight at progressively younger ages, the investigators urged that focus be placed on helping children attain and maintain normal weight to prevent adverse health consequences in the future.

■ COST

The total cost of overweight and obesity was estimated at $117 billion in 2001 and $132 billion in 2002.[19,20] The annual hospital cost related to obesity among children and adolescents was $127 million between 1997 and 1999.[19]

■ CAUSES OF OBESITY

The mechanisms and causes of obesity are poorly understood. Both genetic factors and lifestyle are likely to contribute significantly to variability of body weight in humans.[6] Most experts agree that obesity is the result of chronic

imbalance between caloric intake and caloric expenditure. Simply stating it, obesity is the result of a chronic imbalance between energy intake in the form of food and drink and total energy expenditure. A net deficit in energy balance, either through a reduction in energy intake or an increase in energy expenditure, leads to weight reduction. Conversely, a net excess in energy balance due to a reduction in energy expenditure or an increase in energy intake, leads to weight gain. However, why some people get fat while others don't—even when food intake is similar—is poorly understood.

> Obesity is the result of a chronic imbalance between caloric intake and caloric expenditure. This may be the outcome of a complex interaction between genetic and environmental factors.

Interestingly, a small imbalance in daily energy can lead to significant weight changes over a period of a year. For example, the chemical energy stored in 1 pound (lb) of fat tissue is approximately 3,500 kcal. The average caloric intake of a non-obese adult is approximately 2,465 kcal per day. If caloric intake exceeded expenditure by just 140 kcal a day (i.e., one 12-oz can of Coke per day or any other drink of equivalent caloric value) for 1 year, the result will be a weight gain of approximately 14.6 lbs of adipose tissue.

A chronic energy imbalance that favors weight gain may be the outcome of a complex interaction between genetic and environmental factors.[21,22] However, it is virtually impossible to blame genes for the increase in obesity of epidemic proportion in the United States in the past 20 years, because the gene pool has not changed significantly.[21] It is more likely that the genetic makeup may not necessarily cause obesity, but in the presence of powerful environmental influences, the propensity for obesity is enhanced.

The environmental factors for obesity appear to be over-consumption of calories and reduction in physical activity. Of the two, physical inactivity appears to play the predominant role. According to the 1998 National Institutes of Health (NIH) report on obesity, total caloric intake over the last two decades has not substantially increased while physical activity has decreased significantly.[23]

> The environmental factors for obesity appear to be over-consumption of calories and reduction in physical activity. Of the two, physical inactivity appears to play the predominant role.

■ OBESITY, RISK FACTORS, AND MORTALITY

Cardiovascular Disease

Prior to 1998, obesity was not considered an independent risk factor for CHD. In June 1998, the AHA reclassified overweight and obesity as a major, modifiable risk factor for CHD, comparable in status to the other well-established CHD risk factors.[6]

The findings from several large cohort studies support this view. Data from the Framingham Study show that the degree of obesity was a strong predictor of cardiovascular disease (CVD) for both men and women.[24] Moreover, the influence of obesity on CVD was independent of major CVD risk factors including age, systolic blood pressure (SBP), serum cholesterol, glucose intolerance, left ventricular hypertrophy (LVH), and smoking.

The Nurses' Health Study, with a cohort of over 115,000 middle-aged women free of CVD at baseline, also reported a direct and unequivocal association between the BMI and cardiovascular risk; its findings revealed a direct relationship between BMI and risk of CHD and

mortality. In the 1990 publication, the risk of non-fatal myocardial infarction and CHD mortality was assessed in those with BMI values: < 21; 21 to < 23; 23 to < 25; 25 to < 29; and ≥ 29.[25] As illustrated in **Figure 13.3**, the risk rose progressively with each category of increasing BMI, reaching a 3.3-fold increase in those with the highest BMI (≥ 29).[25] Similarly, in a study of 25,714 men, the relative risk for CVD mortality was 2.0 for men with BMI of 25.0–29.9 (overweight) and 2.6 for obese men (BMI ≥ 30.0) when compared to men of normal weight.[26]

However, not all studies reported a positive association between increased body fat and mortality risk, so the mortality risk association with being overweight or obese remains controversial.[27–29] Some studies reported higher mortality rates in the very lean and very fat, referred to as *J-shaped* or *U-shaped associations*.[5,30–34] Others reported an inverse association, coined as the *obesity paradox*, usually observed in heart failure patients[36,37] and recently reported in non-heart failure veterans.[37] Some studies have even reported no association between body composition and mortality.[31,32,35,38]

The absence of a direct relationship between body weight and mortality may be due to the failure of these studies to control for at least one of confounding factors such as smoking, pre-existing illness, hypertension, and hyperglycemia.[39,40] When adjusted for age only, the finding supported a somewhat of a J-shaped relationship. However, when smokers were excluded, the relationship became direct and more robust. The relative risk for cardiovascular disease death was four times higher in women with BMI ≥ 29.0 kg/m^2 when compared to the leanest women with BMI < 22 kg/m^2. Rates of death due to coronary heart disease were 4.6 and 5.8 times higher in non-smoking women with BMI of 29–31.9 and ≥ 32 kg/m^2, respectively, when compared to those with BMI < 22.0 kg/m^2 (**Figure 13.4**). These findings suggest that the lower mortality risk at the

Figure 13.3 Relative risk of myocardial infarctions in women according to BMI.

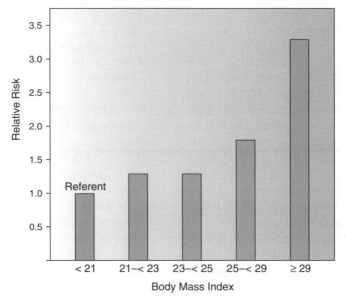

Source: Adapted from Manson JE, et al. *N Engl J Med* 1990;322(13):882–889.

Figure 13.4 Cardiovascular risk of death for women who never smoked according to BMI.

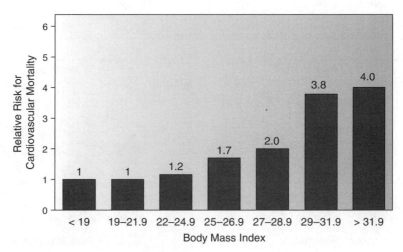

Source: Data from Manson JE, et al. *N Engl J Med* 1995;333(11):677–685.

lower BMI strata was at least in part the consequence of smoking.[5]

Further evidence of the association between smoking, fatness, and mortality was provided by another large prospective study in the United States. During a 14-year follow-up of 457,785 men and 588,369 women, there were 201,622 deaths. The relative risk of death from cardiovascular disease in those with the highest BMI was 2.90 for white men and 2.3 for white women, respectively, as compared with those with a BMI of 23.5 to 24.9. Men and women with a higher BMI had a significant increase in risk of death in all age groups (**Figure 13.5**). The risk associated with a high BMI is greater for whites than for blacks.[41]

To determine whether the risk of death varies according to smoking and disease status, the investigators examined the relationship between BMI and mortality according to smoking status and the presence or absence of a history of disease. The following three major findings emerged[41] (**Figure 13.6**):

- The association between obesity and risk of death was strongest among non-smokers who had no history of disease.

- The association between leanness and risk of death was strongest among current or former smokers with a history of disease.
- The risk of death was intermediate in non-smokers with history of disease and current or former smokers with no history of disease.

Two main conclusions can be drawn from this large study. First, overweight and obesity are associated with a graded increase in risk of death. Second, the higher risk of death observed in lean individuals was the outcome of smoking and/or the pre-existing disease and not leanness itself.

However, controlling for smoking and other risk factors does not completely account for increased mortality in all cases. For example, in one population of approximately 16,000 male veterans, a preliminary analysis revealed a graded inverse relationship between BMI and mortality (unpublished data). This association strengthened after adjusting for cardiorespiratory fitness; it appeared to be stronger in blacks than whites and independent of cardiovascular disease status. In addition, mortality was significantly higher in those with a BMI of < 20.

Figure 13.5　Relative risk of cardiovascular death according to BMI.

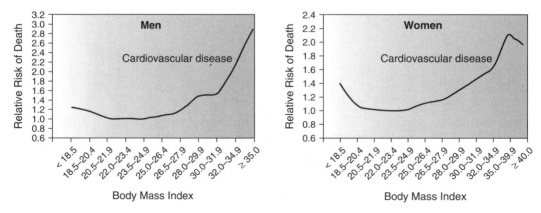

Source: From Calle E, et al. *N Engl J Med* 1999;341(15):1097–1105.

Figure 13.6 Obesity, leanness, and mortality in smokers and nonsmokers with and without disease.

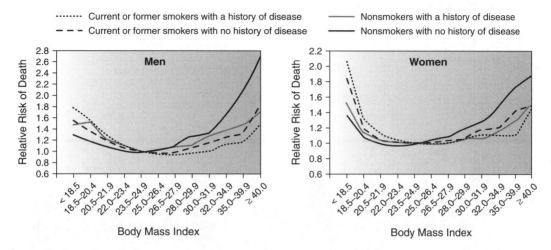

Source: Adapted from Calle E, et al. *N Engl J Med* 1999;341(15):1097–1105.

These observations confirm the notion that in at least some populations, very lean individuals are at a higher risk for mortality. The reason(s) for this is not yet understood.

> Most studies support that overweight and obesity are associated with a graded increase in a risk of death. However, in at least some populations, very lean individuals are at a higher risk for mortality. The reason(s) for this observation is not yet understood.

Obesity and Mortality

As mentioned previously, BMI fails to take body fat distribution into account. Strong evidence supports that the excess accumulation of adipose tissue in the abdomen, (central obesity) is associated with a higher risk for cardiovascular morbidity and mortality than peripheral distribution of body fat.[7] Waist cir-

cumference has been proposed as a surrogate for central obesity. Waist circumference > 102 cm for men and > 88 cm for women is associated with an increased cardiovascular risk.[9,10] However, no large studies have examined and compared the predictive value of BMI and waist circumference.

In a recent large study, the association between BMI, waist circumference, and mortality was assessed in 359,387 individuals from nine European countries who were followed for over 9 years.[42] The conclusions of this study are:

- The J-shape relationship between death and both BMI and waist circumference is evident in both genders.
- The lowest risks of death were observed at a BMI of 25.3 among men and 24.3 among women. Increased risk of death was observed in the lowest and highest BMI categories (**Figure 13.7**).
- When the data were adjusted for BMI, waist circumference was positively

Figure 13.7   Adjusted relative risk of mortality for men and women according to BMI and waist circumference. Note the J-shape with the lowest risk observed at a BMI of 25 to < 26.5 for men and 23.5 to < 25 for women.

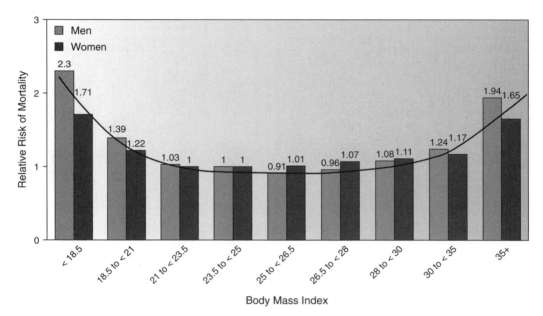

Source: Data from Pischon T, et al. *N Engl J Med* 2008;359:2105–2120.

associated with death. For a given BMI, a 5-cm larger waist circumference was associated with a 17% increase in death for men and 13% in women.

- When general obesity (BMI) was adjusted, the association between waist circumference (abdominal fat) and death was positive and linear (**Figure 13.8**). In addition, the associations tended to be stronger among individuals in lower than higher BMI levels. This observation may explain why the association between BMI and risk of mortality was J-shaped and not linear across the entire range of BMI values.

The overall message of this study is that both BMI (general obesity) and waist circum-

ference (abdominal obesity) are associated with the risk of mortality. However, the use of waist circumference in addition to BMI is useful and should be included, especially in individuals with a low BMI.

Most studies support that overweight and obesity are associated with a graded increase in risk of death. However, in at least some populations, very lean individuals are at higher risk for mortality. According to the findings of a recent study, the distribution of fat (general vs. central obesity) appears to explain part of that observation, suggesting that waist circumference should be considered, especially for individuals with low BMI.

Figure 13.8 Adjusted relative risk of mortality for men and women according to waist circumference adjusted for BMI. Note the linear association between waist circumference and mortality risk.

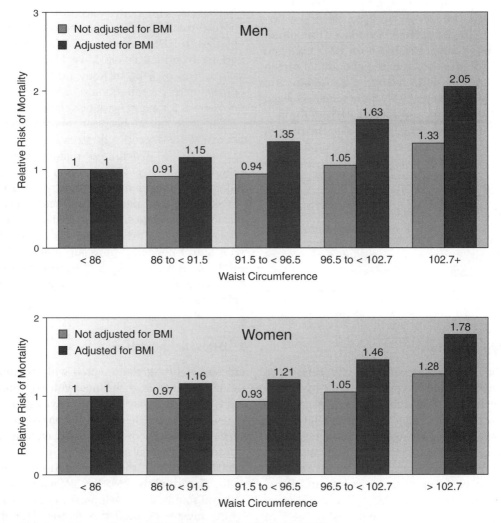

Source: Data from Pischon T, et al. *N Engl J Med* 2008;359:2105–2120.

Other Risk Factors

Obesity not only directly increases the CHD risk but also amplifies it indirectly because of the adverse effects of obesity on several established CHD risk factors. Evidence from multiple studies supports that both BMI $\geq$ 27 and the distribution of fat in the abdominal region of the body (as indicated by a waist-to-hip ratio > 0.85 in women and 0.98 cm in men or a waist circumference of $\geq$ 98 cm and $\geq$ 85 cm for men and women, respectively) are associated with hypertension, diabetes, abnormal lipids, and increased CHD mortality.[5,24,26,41,43–46]

Obesity not only directly increases the CHD risk but also amplifies it indirectly because of the adverse effects of obesity on several established CHD risk factors such as hypertension, lipids and lipoproteins, and diabetes mellitus.

■ Hypertension

Obesity is strongly and directly related to hypertension and the prevalence of hypertension increases as weight increases regardless of age, race, or gender.[47–49] Central fat distribution may be a stronger predictor for developing hypertension than either body weight or BMI.[44,45,50] Conversely, a reduction in body weight even as small as 4.5 kg lowers BP significantly (see Chapter 12).[51,52] In the Dietary Intervention Study in Hypertension, 60% of the obese hypertensive patients who reduced their body weight by an average of 4.5 kg remained normotensive without antihypertensive medication.[53] When weight reduction is added to antihypertensive pharmacologic therapy, a significantly better BP control is achieved.[54]

■ Lipids and Lipoproteins

Obesity is also associated with lipoprotein and lipid abnormalities including lower HDL-cholesterol, and high triglyceride and LDL-cholesterol levels.[46] Conversely, favorable changes in HDL-cholesterol, LDL-cholesterol, and triglycerides levels have been reported with a loss of 5 kg in body fat.[55,56] There is approximately a reduction of 2 mg/dl of total cholesterol for every kg of body weight lost.[57]

The association between obesity and an abnormal lipid profile is stronger when the excess fat is distributed mainly centrally (abdominal obesity). The abnormalities include increased proportion of the more atherogenic small, dense, LDL particles, and higher fasting plasma triglyceride and lower HDL-cholesterol concentrations. Furthermore, the lower HDL-cholesterol concentrations are mainly attributed to fewer HDL_2-cholesterol particles believed to be more protective against atherosclerosis.[58–60]

■ Diabetes Mellitus

Obesity is strongly associated with the development of insulin resistance, glucose intolerance, and diabetes in both developed and developing countries.[61,62] Approximately 90% of patients with type 2 diabetes mellitus are obese.[39] Abdominal obesity may play a more significant role in the manifestation of metabolic abnormalities.[43,63] It also may play an integral role in the development of and is part of the cluster of CHD risk factors identified and designated as metabolic syndrome.[64]

The risk for developing type 2 diabetes rises with the degree of obesity for men and women.[65–67] In the 5-year study of more than 20,000 U.S. male physicians, the relative risk of type 2 diabetes tripled with a BMI > 26.4.[66] In a similar study, the risk for developing type

2 diabetes was elevated significantly (odds ratio = 2.0) in non-diabetic men with a BMI ≥ 27 kg/m^2.[67] In a study of more than 114,000 female nurses followed for 14 years,[65] the increase in relative risk for type 2 diabetes was significantly and directly related to the increase in BMI (**Figure 13.9**). Interestingly, the risk for diabetes increased in women who gained weight during the study and decreased in those who lost weight, suggesting a causal relationship.

The mechanisms mediating the association of excess fat accumulation and type 2 diabetes are not fully understood. Research supports that a combination of genetic factors and molecular mechanisms involving skeletal muscle and fat cells play an integral role in the development of insulin resistance, glucose intolerance, and ultimately diabetes.[68–70]

■ WEIGHT LOSS PROGRAMS

The recent rise in the prevalence of obesity has prompted an acute interest in obesity-related research. Many pharmacologic and non-pharmacologic interventions have been tried and certainly more will follow in the future. Thus far, successful treatment of obesity is limited. In addition, relatively few pharmacologic treatments have been approved by the Food and Drug Administration. These treatments generally induce modest weight loss that is regained soon after discontinuation. Potential

Figure 13.9 Age-adjusted risk for developing type 2 diabetes in women according to BMI.

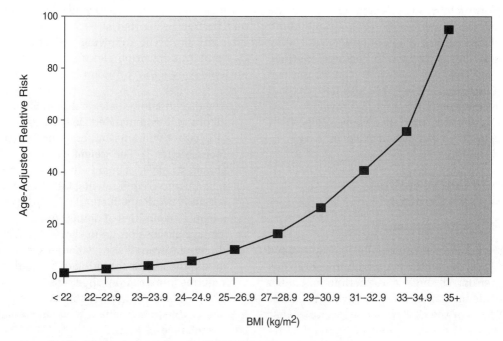

Source: From Colditz GA, et al. *Ann Intern Med* 1995;122(7).

major health risks have been associated with at least some of these medications.

Regardless of the availability of pharmacologic treatments, federal and other health authorities strongly recommend that exercise and sensible eating habits should be emphasized.[21,23] There are several compelling reasons for this recommendation:

1. The combination of proper exercise and diet provide the most effective way to prevent obesity.
2. Exercise is the most consistent factor in maintaining post-therapy weight losses.
3. It is the most efficacious and cost-effective therapy with minimum, if any, side effects.
4. It can be used in conjunction with pharmacologic therapy and improve the outcome.
5. It has a positive impact on overall health.

Unfortunately, only 42% of patients are being counseled by a healthcare professional about weight loss[71] and only 34% of patients are being counseled by physicians to begin or continue exercise. This is true despite the strong evidence of exercise-related health benefits and recommendations by the U.S Preventive Services Task Force that physicians advise their able patients to increase physical activity.[72]

Dietary Interventions for Weight Control

■ Caloric Restrictions

Weight reduction is principally determined and directly related to the net deficit in energy balance, either through a reduction in energy intake or an increase in energy expenditure regardless of the diet composition.[73] Because the chemical energy stored in 1 pound of fat tissue is approximately 3,500 kcal, a deficit of 1,500 kcal per day theoretically will lead to 3 pounds of fat loss in 1 week. This is an enticing proposition for the obese patient, and gave rise to a number low-calorie (< 1,200 kcal/day) and even very-low calorie (< 800 kcal/day) diet programs worldwide.

The rapid reduction of body weight achieved by starvation or semi-starvation diets and their popularity are not surprising. Unfortunately, most of these diets have little or no scientific merit and are rather limited in promoting safe and effective weight reduction and maintenance. In fact, they can be very unhealthy and potentially dangerous. Thus, dramatic and rapid weight loss (beyond 1 kg per week) should be discouraged. According to the American College of Sports Medicine, the daily caloric restriction should be between 500 and 1,000 kcal, with a caloric intake not lower than 1,200 kcal/day, and weight reductions of no more than 1 kg or approximately 2 lbs per week.[12,74,75] This results in smaller losses of water, electrolytes, minerals, glycogen stores, and fat-free tissue and is less likely to cause malnutrition.[48] The following are characteristics and guiding principles for a responsible and safe weight loss program.[12,74-76]

- The diet should be safe. It should include all of the Recommended Daily Allowances (RDAs) for vitamins, minerals, and protein (see Chapter 3). The weight loss diet should supply less energy than the patient's maintenance requirements, but maintain essential nutrients. It should also provide adequate quantities of dietary fiber.
- The weight loss program should be directed toward a slow, steady weight loss unless the health condition of the patient requires more rapid weight loss.
- The diet must be as palatable and acceptable to the patient to aid in patient compliance.
- The program should include a strategy for weight maintenance after the weight loss

phase. It is of little benefit to lose a large amount of weight only to regain it later. The dietary strategy therefore should be associated with behavior modification and increased physical exercise.

- A medical assessment of the general health of the patient and medical conditions that might be affected by dieting and weight loss is a *sine qua non* prior to each dietary strategy. Also, medical advice on the appropriateness of weight loss is of utmost importance, as is the definition of a sensible goal of weight loss tailored to each individual.

In summary, it is imperative to keep in mind the two major objectives of any weight reduction program:

1. Provide healthy and effective nutrition for the individual
2. Reduce body fat while maintaining lean body mass

More importantly, some responsible perspective must be given to the effects that diet has on the cardiovascular system and the premature development of CHD. Finally, in the desperate and obsessive quest to lose weight, it is important to emphasize that the hype must be tempered by the very sobering fact that most of the weight lost during the dieting period is gained back within 1 to 5 years.[77]

Most of the weight lost by dieting alone is gained back within 1 to 5 years.

■ Dietary Manipulations

Diet composition modifications are based on the assertion that restriction of one energy source (i.e., carbohydrates) will create a deficit and force the body's metabolism to shift to predominantly burn fat for energy. Based on this assertion, low carbohydrate, high fat/high protein diets have gained an overwhelming popularity. These diets dismiss the notion that caloric intake is important in weight gain or loss and propose that carbohydrates are the villains in obesity.

There is some support that in at least some populations, weight losses are initially greater with a high-fat, low-carbohydrate diet than the more traditional low-fat, high-carbohydrate diets.[78,79] However, the greater weight loss is likely the result of fewer calories consumed by those on a high-fat diet and not due to any metabolic advantage of such diet that enables weight loss even at a greater consumption of calories.[78–81] Even so, it is prudent to view these reports with caution. Both studies were short term, so the long-term effects of high-fat, low-carbohydrate diets on the risk of heart disease remains uncertain.

A more balanced approach to weight reduction is a moderate restriction in total energy intake by reducing both fat and carbohydrate intake. Because weight loss is determined by caloric restriction, such an approach leads to a greater reduction in body weight, with lower losses in lean body mass and micronutrients than diets that restrict only dietary fat or carbohydrate intake.[82] Finally, a diet recommended for the prevention and treatment of heart disease, diabetes, and cancer should be emphasized for the prevention and treatment of obesity. Overwhelming evidence favors a balanced diet that is low in simple sugars, saturated fat, and red meat, while high in fiber and complex carbohydrates, particularly in fruits, vegetables, legumes, and cereals. This is similar to the Mediterranean diet. In the Lyon Heart Study,[83] a Mediterranean-style diet resulted in a 76% reduction in cardiovascular events after a 5-year period.

Physical Activity and Weight Loss

The rationale that chronic exercise promotes a reduction in body fat is based on the premise that exercise increases total daily energy expenditure without a corresponding increase in energy intake.[84]

The emphasis here is on the corresponding increase in energy intake. It is now well accepted that exercise alone results in modest but favorable changes in body weight and body fat distribution. A meta-analysis reported an exercise-induced weight reduction of 0.2 kg per week.[85] This exercise-induced weight reduction is achieved by long-term aerobic exercises or physical activity of sufficient intensity, duration, and frequency. However, when the energy intake is held constant, exercise alone can achieve significant and more impressive weight losses.[84] This was shown in at least one study where the investigators achieved 7.6 lbs of weight loss over a period of 3 months when an energy deficit of 700 kcal per day was achieved by exercise only and caloric intake was held constant to pre-exercise levels.[86]

The effectiveness of exercise to induce weight loss is directly related to the total number of kcal expanded.[87] In this regard, the duration of exercise becomes important. In a recent 18-month exercise study, overweight women exercising more than 200 minutes per week realized a significantly greater weight reduction (−13.1 kg) than those exercising 150 to 200 minutes/week (−8.5 kg), or less than 150 minutes/week (3.5 kg). The investigators concluded that a dose-response relationship existed between amount of exercise and long-term weight loss, and that a minimum of 150 minutes of exercise per week may be necessary for enhanced weight loss.[88]

Although the exercise-induced losses in body weight may be viewed as relatively small and disappointing by some, it is worth point-ing out that weight loss must be viewed as a long-term process. After all, excess weight accumulation did not occur overnight. In this regard, long-term exercise-induced weight is promising. In an 8-week-diet or diet-plus-exercise program consisting of 35 to 60 minutes of aerobic activity 3 days per week, weight losses were similar in both groups. However, those who did not exercise during the 18-month follow-up period gained about 60% of the weight back in 6 months and 92% of the weight back at 18 months. For those who continued to exercise during the 18-month follow-up period, body weight did not change significantly (**Figure 13.10**).[89] Finally, increased physical activity combined with a prudent diet and behavior modification is likely to be a more effective a way to maximize weight loss.[90,91] Furthermore, the exercise program should focus on long duration and low intensity, tailored for expending calories rather than improving fitness.[90]

Author's Note

Does Exercise Increase Appetite?

If exercise increases energy expenditure, why is it that it does not increase energy intake? In fact, initially exercise does increase energy intake. That is why the most effective way to lose weight through exercise is to also control energy intake.

However, in the long run, exercise creates an energy deficit. Why this occurs is not quite clear. Perhaps it is related to the intrinsic response of the body or any parts of it exposed to the stimulus (stress) to become more efficient in order to handle and overcome the stress imposed upon it. In the case of excess body fat, the regularly performed exercise requires that the muscles become more efficient in carrying the body through the exercise process. For this, muscles must get stronger (and they do) and excess weight (fat) must be shed.

Figure 13.10 Weight loss with diet or a combination of exercise and diet. Note that the initial weight loss was similar in both groups. However, only the diet combined with exercise group maintained weight losses during the 18 months of follow-up.

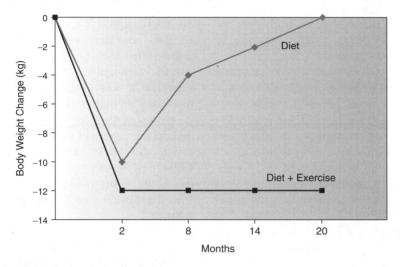

Source: Adapted from Pavlou KN, et al. *Am J Clin Nutr* 1989;49(5 Suppl):1115–1123.

The American College of Sports Medicine states that exercise has to be a key component in any weight loss program. If exercise is not included, the program is incomplete and likely to fail.

■ Exercise Programs

When designing an exercise program for the obese patient to promote long-term weight loss, several factors should be considered. Obese patients are likely to have other cardiovascular risk factors and health-related conditions, including type 2 diabetes mellitus, hypertension, dyslipidemia, and even subclinical CHD. They also may have musculoskeletal problems, heat intolerance, difficulty breathing, and movement restrictions, feel uncomfortable exercising due to their weight, and lack motivation. It is strongly recommended that the obese patient undergo a detailed medical evaluation before engaging in any exercise. An exercise tolerance test to rule out CHD is recommended especially for patients over the age of 40, with family history of CHD, or multiple risk factors.

Recommendations for exercise intensity should be tailored to meet individual patient needs and abilities. For patients with moderate or severe obesity (classes II and III), the exercise program should emphasize non–weight-bearing or low-impact activities such as stationary biking, walking, swimming, and other water exercises. The exercise intensity should be low and progressively increased to moderate levels. Patients of relatively poor fitness levels and over the age of 50 should be advised to begin exercising at low intensities (heart rate of approximately 95 bpm to 100 bpm). As the fitness level of such patients improves, the exercise intensity can be increased progressively.

For patients under the age of 50 or for those who are in a relatively good physical condition and not restricted by body weight (overweight to obese class I), exercising at a low intensity may not present a challenge and patients may discontinue the program. Such individuals may be better served if the exercise intensity is moderate (approximately 110–130 bpm). As fitness increases, his or her resting heart rate is likely to decrease. The exercise heart rate should then be recalculated based on the heart rate reserve method discussed in Chapter 2.

Periodic and progressive adjustments in the exercise intensity should be made when necessary. Exercise intensity should rise progressively every 2 to 4 weeks of regular exercise. It is recommended that increases are in the increments of approximately five heartbeats per minute, but not to exceed the upper limits of safe exercise (80% of the predicted maximum heart rate [PMHR]). For example, a patient whose lower limit of exercise heart rate is 100 bpm can increase it to 105 bpm after 2 to 4 weeks of regular exercise.[92]

Exercise-induced weight loss is the result of the interaction between exercise intensity, frequency, duration, and length of training. Because the primary fuel on low intensity, long-duration exercises is fat, the traditional thinking was that this type of exercise may be more suitable for fat reduction. However, the common factor in exercise-induced weight reduction appears to be caloric expenditure. In general, regardless of the type, duration, frequency, or preferred fuel, exercises with similar caloric expenditures are likely to yield similar losses in body weight.

It is also important to emphasize that low rather than high intensity exercise should be encouraged for the following reasons: (1) patients are more likely to participate in a low rather than high intensity exercise; and (2) the risk-benefit ratio for low intensity exercise is substantially lower than that for exercises of higher intensities. Finally, exercise prescription for body fat reduction and weight management should adhere to the following guidelines provided by the American College of Sports Medicine.[12,75] The duration required for different activities to expand 300 kcal for different body weights is provided in **Table 13.4**.

- Obese patients should be encouraged to initiate an exercise program of low-to-moderate intensity, and long duration to reduce the risk for cardiovascular complications and orthopedic injuries.
- The frequency should be most days of the week with preferably some activity performed every day.
- The duration of exercise should be sufficient to cause the expenditure of 200 to 300 kcal per exercise session. Exercise programs should be adjusted to promote progressively higher caloric expenditure of 300 to 500 kcal per session or 1,000 to 2,000 kcal per week as the obese patient develops confidence, muscular strength, and cardiovascular endurance. The duration needs to be continuous to produce benefits.
- A daily accumulation of 30 to 60 minutes of exercise and a minimum of 150 minutes per week is preferred. Durations longer than the minimum 150 minutes yield greater losses. Some work supports that exercise durations > 200 minutes may be needed

Table 13.4 Minutes of Continuous Activity Necessary to Expand 300 kcal Based on Body Weight

Activity	120	130	140	150	160	170	180	190	200	210	220	230	240	250
Stationary cycling	66	61	57	53	50	47	44	42	40	38	36	35	33	32
Cycling (leisure)	83	76	71	66	62	58	55	52	50	47	45	43	41	40
Walking														45
3.0 mph	94	87	81	76	71	67	63	60	57	54	52	49	47	
3.5 mph	83	76	71	66	62	58	55	52	50	47	45	43	41	40
Swimming	41	38	35	33	31	29	28	26	25	24	23	22	21	20
Yoga	83	76	71	66	62	58	55	52	50	47	45	43	41	40
Resistance exercise	55	51	47	44	41	39	37	35	33	31	30	29	28	26
High impact aerobic dance	55	51	47	44	41	39	37	35	33	31	30	29	28	26
Low impact aerobic dance	66	61	57	53	50	47	44	42	40	38	36	35	33	32
Golf (walking)	73	68	63	59	55	52	49	46	44	42	40	38	37	35
Raking a lawn	83	76	71	66	62	58	55	52	50	47	45	43	41	40
Lawn mowing	73	68	63	59	55	52	49	46	44	42	40	38	37	35

Source: Jakicic JM, Clark K, Coleman E, et al. American College of Sports Medicine Position Stand on appropriate intervention strategies for weight loss and prevention of weight regain for adults. *Med Sci Sports Exerc* 2001;33(12):2401–2516.

for greater reduction and maintenance of weight.[93] For those unable to sustain longer exercise periods, intermittent bouts (10-minute minimum) can be implemented at different times throughout the day.

- For those with low cardiorespiratory fitness, the duration of exercise can begin with as little as 5-minute bouts with rest between bouts. The duration can increase progressively over a period of weeks until the desired goal is achieved. The rate of progression should be specific for each patient.
- The first choice of exercise should be walking. It is the safest form of exercise and requires no instructions. Cycling, water exercises, or stair climbing also could be considered if the patient feels comfortable and after some instruction is provided to the patient.

Spot Reducing

One of the most misleading claims made about weight loss is that fat can be "trimmed-off" from a particular area of the body, otherwise known as *spot reducing*. The areas of the body that most people are concerned with are the waist and the thighs. The exercises recommended for the waist are sit-ups and for the thighs, a number of leg exercises that concentrate on that particular area of interest. Over the years, these two areas of the body have claimed a number of exercise devices, millions of dollars, and many disappointments. Why? Spot reduction is a myth. It simply does not work. Here are the reasons:

1. The body does not discriminate where the fat comes from to use for energy. The fat comes from the entire body and not from a particular site.
2. The exercises (sit-ups, leg lifts, etc.) are not aerobic. In addition, they are not demanding enough (energy-wise) to activate the use of large quantities of fat stores for energy.

Sit-ups, however, provide a great way to firm up the abdominal muscles and improve health by several ways. Strengthening the abdominal muscles improves posture, and reduces lower back pain and the incidence of back injuries. Similarly, leg exercise will increase leg strength, reduce leg fatigue, and firm up the legs. Combining these exercises with a brisk walk or jog and low fat diet provides a good combination to reduce body fat and accentuate the leg and stomach muscles.

not really matter how much we chew it. I partially agree with both of these arguments. However, climbing the stairs or just walking spends calories. I don't know about you, but I'd rather spend calories (even a few) rather than store them as fat. Think that 100 kcal a day translates to 36,500 calories in 1 year, which is the equivalent of about 10 pounds of fat. On the other hand, walking 1 mile requires about 100 kcal. "To be or not to be" shaped by 10 pounds of extra fat at the end of each year is each individual's choice.

Regarding chewing, evidence suggests that those who eat in a hurry usually consume more calories than when slowing down and chewing a bit longer. The taste of the food in the mouth and the volume of it in the stomach are parts of the feedback mechanism to signal that we have eaten enough. It is likely that shoving half-chewed food down the throat bypasses or at least hinders that mechanism.

Figure 13.11 The adjusted risk of mortality is significantly higher in fit individuals for each category of body weight.

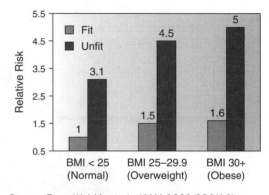

Source: From Wei M, et al. *JAMA* 1999;282(16): 1547–1553.

■ BODY WEIGHT AND MORTALITY

Despite the relatively low weight reduction associated with increased physical activity, findings from large epidemiologic studies support that increased physical activity or higher fitness levels are associated with a significant reduction in the risk of cardiovascular disease and all-cause mortality regardless of weight losses. In a study of 25,714 men followed up to 10 years, the investigators reported that mortality rates were two to three times higher in obese men compared to normal weight men. However, for each category of body weight (normal weight, overweight, or obese), higher fitness levels were associated with lower risk of mortality (**Figure 13.11**). When compared to other risk factors (blood cholesterol, hypertension, and smoking), being low fit carried a similar

risk in every body weight category for cardiovascular and all-cause mortality (**Figure 13.12**). Based on these findings, Manson and co-investigators concluded that it is as important for clinicians to assess the fitness status of an obese patient as it is to evaluate blood pressure, inquire about smoking habits, and measure fasting plasma glucose and cholesterol levels.[25]

In an even larger study of 116,564 women, higher levels of physical activity were beneficial at all categories of body weight. After adjusting for age, smoking status, parental history of coronary heart disease, menopause, hormonal use, and alcohol consumption, higher levels of physical activity did not eliminate the higher risk of mortality associated with overweight and obesity. However, the relative risk for cardiovascular and all-cause mortality was significantly higher in women whose physical activity level was less than one hour a week (**Table 13.5**).[94] This finding supports that increased levels of physical activity attenuated the mortality risk in all categories of adiposity.[85]

Figure 13.12 Low fitness carries similar risk in every body weight category for cardiovascular and all-cause mortality as the traditional cardiovascular risk factors. (a) BMI 18.5–24.9; (b) BMI 25–29.9); (c) (BMI ≥ 30).

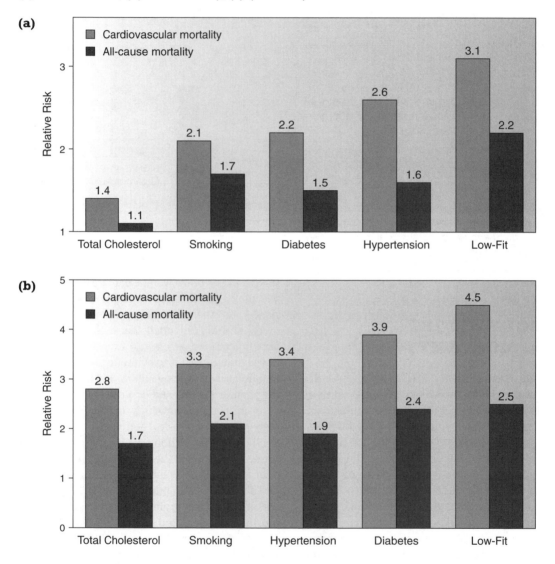

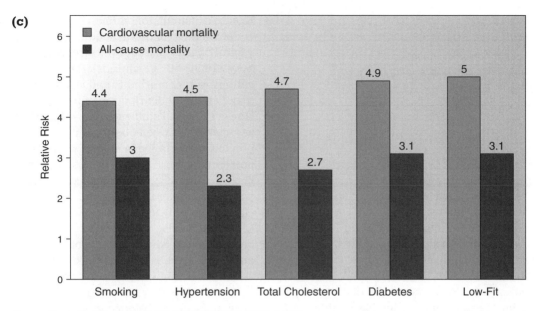

Source: From Wei M, et al. *JAMA* 1999;282(16):1547–1553.

Table 13.5 All-Cause and Cardiovascular Disease Mortality According to BMI and Physical Activity

BMI	Physical Activity (hours/week)		
	≥ 3.5	1.0–3.4	< 1.0
All-Cause Mortality			
< 25 Relative Risk	1	1.18	1.55
25–29.9 Relative Risk	1.28	1.33	1.64
≥ 30 Relative Risk	1.91	2.05	2.42
Cardiovascular Mortality			
< 25 Relative Risk	1	1.51	1.89
25–29.9 Relative Risk	1.58	2.06	2.52
≥ 30 Relative Risk	2.87	4.26	4.73

Source: Adapted from Hu FB, Willett CW, Li T, et al. Adiposity as compared with physical activity in predicting mortality among women. *N Engl J Med* 2004;351(26):2694–2703.

Data support that assessing the fitness status of an obese patient is as important as it is to evaluate blood pressure, inquire about smoking habits, and measure fasting plasma glucose and cholesterol levels.

■ SUMMARY

- Obesity is defined as the accumulation of excess body fat, usually ≥ 25% of the total body weight for men and ≥ 33% for women. The prevalence of obesity has risen significantly in both genders during the past 2 decades. In children and adolescents, the prevalence of obesity during the same time period has doubled.
- The mechanisms and causes of obesity are poorly understood. Obesity simply is the result of chronic imbalance between energy intake in the form of food and drink, and total energy expenditure. Body weight is principally determined and directly related to the net deficit in energy balance, either through a reduction in energy intake or an increase in energy expenditure regardless of the diet composition.
- Both genetic factors and lifestyle are likely to contribute significantly to the variability of body weight in humans. It is more likely that the genetic makeup may not necessarily cause obesity, but in the presence of powerful environmental influences, the propensity for obesity is enhanced.
- Both overweight and obesity are considered leading risk factor of diabetes, hypertension, coronary heart disease, and premature mortality in the developed nations.

- Excess accumulation of fat in the abdomen area (android, abdominal, or central obesity) has an even stronger association with a higher risk for cardiovascular morbidity and mortality than peripheral distribution of body fat.
- However, not all studies agree with the association between obesity and premature mortality. In at least some populations, low BMI has been shown to increase mortality. This so-called *obesity paradox* is under investigation.
- Obesity not only increases directly the CHD risk but also amplifies it indirectly because of the adverse effects of obesity on several established CHD risk factors. Obesity is strongly associated with the development and prevalence of hypertension, insulin resistance, glucose intolerance, and diabetes in both developed and developing countries.
- Weight reduction has become an obsession and lucrative business in the developed countries. Many diet regimens, products, and methods (some unorthodox) have been proposed for weight reduction.
- Rapid reduction of body weight can be achieved by starvation or semi-starvation diets. Unfortunately, most of these diets have little or no scientific merit and are rather limited in promoting safe and effective weight reduction and maintenance. In fact, they can be very unhealthy and potentially dangerous.
- The major objectives of any weight reduction program are to provide healthy and effective nutrition for the individual and to reduce body fat while maintaining lean body mass. More importantly, some responsible perspective must be given to the effects that diet has on the cardiovascular system and the premature development of CHD.

- Chronic exercise of adequate intensity and duration can promote a reduction in body fat by increasing total daily energy expenditure. However, increased physical activity combined with a prudent diet and behavior modification is likely to be a more effective a way to maximize weight loss.
- Exercise programs should focus on long duration and low intensity, tailored for expending calories rather than improving fitness.
- Exercise-induced weight reduction occurs throughout the body. The effects of exercise on body weight cannot be directed to a particular area of the body (spot reducing) by performing exercise directed to that part of the body.
- Increased physical activity attenuates the higher risk of cardiovascular and all-cause mortality associated with overweight and obesity.
- The relative risk for mortality associated with low fitness is similar to the risk of high blood cholesterol, diabetes, hypertension, and smoking.

■ REFERENCES

1. Seidell JC. Time trends in obesity: an epidemiological perspective. *Horm Metab Res* 1997;29(4):155–158.
2. World Health Organization (WHO). *Obesity: Preventing and Managing the Global Epidemic*. Geneva: WHO/NUT/NCD; 1998.
3. Eckel RH, Krauss RM. American Heart Association call to action: obesity as a major risk factor for coronary heart disease. AHA Nutrition Committee. *Circulation* 1998;97(21): 2099–2100.
4. Lee IM, Manson JE, Hennekens CH, Paffenbarger RS Jr. Body weight and mortality: a 27-year follow-up of middle-aged men. *JAMA* 1993;270(23):2823–2828. (see comment).
5. Manson JE, Willett WC, Stampfer MJ, et al. Body weight and mortality among women. *N Engl J Med* 1995;333(11):677–685. (see comments)
6. Stevens J, Cai J, Pamuke R, et al. The effect of age on the association between body-mass index and mortality. *N Engl J Med* 1998;338 (1):1–7. (see comments)
7. Kannel WB, Cupples LA, Ramaswami R, et al. Regional obesity and risk of cardiovascular disease; the Framingham Study. *J Clin Epidemiol* 1991;44(2):183–190.
8. Suk SH, Sacco RL, Boden-Albala B, et al. Abdominal obesity and risk of ischemic stroke: the Northern Manhattan Stroke Study. *Stroke* 2003;34(7):1586–1592.
9. Rosenbaum M, Leibel RL, Hirsch J. Obesity. *N Engl J Med* 1997;337(6):396–407.
10. van der Kooy K, Leenen R, Seidell JC, et al. Waist-hip ratio is a poor predictor of changes in visceral fat. *Am J Clin Nutr* 1993;57(3): 327–333.
11. National Center for Health Statistics. *Health, United States, 2007*. With *Chartbook on Trends in the Health of Americans*. Hyattsville, MD: US Department of Health and Human Services, Centers for Disease Control and Prevention, National Center for Health Statistics; 2007. Available at www.cdc.gov/nchs/hus.htm. Accessed April 1, 2007.
12. Jakicic JM, Clark K, Coleman E, et al. American College of Sports Medicine position stand. Appropriate intervention strategies for weight loss and prevention of weight regain for adults. *Med Sci Sports Exerc* 2001;33(12): 2145–2156.
13. Ogden CL, Carroll MD, Flegal KM, et al. High body mass index for age among US children and adolescents, 2003–2006. *JAMA* 2008;299: 2401–2405. (see comment)
14. Flegal KM, Graubard BI, Williamson DF, Gail MH. Excess deaths associated with underweight, overweight, and obesity. *JAMA* 2005; 293(15):1861–1867. (see comments)
15. Allison DB, Fontaine KR, Manson JE, et al. Annual deaths attributable to obesity in the United States. *JAMA* 1999;282(16):1530–1538.

16. Troiano RP, Flegal KM. Overweight children and adolescents: description, epidemiology, and demographics. *Pediatrics* 1998;101(3 Pt 2):497–504.

17. Rossner S. Obesity: the disease of the twenty-first century. *Int J Obes Relat Metab Disord* 2002;26(Suppl 4):S2–S4.

18. Baker JL, Olsen LW, Sorensen TI. Childhood body-mass index and the risk of coronary heart disease in adulthood. *N Engl J Med* 2007;357(23):2329–2337.

19. Centers for Disease Control and Prevention. Preventing obesity and chronic diseases through good nutrition and physical activity. 2005. Available at www.cdc.gov/nccdphp/publications/factsheets/prevention/obesity.htm. Accessed April 1, 2009.

20. Rosamond W, Flegal K, Furie K, et al. Heart disease and stroke statistics—2008 update: a report from the American Heart Association Statistics Committee and Stroke Statistics Subcommittee. *Circulation* 2008;117(4): e25–146.

21. Koplan JP, Dietz WH. Caloric imbalance and public health policy. *JAMA* 1999;282(16): 1579–1581.

22. Pérusse L, Chagnon YC, Weisnagel J, Bouchard C. The human obesity gene map: the 1998 update. *Obes Res* 1999;7(1):111–129.

23. National Institute of Health (NIH), National Heart, Lung and Blood Institute. *Clinical Guidelines on the Identification, Evaluation and Treatment of Overweight and Obesity in Adults*. Bethesda: NIH; 1998. Available at http://hp2010.nhlbihin.net/oei_ss/download/pdf/CORESET1.pdf. Accessed April 1, 2009.

24. Hubert HB, Feinleib M, McNamara PM, Castelli WP. Obesity as an independent risk factor for cardiovascular disease: a 26-year follow-up of participants in the Framingham Heart Study. *Circulation* 1983;67(5):968–977.

25. Manson JE, Colditz GA, Stempfer MJ, et al. A prospective study of obesity and risk of coronary heart disease in women. *N Engl J Med* 1990;322(13):882–889. (see comments)

26. Wei M, Kampert JB, Barlow CE, et al. Relationship between low cardiorespiratory fitness and mortality in normal-weight, overweight, and obese men. *JAMA* 1999;282(16): 1547–1553.

27. Blair SN, LaMonte MJ. Commentary: current perspectives on obesity and health: black and white, or shades of grey? *Int J Epidemiol* 2006;35:69–72.

28. Zamboni M, Mazzali G, Zoico E, et al. Health consequences of obesity in the elderly: a review of four unresolved questions. *Int J Obes* 2005;29:1011–1029.

29. Andres R. Beautiful hypothesis and ugly facts: the BMI-mortality association. *Obes Res* 1999;7:417–419.

30. Folsom AR, Kaye SA, Sellers TA, et al. Body fat distribution and 5-year risk of death in older women. *JAMA* 1993;269(4):483–487. (Erratum 1993;269[10]:1254).

31. Stevens J, Keil JE, Rust PF, et al. Body mass index and body girths as predictors of mortality in black and white women. *Arch Intern Med* 1992;152(6):1257–1262. (see comment).

32. Tuomilehto J, Sulonen JT, Marti B, et al. Body weight and risk of myocardial infarction and death in the adult population of eastern Finland. *Br Med J (Clin Res Ed)* 1987;295(6599): 623–627.

33. Harris T, Cook EF, Garrison R, et al. Body mass index and mortality among nonsmoking older persons. The Framingham Heart Study. *JAMA* 1988;259(10):1520–1524.

34. Hanson RL, McCance DR, Jacobsson LTH, et al. The U-shaped association between body mass index and mortality: relationship with weight gain in a Native American population. *J Clin Epidemiol* 1995;48:903–916.

35. Vandenbroucke JP, Mauritz BM, de Bruin A, et al. Weight, smoking, and mortality. *JAMA* 1984;252(20):2859–2860.

36. Garn SM, Hawthorne VM, Pilkington JJ, Pesick SD. Fatness and mortality in the west of Scotland. *Am J Clin Nutr* 1983;38: 313–319.

37. McAuley P, Myers J, Abella J, Froelicher VF. Body mass, fitness and survival in veteran patients: another obesity paradox? *Am J Med* 2007;120:518–524.

38. Sui X, LaMonte MJ, Laditka JN, et al. Cardiorespiratory fitness and adiposity as mortality predictors in older adults. *JAMA* 2007;298:2507–2516.

39. Garrison RJ, Feinleib M, Castelli WP, McNamara PM. Cigarette smoking as a confounder of the relationship between relative weight and long-term mortality. The Framingham Heart Study. *JAMA* 1983;249(16):2199–2203.

40. Manson JE, Stampfer JM, Hennekens CH, Willet WC. Body weight and longevity. A reassessment. *JAMA* 1987;257(3):353–358.

41. Calle EE, Thun MJ, Petrelli JM, et al. Body-mass index and mortality in a prospective cohort of U.S. adults. *N Engl J Med* 1999;341(15):1097–1105. (see comment).

42. Pischon T, Boeing H, Hoffmann K, et al. General and abdominal adiposity and risk of death in Europe. *N Engl J Med* 2008;359(20):2105–2120. (see comments).

43. Bjorntorp P. Abdominal obesity and the metabolic syndrome. *Ann Med* 1992;24(6):465–468.

44. Bjorntorp P. Abdominal fat distribution and disease: an overview of epidemiological data. *Ann Med* 1992;24(1):15–18.

45. Pouliot MC, Després JP, Lemieux S, et al. Waist circumference and abdominal sagittal diameter: best simple anthropometric indexes of abdominal visceral adipose tissue accumulation and related cardiovascular risk in men and women. *Am J Cardiol* 1994;73(7):460–468.

46. Pouliot MC, Després JP, Nadeau A, et al. Visceral obesity in men. Associations with glucose tolerance, plasma insulin, and lipoprotein levels. *Diabetes* 1992;41(7):826–834.

47. Hsu PH, Mathewson FA, Rabkin SW. Blood pressure and body mass index patterns: a longitudinal study. *J Chronic Dis* 1977;30(2):93–113.

48. Kannel WB, Hjortland MC, McNamara PM, Gordon T. Menopause and risk of cardiovascular disease: the Framingham Study. *Ann Intern Med* 1976;85(4):447–452.

49. Stamler R, Stamler J, Reidlinger WF, et al. Weight and blood pressure. Findings in hypertension screening of 1 million Americans. *JAMA* 1978;240(15):1607–1610.

50. Shear CL, Friedman DS, Burke GL, et al. Body fat patterning and blood pressure in children and young adults. The Bogalusa Heart Study. *Hypertension* 1987;9(3):236–244.

51. The effects of nonpharmacologic interventions on blood pressure of persons with high normal levels. Results of the Trials of Hypertension Prevention, Phase I. *JAMA* 1992;267(9):1213–1220. (Erratum 1992;267[17]:2330; see comments).

52. Effects of weight loss and sodium reduction intervention on blood pressure and hypertension incidence in overweight people with high-normal blood pressure. The Trials of Hypertension Prevention, phase II. The Trials of Hypertension Prevention Collaborative Research Group. *Arch Intern Med* 1997;157(6):657–667. (see comments).

53. Langford HG, Blaufox MD, Oberman A, et al. Dietary therapy slows the return of hypertension after stopping prolonged medication. *JAMA* 1985;253(5):657–664.

54. Davis BR, Blaufox MD, Oberman A, et al. Reduction in long-term antihypertensive medication requirements. Effects of weight reduction by dietary intervention in overweight persons with mild hypertension. *Arch Intern Med* 1993;153(15):1773–1782.

55. Wood PD, Stephanick ML, Dreon DM, et al. Changes in plasma lipids and lipoproteins in overweight men during weight loss through dieting as compared with exercise. *N Engl J Med* 1988;319(18):1173–1179.

56. Wood PD, Stephanick ML, Williams PT, Haskell WL. The effects on plasma lipoproteins of a prudent weight-reducing diet, with or without exercise, in overweight men and women. *N Engl J Med* 1991;325(7):461–466.

57. Dattilo AM, Kris-Etherton PM. Effects of weight reduction on blood lipids and lipoproteins: a meta-analysis. *Am J Clin Nutr* 1992;56(2):320–328.

58. Després JP, Ferland M, Moorjani S, et al. Role of hepatic-triglyceride lipase activity in the association between intra-abdominal fat and

plasma HDL cholesterol in obese women. *Arteriosclerosis* 1989;9(4):485–492.

59. Ostlund RE Jr, Staten M, Kohrt WM, et al. The ratio of waist-to-hip circumference, plasma insulin level, and glucose intolerance as independent predictors of the HDL2 cholesterol level in older adults. *N Engl J Med* 1990; 322(4):229–234.

60. Terry RB, Wood PD, Haskell WL, et al. Regional adiposity patterns in relation to lipids, lipoprotein cholesterol, and lipoprotein subfraction mass in men. *J Clin Endocrinol Metab* 1989;68(1):191–199.

61. Brancati FL, Kao WH, Folsom AR, et al. Incident type 2 diabetes mellitus in African American and white adults: the Atherosclerosis Risk in Communities Study. *JAMA* 2000;283 (17):2253–2259. (see comment)

62. Folsom AR, Kushi LH, Anderson KE, et al. Associations of general and abdominal obesity with multiple health outcomes in older women: the Iowa Women's Health Study. *Arch Intern Med* 2000;160(14):2117–2128.

63. Després JP. Abdominal obesity as important component of insulin-resistance syndrome. *Nutrition* 1993;9(5):452–459.

64. Reaven GM. Banting lecture 1988. Role of insulin resistance in human disease. *Diabetes* 1988;37(12):1595–1607.

65. Colditz GA, Willett WC, Rotnitzky A, Manson JE. Weight gain as a risk factor for clinical diabetes mellitus in women. *Ann Intern Med* 1995;122(7):481–486. (see comments).

66. Manson JE, Nathan DM, Krolewski AS, et al. A prospective study of exercise and incidence of diabetes among US male physicians. *JAMA* 1992;268(1):63–67.

67. Wei M, Gibbons LW, Mitchell TL, et al. The association between cardiorespiratory fitness and impaired fasting glucose and type 2 diabetes mellitus in men. *Ann Intern Med* 1999; 130(2):89–96.

68. Kahn BB, Flier JS. Obesity and insulin resistance. *J Clin Invest* 2000;106(4):473–481.

69. Kraus W. Insulin resistance syndrome and cardiovascular disease: genetics and connections to skeletal muscle function. *Am Heart J* 1999;138(5 Pt 1):S413–S416.

70. Ryder JW, Gilbert M, Zierath JR. Skeletal muscle and insulin sensitivity: pathophysiological alterations. *Front Biosci* 2001;6:D154–D163.

71. Galuska DA, Will JC, Serdula MK, Ford ES. Are health care professionals advising obese patients to lose weight? *JAMA* 1999;282(16): 1576–1578. (see comment).

72. Wee CC, McCarthy EP, Davis RB, et al. Physician counseling about exercise. *JAMA* 1999;282(16):1583–1588. (see comment).

73. Hill JO, Drougas H, Peters JC. Obesity treatment: can diet composition play a role? *Ann Intern Med* 1993;119(7 Pt 2):694–697.

74. U.S. Department of Health. *Choosing a Safe and Successful Weight-loss Program.* NIH Publication No.94-3700. 1993. Available at www.nhlbi.nih.gov/health/public/heart/ obesity/lose_wt/wtl_prog.htm. Accessed April 2, 2009.

75. Whaley M, Otto RM, eds. *ACSM's Guidelines for Exercise Testing and Prescription,* 7th ed. New York: Lippincott Williams & Wilkins; 2006.

76. Garrow J. *Obesity and Related Disorders.* New York: Churchill Livingston; 1998: 145–183.

77. Wadden TA. Treatment of obesity by moderate and severe caloric restriction. Results of clinical research trials. *Ann Intern Med* 1993;119(7 Pt 2):688–693.

78. Foster GD, Wyatt HR, Hill JO, et al. A randomized trial of a low-carbohydrate diet for obesity. *N Engl J Med* 2003;348(21):2082–2090. (see comments).

79. Samaha FF, Iqbal N, Seshadri P, et al. A low-carbohydrate as compared with a low-fat diet in severe obesity. *N Engl J Med* 2003;348(21): 2074–2081. (see comments).

80. Anderson JW, Konz EC, Jenkins DJ. Health advantages and disadvantages of weight-reducing diets: a computer analysis and critical review. *J Am Coll Nutr* 2000;19(5): 578–590.

81. Freedman MR, King J, Kennedy E. Popular diets: a scientific review. *Obes Res* 2001;9 (Suppl 1):1S–40S.

82. Schlundt DG, Hill JO, Pope-Cordle J, et al. Randomized evaluation of a low fat ad libitum

carbohydrate diet for weight reduction. *Int J Obes Relat Metab Disord* 1993;17(11): 623–629.

83. de Lorgeril M, Salen P, Martin JL, et al. Mediterranean diet, traditional risk factors, and the rate of cardiovascular complications after myocardial infarction: final report of the Lyon Diet Heart Study. *Circulation* 1999;99(6):779–785. (see comments).

84. Ross R, Freeman JA, Janssen I. Exercise alone is an effective strategy for reducing obesity and related comorbidities. *Exerc Sport Sci Rev* 2000;28(4):165–170.

85. Miller WC, Koceja DM, Hamilton EJ. A meta-analysis of the past 25 years of weight loss research using diet, exercise or diet plus exercise intervention. *Int J Obes Relat Metab Disord* 1997;21(10):941–947.

86. Ross R, Dagone D, Jones PJ, et al. Reduction in obesity and related comorbid conditions after diet-induced weight loss or exercise-induced weight loss in men. A randomized, controlled trial. *Ann Intern Med* 2000;133(2): 92–103.

87. Ballor DL, Keesey RE. A meta-analysis of the factors affecting exercise-induced changes in body mass, fat mass and fat-free mass in males and females. *Int J Obes* 1991;15(11): 717–726.

88. Jakicic JM, Winters C, Lang W, Wing RR. Effects of intermittent exercise and use of home exercise equipment on adherence, weight loss, and fitness in overweight women: a randomized trial. *JAMA* 1999;282(16): 1554–1560.

89. Pavlou KN, Krey S, Steffee WP. Exercise as an adjunct to weight loss and maintenance in moderately obese subjects. *Am J Clin Nutr* 1989;49(5 Suppl):1115–1123.

90. Brochu M, Poehlman ET, Ades PA. Obesity, body fat distribution, and coronary artery disease. *J Cardiopulm Rehabil* 2000;20(2): 96–108.

91. Savage PD, Lee M, Harvey-Berino J, et al. Weight reduction in the cardiac rehabilitation setting. J *Cardiopulm Rehabil* 2002;22(3): 154–160.

92. Kokkinos PF, Narayan P, Papademetriou V. Exercise as hypertension therapy. *Cardiol Clin* 2001;19(3):507–516.

93. Schoeller DA, Shay K, Kushner RF. How much physical activity is needed to minimize weight gain in previously obese women? *Am J Clin Nutr* 1997;66(3):551–556.

94. Hu FB, Willett CW, Li T, et al. Adiposity as compared with physical activity in predicting mortality among women. *N Engl J Med* 2004;351(26):2694–2703.

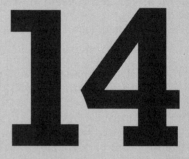

Cardiovascular Risk of Injury or Death from Physical Activity

■ **Overtraining**
  Warning Signs and Symptoms of
    Overtraining
  Best Time to Exercise
  Sleep and Exercise
■ **Summary**

T he purpose of this chapter is to foster a deeper understanding of the potential injury inherent in physical activity or structured exercise programs. This is important if doctors are to encourage large populations to become more physically active. Such an understanding also will help the scientists to tailor exercise programs that minimize risk and maximize health benefits.

Injury during or as a result of exercise is not a new phenomenon. The first death mentioned as a result of physical exertion is recorded by the Greeks.

Legend has it that Phidippides, a messenger, ran from the battlefield of Marathon to Athens (approximately 26 miles) to carry the news to the Athenians that they were victorious against the invading Persians. He reached Athens in perhaps 3 hours, delivered his message, and died shortly thereafter from exhaustion.

Was it the 26-mile run that killed Phidippides? Not likely! Less known are the facts that, only days prior to the battle at Marathon, Phidippides had been sent to Sparta to ask for help. He ran the rugged, mountainous 140-mile course in about 36 hours to deliver the message. Afterwards, Phidippides ran that same 140-mile trail back to Athens with the disappointing news that the Spartans refused to send warriors to help. A few days later he was in the battle of Marathon where, in all likelihood, Phidippides had been carrying messages back and forth to the different generals on the field during the day's battle. It was at the end of that last day when he was charged with running to Athens to deliver the victorious news.

Although we cannot know exactly what killed Phidippides, the story has prompted some to proclaim that the human body is not designed to withstand the punishing 26-mile run and inspired others to test the possibility that we are designed to run this and more. The numerous modern marathon and ultra-marathon races run by millions of runners annually are proof that humans are capable of such a task when trained properly. On the other hand, the occasional death of a runner reminds us of our vulnerabilities.

Over the years we have come to realize that there is an inherent risk for injury when the body is exposed to the stress that is concomitant with physical activity or exercise. That is, the likelihood of injury increases by the simple fact that the body is exposed to greater physical stresses. We also have realized that the human body possesses an inherent capacity to adapt to these stresses. By doing so, it becomes more resilient to the stress as well as to the potential injury carried by the stress.

This can be illustrated by using an analogy with the sun. Exposure to the sun stimulates certain skin cells (melanocytes) to produce melanin, a biological substance that gives the skin its natural color and also acts as a sunscreen, protecting the skin from ultraviolet light. As more melanin is produced, the skin becomes darker and more resilient to sunburn and other harmful effects of ultraviolet light.

Similarly, proper exercise allows the body to adapt to the physical stress, so that as the duration, intensity, and frequency (volume) of exercise progressively increase, the body becomes more resilient to the potential risk of injury inherent to the exercise. In fact, the risk of injury during physical activity is much higher in those not accustomed to that activity (sedentary) compared to those who maintain a physically active lifestyle. In short, exercise or physical exertion can be considered as a two-edged sword: it can increase the short-term risk of sudden death and also protect against it when proper exercise is performed regularly.

Because exercise can protect against injury, the goal of any exercise program should be to lower the risk to an absolute minimum while maximizing the exercise-related benefits. When the risk increases, exercise needs to be re-evaluated and adjusted. The probability, severity, and type of injury are dictated by a number of factors discussed in this chapter. The reader is encouraged to become very familiar with the risk of injury and even death associated with exercise or physical activity, especially in individuals with cardiovascular and other chronic diseases.

■ ETIOLOGY OF CARDIOVASCULAR RISKS

The acute cardiovascular changes that occur during physical exertion foster the likelihood of a cardiovascular event when the cardiovascular system is compromised. For example, during physical activity or exercise, the heart rate and systolic blood pressure (SBP) increase (see Chapter 12). This in turn causes the oxygen demand of the myocardium to rise. In the case of significant coronary artery disease that limits coronary blood flow, ischemia may ensue, which may lead to malignant arrhythmias and even death.

Another possibility is plaque rupture within the coronary arteries, first proposed by Black and coworkers.[1] The investigators reported acute plaque rupture in 13 individuals who died or suffered a myocardial infarction (MI) during vigorous exertion. The reasons for plaque rupture during strenuous physical activity are not well understood. Black postulated that during physical work, the myocardial contractions in the blood vessels become more vigorous. This

places a greater excursion of blood through the coronary arteries because of the increase in end-diastolic volume and reduction in end-systolic volume. This along with the increased "twisting and bending" of the coronary arteries with each contraction during vigorous exercise might contribute to plaque rupture (coined *Blacks' crack in the plaque*), resulting in myocardial infarction and sudden cardiac death.

■ MYOCARDIAL INFARCTION AND SUDDEN CARDIAC DEATH

Almost all exercise-related deaths in previously asymptomatic adults without prior history of coronary heart disease have been the result of atherosclerotic plaque rupture in one of the coronary arteries that led to an acute coronary thrombosis.[2] These events have been substantiated by coronary angiography in athletes within hours following exercise[3] and also in those shoveling snow[4] or engaging in other physically demanding activities.[5]

Because the most common cause of cardiac complications is atherosclerotic coronary artery disease, the risk of exercise varies according to the population. In older populations where the prevalence of coronary atherosclerotic disease is high, the risk of death during exercise or physical exertion will be correspondingly high.[6]

Despite this risk, the exercise-related cardiac event is relatively rare even in such populations. One widely known study on the incidence of exercise-related deaths is the Rhode Island study.[7] Thompson and colleagues collected data on all deaths in joggers during a 5-year period from 1975 to 1980. There was one death per year for every 7,620 male joggers between the ages of 30 and 65 years. When those with known coronary heart disease were excluded, the death rate was one death per year for every 15,240 male joggers. In general, the estimated rate of sudden cardiac death is very low. Others estimated the rate of sudden death during exercise to be between 0 and 2 per 100,000 hours of exercise in the general population and 0.13 to 0.61 per 100,000 hours in cardiac rehabilitation programs.[8,9]

Fitness of the Individual and Risk of Sudden Cardiac Death

Study findings support that physically active individuals are less likely to suffer a sudden cardiac event during physical exertion (**Figures 14.1** and **14.2**). The risk for a myocardial infarction attributed to exercise and the role of the fitness status of the individual also were assessed by several studies in the United States[10–12] and Europe.[13] Mittleman and colleagues[10] examined the relative risk of those who survived a myocardial infarction during or within 1 hour after exercise. The investigators concluded the following:

Figure 14.1   The relative risk of myocardial infarction within 1 hour of exercise according to physical activity.

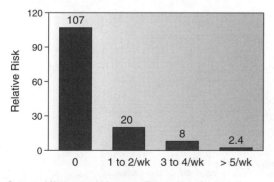

Source: Mittleman MA, et al. Triggering of acute myocardial infarction by heavy physical exertion. Protection against triggering by regular exertion. *N Engl J Med* 1993;329(23):1677–1683.

Figure 14.2   The relative risk of exercise-related myocardial infarction according to physical activity status

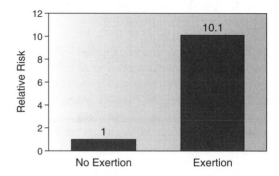

Source: Giri S, et al. Clinical and angiographic characteristics of exertion-related acute myocardial infarction. *JAMA* 1999;282(18):1731–1736.

- The relative risk for a myocardial infarction was 5.6-fold higher during vigorous compared to less vigorous exercise. Activities included jogging (30%), yard work (52%) consisting of chopping wood or gardening, and lifting and pushing (18%).
- Diabetics had an 18.9 times higher risk of a myocardial infarction during exercise than at rest.
- In sedentary individuals, the relative risk of a myocardial infarction was 107-fold higher during exercise than at rest.
- The relative risk of myocardial infarction in individuals who engaged in physical activity five or more times per week was 2.4-fold higher during exercise compared to rest.
- However, when compared to the exercise-related mortality risk of the inactive individuals in this study, the relative risk of those who engaged in physical activity five or more times per week was approximately 45 times higher (Figure 14.1).

Giri and colleagues[11] also examined the risk for an MI in active and sedentary individuals who underwent angioplasty as a treatment for their myocardial infarction. These investigators reported the following:

- The overall risk of a myocardial infarction during physical exertion was 10 times higher compared to rest (Figure 14.2).
- The risk was among the sedentary individuals was 30.5 times higher.
- The risk in the physically active individuals was not raised significantly (**Figure 14.3**).

In the German population, the findings were similar. The relative risk of an MI during physical exertion was 2.1-fold higher compared to resting individuals.[13] However, the risk in physically inactive individuals was over five times higher when compared to the physically active (**Figure 14.4**).

The Physicians' Health Study,[12] examined male physicians (N = 21,481) who were ini-

tially free of cardiovascular disease and who provided baseline information on their habitual level of exercise. Investigators compared the risk of sudden death during and up to 30 minutes after an episode of vigorous exertion with the risk incurred during periods of either no or light exertion. In addition, they evaluated whether the risk of sudden death associated with vigorous exertion was attenuated by habitual vigorous exercise. The follow-up period was 12 years. Albert and colleagues reported a significant transient increase in the relative risk of sudden death during and up to 30 minutes after vigorous exertion. However, the absolute risk of sudden death was extremely low during any particular episode of vigorous exertion was one sudden death per 1.51 million episodes of exertion. They concluded that habitual vigorous exercise diminishes the risk of sudden death during vigorous exertion.

Collectively, findings of these studies strongly support that the risk of cardiac events

Figure 14.3   The relative risk of exercise-related myocardial infarction according to physical activity status. Note that the increase in exercise-related risk occurs in the two least active groups whereas the risk is diminished and even eliminated in individuals engaging in moderate levels of physical activity.

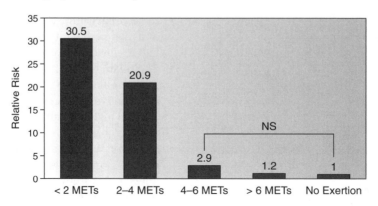

Source: Giri S, et al. Clinical and angiographic characteristics of exertion-related acute myocardial infarction. *JAMA* 1999;282(18):1731–1736.

Figure 14.4 The relative risk of exercise-related myocardial infarction according to physical activity status. Again, the risk is substantially lower in physically active compared to inactive individuals.

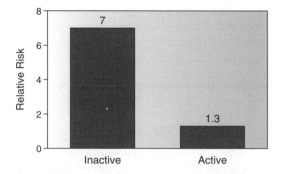

Source: Willich SN, et al. Physical exertion as a trigger of acute myocardial infarction. Triggers and Mechanisms of Myocardial Infarction Study Group. *N Engl J Med* 1993;329(23):1684–1690.

increases as a result of physical exertion or exercise. However, the risk is substantially diminishes and (in some studies) is eliminated if the individual is physically active.

Exercise is associated with a transient increase in the risk of a cardiac event. For example, for men with coronary artery disease, the risk of sudden death during exercise increases about sixfold. However, the risk for overall mortality for exercisers is half that of sedentary individuals. Therefore, the long-term benefits of exercise outweigh the risk of being sedentary.

The estimated rate of sudden death during exercise ranges from 0 to 2 per 100,000 hours of exercise in the general population and 0.13 to 0.61 per 100,000 hours in cardiac rehabilitation programs.

Exercise-Related Cardiac Events in Young Athletes

Exercise-related cardiac events as a result of coronary heart disease is rare in young people. When it occurs, it is the result of genetic abnormalities in low density lipoprotein (LDL).[14] The major cause of death in this age group is congenital cardiac abnormalities (**Table 14.1**). Of those, hypertrophic cardiomyopathy accounts for 56% of the cases.[15]

The potential cardiovascular complications of exercise can be summarized as follows: Exercise or habitual physical activity reduces coronary heart disease events, but vigorous activity can acutely and transiently increase the risk of sudden cardiac death and acute MI in susceptible persons. Exercise-associated acute cardiac events generally occur in individuals with structural cardiac disease. Hereditary or congenital cardiovascular abnormalities are predominantly responsible for cardiac events among young individuals, whereas atherosclerotic disease is primarily responsible for these events in adults. The absolute rate of exercise-related sudden

Table 14.1 Common Cardiac Causes of Death in High School and College Athletes

Cardiac Causes of Death	Percent
Hypertrophic cardiomyopathy	56
Coronary artery abnormalities	11
Myocarditis	7
Aortic stenosis	6
Cardiomyopathy	6
Atherosclerotic coronary disease	2
Aortic rupture	2

Source: Van Camp SP, Bloor CM, Mueller FO, et al. Nontraumatic sports death in high school and college athletes. *Med Sci Sports Exerc* 1995;27(5):641–647.

cardiac death varies with the prevalence of disease in the study population. The incidence of both acute myocardial infarction and sudden death is greatest in the habitually least physically active individuals. Maintaining physical fitness through regular physical activity may help to reduce events because a disproportionately higher number of events occur in the least physically active subjects who perform unaccustomed physical activity.[16]

■ MINIMIZING THE RISK

The risk of exercise-related injuries only can be minimized. They cannot be eliminated. The goal of any exercise program should be to lower the risk of exercise to an absolute minimum and maximize the benefits. When the risk increases, exercise needs to be re-evaluated and adjusted.

It is important to mention that no strategies have been adequately studied that evaluate their ability to reduce exercise-related acute cardiovascular events.[16] However, the risk can be attenuated by systematically controlling all factors that potentially increase the risk of injury. For example, maintaining physical fitness through regular physical activity may help to reduce events because a disproportionate number of events occur in the least physically active subjects performing unaccustomed physical activity. Other strategies, such as screening patients before participation in exercise, excluding high-risk patients from certain activities, promptly evaluating possible prodromal symptoms, training fitness personnel how to cope with emergencies, and encouraging patients to avoid high-risk activities, appear prudent but have not been systematically evaluated.[16]

Despite the lack of strong evidence on exercise-related risk prevention, the limited data available and certain intuitive approaches to reduce the risk are presented.

Type of Exercise Performed

For certain populations, particular types of exercise can cause more injury than others. For example, jogging may not be the recommended type of exercise for an obese person. A more appropriate form of exercise may be walking or swimming, starting slowly and building up speed and distance over a period of weeks to months. More information about the types of exercise for different populations and those with a specific disease is discussed later in this chapter.

Intensity of Exercise

Very little information is available on the intensity and risk of injury relationship, so no clear conclusion can be made. As a general rule, studies have found that the more intense the exercise, the higher the risk for injury. One study found that a runner's best time on a 10-mile run was associated with a higher risk of injury. However, when adjusted for the total distance, the association was no longer statistically significant.[17]

It is important to keep in mind that exercise need not be intense for health benefits to occur. In fact, the proportional increase of health benefits is substantially higher at lower rather than higher intensities, regardless of the risk for injury.

Duration of Exercise

There is also a lack of information about the relationship between exercise duration and injury. The findings of one study suggest that the injury incidence rate appears to be higher when running for more than 45 minutes per session.[18]

An important point to make is that optimum exercise benefits are realized at durations between 20 and 40 minutes per session. In fact, benefits begin to plateau with exercise lasting over 40 minutes, with little to no benefits beyond 60 minutes.

Frequency of Exercise

Exercising once a week is not enough to induce any health benefits and may even increase the risk for injury. At least one study found twice the risk of injury in those attending aerobics class once a week compared to those attending class four times per week.[17] One reason may be that the stimulation for the body to adapt to changes is not adequate. This can lead to the false sense that the participant can tolerate more exercise than he or she actually can endure. This becomes very evident when exercising in hot environments. The "weekend athlete" is usually more prone to heat-related injuries than the seasoned athlete. More on heat-related injury and exercise is presented later in this chapter.

There is also some evidence to support that the risk is similar when running two, three, or four sessions per week.[18] It is my personal opinion that exercising more than six times per week maybe counterproductive for most people. This is based on the notion that the body is not allowed enough time to recover and make the necessary adaptations. As a result, muscle strains, pulls, and even bone fractures are more likely.

The number of exercise sessions per week is also influenced by the individual's weekly schedule, sleep, age, diet, level of fitness, and a number of other factors. It is also a good practice to stop exercising for 1 week of every 12 weeks of consistent exercise.

Engaging in physical activity once a week is not enough and perhaps injurious and every day is too much. It appears that a prudent approach for most people is to engage in exercise at least two to five times a week.

Cumulative Distance Run

There is consistent evidence to support that the amount of distance run per week is associated with increased risk of injury.[19,20] The risk increases after about 20 miles per week and remains significant even after adjusting for other factors related to running.[17,21] Based on this observation, one can extrapolate that progressively running four to five times per week at a distance of 4 to 5 miles per session appears to be within a relatively safe domain.

The Presence of Disease

The presence of a disease can diminish the body's capacity to do work and therefore increases the risk of injury during physical work. Particular attention should be given to those with chronic illness who wish to become more physically active.

The good news is that, if challenged properly, the body will respond by becoming more resilient to injury. The final outcome is that the exercise may not "cure" the disease, but it makes the body more capable of coping with the disease.

It is important to keep in mind that physical activity or exercise represents stress for the body. Increased stress (any stress) has the inherent potential to cause harm. However, keep in mind that the risk of death during exercise is extremely low and the benefits are high. One can think of exercise as the armor worn by the ancient and modern warriors. The armor does not guarantee full immunity from injury or death during the battle. It only increases protection, and by doing so decreases the risk of injury. Given the choice, no warrior of sound mind would go to a battle without it. Similarly, exercise does not guarantee immortality, only protection against premature mortality.

■ EXERCISE IN HOT ENVIRONMENTS AND RELATED HEALTH RISKS

Heat-related illnesses are likely to occur in hot, humid environments. They are the result of the inability of the body to dissipate heat rapidly.[22] Heat is eliminated by the difference in temperature between the body and the environment. This is accomplished by sweating and evaporation of moisture on the skin that results in cooling. Generally, an increase in the ambient temperature results in a proportional increase in the rate of sweating.

Heat produced by working muscles and other interior tissues is transferred to the skin via blood circulation. When the ambient temperature is less than body temperature, heat dissipates to the surrounding environment thereby cooling the blood, which cools the internal organs.

When the ambient temperature is higher than body temperature, the body actually gains heat. In this case, sweating and evaporation becomes the only means for heat dissipation. However in humid conditions, evaporation diminishes. This causes more sweating and a greater loss of water without the cooling effect.

Under such environmental conditions, especially when exercising or working and without adequate hydration, excessive water loss can occur that results in dehydration and overheating. This is more common among those who are in poor physical condition or in individuals who are not acclimated to the hot environment. Excessive water loss of about 6% to 10% of body weight regardless of the reason, will lead to the following heat-related illnesses:

1. Muscle cramping, resulting from excessive sodium (salt) loss.
2. Heat exhaustion, due to a large volume of water loss. Symptoms include: paleness, heavy sweating, dizziness, fainting, nausea, and vomiting.
3. Heat stroke (the most serious of the three) is a life-threatening form of hyperthermia caused by dehydration and an inability of the body to dissipate heat. Onset of symptoms may be sudden. Symptoms can mimic a heart attack, but include nausea, vomiting, weakness, dizziness, headache, aches, and muscle cramping. There is no sweating and the skin may be flushed red and dry despite high body temperatures. The individual may have difficulty breathing, a rapid pulse, appear disoriented and confused, and have a seizure or even go into a coma.

Dehydration and Arrhythmias

In addition to the heat-related illnesses mentioned, dehydration can present an even greater risk for individuals with cardiovascular disease (CVD) for two reasons. First, the workload of the heart increases as the demand for blood to maintain a constant core temperature increases. Second, the loss of water can lead to electrolyte imbalance. Consequently, the propensity for arrhythmias increases. Both conditions increase the risk for a serious cardiac event.

Additional Risk Factors

It is important to remember that the strain on the body imposed by a hot environment not only depends on the environmental temperature but in a number of other factors. The following have been identified as likely to increase the risk of heat-related illness.

- Age
- Overweight
- Dehydration
- Lack of acclimatization

- Poor fitness
- Exercise intensity (the higher the intensity, the higher the risk)
- Alcohol consumption
- Certain medications that promote that promote excessive discharge of urine (diuretics)
- Caffeine consumption or other supplements that promote excessive discharge of urine
- Tight-fitting, dark clothing

Clothing worn during exercise should be of a light-color, cotton (or other moisture-wicking) material, and loose. It should not restrict movement. Clothing that interferes with sweat evaporation must not be worn. Suits made of plastic or other non-natural fibers (e.g., polyester) that hinder sweat evaporation must be avoided.

To minimize the risk of heat-related injuries, the following should be considered:

1. Exercising in the heat should be avoided (**Table 14.2**). Note that moisture in the air increases the body's heat stress. When humidity is high (over 80%), even temperatures carrying a moderate risk can be dangerous.
2. If exercising or working in hot environments cannot be avoided, proper hydration must be practiced. Plenty of fluids should be consumed before exercise and afterwards.

3. Avoid exercising in the middle of the day (11:00 AM to 2:00 PM), because the temperature during that period is generally the highest in the day.
4. Proper clothing (light-colored, cotton or other moisture-wicking fabric) should be worn.

The Heat-Stress Index

Another way to look at the strain of heat on the body is to consider temperature plus humidity. The risk of heat-related injuries increases when the temperature plus humidity add to 90° or above (**Table 14.3**).

■ Water Replacement

How much water does one need when exercising in hot environments? There is no straightforward answer to this question. Normally, adults drink about 1.2 liters of water each day (or approximately 41 oz, which is 5 to 6 cups. However, in hot and humid environments, the need and desire for water increases significantly. This is particularly true when one exercises in a hot and humid environment. As stated earlier in this chapter, cooling of the body is accomplished to a major degree by the evaporation of sweat. In a hot environment, the sweat rate increases dramatically. If the environment is also high in humidity, then the sweat rate is even higher. As one sweats, the volume of

Table 14.2 Exercise Guidelines for Hot Environments

Temperature (°F)	Risk of Heat Injury and Recommendations
Below 65°	Low risk.
65° to 73°	Moderate risk. Avoid strenuous exercise, especially if not acclimated.
73° to 82°	High risk. Avoid all outdoor physical activity.
Above 82°	Very high risk. Avoid all outdoor physical activity.

Table 14.3 Heat-Stress Index	
Temperature (°F) **+ Humidity (%)**	**Risk of Heat Injury**
90–105	Possibility of heat cramps
105–130	Heat cramps or heat exhaustion likely; heat stroke possible
130 or more	Heat stroke a definite risk

water in the body decreases. This has serious consequences in physical performance and overall health. A loss of 4% to 5% of body weight in water diminishes the body's capacity to do hard work by 20% to 30%. A loss of 10% to 20% of body weight in water leads to heat stroke, and possibly death.

When exercising in a hot environment, one needs to keep in mind that thirst is not a sufficient or reliable indicator to the need for water. Plenty water must be taken before the event and during an exercise session or athletic event to prevent dehydration. Although this is now common knowledge among athletes, too often the information is not applied correctly.

Exercise, Sweating, and Weight Loss

There was (and perhaps still is) a widespread misconception that weight loss can be expedited through excessive sweating during exercise. This notion was supported by the fact that the actual scale weight is lower immediately after exercise. But this phenomenon is not a mystery. The loss of water through sweat during exercise translates into a lower reading on the scale.

However, this is not a *true* weight loss—the loss of weight is not due to loss of body fat. It is only due to the loss of water, which is replen-ished within a few minutes after drinking water.

Not only is there no actual weight loss from excessive sweating, but the health problems mentioned previously (muscle cramping, heat exhaustion, heat stroke) are very likely to occur, especially when a rubber suit or similar nonbreathable fabric clothing is worn that does not allow the sweat to evaporate. Clothing that don't allow sweat to evaporate must never be worn when exercising or doing physical work.

Proper Clothing for Exercise

The environment should be a strong factor in choosing proper clothing for exercise. In hot weather, clothing should be made of cotton or other types of breathable fabric to maximize air circulation and sweat evaporation. In cold weather, layers of clothing are more effective in keeping you warm than a single heavy garment. Wearing a turtleneck sweater and a hat will keep your neck and head warm, and is recommended because we lose considerable heat from the neck and head areas. A windbreaker jacket is an excellent choice to protect you from the wind and even a light rain. For the legs, clothing should not be too heavy because exercise keeps the legs relatively warm.

Recently, synthetic materials have been developed for use in exercise clothing. The concept is to wick moisture away from the body and therefore keep you cooler and more comfortable when exercising in hot environments. The feel and look of such exercise garments is a personal choice. So long as such exercise garments improve heat dissipation in hot environments and reduce heat losses in cold environments, such garments are recommended.

A good pair of walking or jogging shoes is a must. Good shoes will protect against leg and foot injuries. Almost all shoe manufacturers provide adequate shoes for exercise. However, some shoes are softer than others, some are wider, and others provide more support for different parts of the foot. It is a good idea to try different types of shoes before deciding on the one that will be the best fit for the particular type of exercise or sport.

■ OVERTRAINING

There was time when the "fitness gurus" preached that exercise had to be vigorous or there was no reason to exercise. "No pain, no gain" was their motto. This attitude drove a number of ambitious people into overtraining and all of the pitfalls that went with it.

Overtraining occurs when either the frequency, intensity, duration of exercise, or all are violated. Overtraining is a serious problem. Not only does it decrease performance, but it also increases the chance for injury and may even lead to serious illness. Overtraining is worse than not exercising at all.

Warning Signs and Symptoms of Overtraining

There are signs and symptoms that are likely to develop with overtraining. Although these symptoms may vary from one person to another, a general understanding of these symptoms can be helpful for every athlete to know. If any of these symptoms are present following several weeks of hard training and no rest, the athlete should stop training immediately for at least 3 days. If no improvement is evident at the end of a week, a physician should be consulted. Symptoms of overtraining include:

1. Stiffness and soreness in the muscles, tendons, or joints that lasts for several days longer than usual.
2. Decrease in performance.
3. Persistent fatigue and sluggishness over several days.
4. An elevation in the resting heart rate by 6 to 12 bpm.
5. Excessive irritability, anxiety, nervousness.
6. Frequent sore throats and colds.
7. Loss of appetite.
8. Diarrhea or constipation.
9. Loss of interest in the sport or activity.
10. Uneasy sleep and nightmares.
11. Elevated white blood cell count.

Best Time to Exercise

The time of the day to initiate exercise is usually a matter of preference for most people. Others may have limited choices because of job and/or or family responsibilities. There are positive and negative aspects for exercising at different times in the day. These are discussed briefly.

Because exercise increases alertness and induces a natural emotional "high" for approximately 4 hours afterwards, some people believe that the best time to exercise is in the afternoon hours. They feel like the afternoon exercise period rejuvenates them from the morning's work and allows them to stay alert late into the day.

This is generally true. However, avoid exercising in the middle of the day (11:00 AM to 2:00 PM) when the weather is hot. Air pollution is the highest during that time, especially during hot, humid weather. If you must exercise during the midday hours, it would be preferable to exercise in indoors in a temperature-regulated (cooled) environment, perhaps a gym.

Sleep and Exercise

Just as exercise affects alertness and mood, it also affects sleep. It is interesting that although exercise will keep you alert for hours, it will also help you to fall asleep quickly. Usually the sleep is deep and restful. Keep in mind that unlike sleeping pills, there are no side effects with exercise, so one does not have nightmares. With regular exercise (providing that you don't exercise too late at night), you can look forward into a good night's sleep and being rested and alert the next day.

A Final Note

It is important to keep in mind that physical activity or exercise represents "stress" for the body. Increased stress (any stress) has the inherent potential to cause harm. However, let us keep in mind that the risk of death during exercise is extremely low, while the benefits are high. One can think of exercise as the armor worn by the ancient and modern warriors. The armor does not guarantee full immunity from injury or death during the battle. It only increases protection and by doing so, decreases the risk of injury. Given the choice, no warrior of sound mind would go to the battle without it. Similarly, exercise does not guarantee immortality, only protection against premature mortality.

■ SUMMARY

- There is an inherent risk of injury when the body is exposed to physical stress (physical activity or exercise). There is also an inherent capacity possessed by the body to adapt to the stress exposed and become more resilient. The goal of any exercise program thus should be to lower the risk imposed by exercise to absolute minimum and maximize the exercise-related benefits.

- Exercise is associated with a small and transient increase in risk for a cardiac event. However, the risk is substantially diminished and in some studies eliminated if the individual is physically active.

- In general, practicing moderation is the best approach to reduce the risk of an exercise-related cardiac event.

- Exercise-related cardiac events as a result of coronary heart disease are rare in young subjects. When it occurs, it is the result of genetic abnormalities.

- The most important factors that contribute to the risk of musculoskeletal injuries include the intensity of the activity and the cumulative weekly mileage or total exposure to the activity.

- Heat-related illnesses are likely to occur in hot and humid environments. They are the result of the inability of the body to dissipate heat. In addition to the obvious (i.e., avoid exercising in extremely hot temperatures), proper hydration, and wearing light-colored cotton or other moisture-wicking clothing is recommended for reducing the risk of heat-related illness.

- Individuals with CVD are at a relatively higher risk when exercising in the heat.

- Overtraining is a serious problem. It is likely to occur when either the frequency, intensity, duration of exercise, or all three factors are violated. Not only will it decrease performance, but it also increases the chance for injury and even serious illness. Overtraining is worse than not exercising at all.

- The time of day to exercise varies among individuals and there is no best time. However, exercise increases alertness for several hours afterwards. For this reason, it is not advisable to exercise late in the evening because it may interfere with falling asleep. On the other hand, exercise helps you to fall asleep quickly and the quality of sleep is deep and restful.

■ REFERENCES

1. Black A, Black MM, Gensini G. Exertion and acute coronary artery injury. *Angiology* 1975;26(11):759–783.
2. Davies MJ, Thomas AC. Plaque fissuring: the cause of acute myocardial infarction, sudden ischaemic death, and crescendo angina. *Br Heart J* 1985;53(4):363–373.
3. Ciampricotti R, Deckers JW, Travane R, et al. Characteristics of conditioned and sedentary men with acute coronary syndromes. *Am J Cardiol* 1994;73(4):219–222.
4. Hammoudeh AJ, Haft JI. Coronary-plaque rupture in acute coronary syndromes triggered by snow shoveling. *N Engl J Med* 1996;335(26):2001.
5. Burke AP, Farb A, Malcolm GT, et al. Plaque rupture and sudden death related to exertion in men with coronary artery disease. *JAMA* 1999;281(10):921–926.
6. Thompson P. The cardiovascular risks of exercise. In: *Exercise & Sports Cardiology.* New York: McGraw-Hill; 2001:127–145.
7. Thompson PD, et al. Incidence of death during jogging in Rhode Island from 1975 through 1980. *JAMA* 1982;247(18):2535–2538.

8. Haskell WL. Cardiovascular complications during exercise training of cardiac patients. *Circulation* 1978;57(5):920–924.
9. Van Camp SP, Peterson RA. Cardiovascular complications of outpatient cardiac rehabilitation programs. *JAMA* 1986;256(9):1160–1163.
10. Mittleman MA, Maclure M, Tofler GH, et al. Triggering of acute myocardial infarction by heavy physical exertion. Protection against triggering by regular exertion. Determinants of Myocardial Infarction Onset Study Investigators. *N Engl J Med* 1993;329(23):1677–1683. (see comments)
11. Giri S, Thompson PD, Kiernan JF, et al. Clinical and angiographic characteristics of exertion-related acute myocardial infarction. *JAMA* 1999;282(18):1731–1736.
12. Albert CM, Mittleman MA, Chae CU, et al. Triggering of sudden death from cardiac causes by vigorous exertion. *N Engl J Med* 2000;343(19):1355–1361. (see comments).
13. Willich SN, et al. Physical exertion as a trigger of acute myocardial infarction. Triggers and Mechanisms of Myocardial Infarction Study Group. *N Engl J Med* 1993;329(23):1684–1690.
14. Maron BJ, Roberts WC, McAllister HA, et al. Sudden death in young athletes. *Circulation* 1980;62(2):218–229.
15. Van Camp SP, Bloor CM, Mueller FO, et al. Nontraumatic sports death in high school and college athletes. *Med Sci Sports Exerc* 1995;27(5):641–647.
16. Thompson PD, Franklin BA, Balady GJ, et al. Exercise and acute cardiovascular events placing the risks into perspective: a scientific statement from the American Heart Association Council on Nutrition, Physical Activity, and Metabolism and the Council on Clinical Cardiology. *Circulation* 2007;115(17):2358–2368.
17. Marti B, Vader JP, Minder CE, Abelin T. On the epidemiology of running injuries. The 1984 Bern Grand-Prix study. *Am J Sports Med* 1988;16(3):285–294.
18. Pollock ML, Gettman LR, Milesis CA, et al. Effects of frequency and duration of training

on attrition and incidence of injury. *Med Sci Sports* 1977;9(1):31–36.

19. Jones BH, Cowan DN, Knapik JJ. Exercise, training and injuries. *Sports Med* 1994;18(3): 202–214.

20. Koplan JP, Rothenberg RB, Jones EL. The natural history of exercise: a 10-year follow-up of a cohort of runners. *Med Sci Sports Exerc* 1995;27(8):1180–1184.

21. Lysholm J, Wiklander J. Injuries in runners. *Am J Sports Med* 1987;15(2):168–171.

22. Selected issues in injury and illness prevention and the team physician: a consensus statement. *Med Sci Sports Exerc* 2007;39(11): 2058–2068.

Glossary

Absolute refractory period The time during which the cardiac muscle cells are absolutely unexcitable; if another stimulus comes along, they will not depolarize regardless of the strength of that stimulus.

Absolute risk reduction The difference between two event rates.

Absolute risk The risk of developing a disease over a time period.

Acetylcholine A neurotransmitter that stimulates an impulse that reaches the muscle and spreads quickly throughout the muscle fibers.

Acetylcholine The mediator for the parasympathetic system.

Actin A protein contained in myofibrils and is involved in muscle contraction by bonding tightly with myosin.

Action potential A sequence of changes in the membrane permeability for sodium and potassium that alters the resting state of cells and subsequently the resting potential.

Adenosine diphosphate (ADP) The resulting compound, containing two phosphate molecules, after considerable free energy is released when one of the phosphate bonds in ATP is broken.

Adenosine triphosphate (ATP) The energy compound, containing three phosphate molecules, which all living cells use for their functions. The nucleotide ATP transports chemical energy within the cell for metabolism, and is consumed by many enzymes; it is involved in cellular processes such as cell division, motility, and biosynthetic reactions. After it is used in these processes ATP becomes its precursors (ADP and AMP) so it is constantly being recycled.

Adrenaline Another name for the epinephrine hormone.

Adventitia The connective tissue sheath that surrounds the blood vessel and binds it to surrounding tissue.

Aerobic exercises or activities Repetitive movements of relatively low intensity using large muscle groups (walking or cycling) that last over a relatively long period of time (generally 5 minutes or more).

Aerobic metabolism The process of energy formation (ATP) by the use of oxygen.

Afterload The ventricular wall tension generated by the left ventricle during systole; it is approximately equal to the systolic blood pressure.

All-or-none law States that when stimulated, either all or none of the cardiac muscle fibers will contract.

Alpha cells Pancreatic cells that release glucagon.

Amino acids The building blocks of proteins.

Anaerobic exercises or activities Activities characterized by bursts of intense effort (maximum or near maximum) lasting only a short time.

Anaerobic metabolism The process of energy formation (ATP) without the use of oxygen.

Anaerobic threshold Another term for lactate threshold.

Anterior wall of the heart The area of the heart comprised of the right atrium and ventricle.

Aorta The main trunk of the systemic arterial tree of blood vessels. It rises from the heart and is comprised of the ascending, arch, and descending aorta.

Aortic valve The valve situated at the root of the aorta. It allows oxygen-rich blood to flow from the left ventricle into the aorta and out to the body; the flap of the valve closes after every heart beat so that blood cannot wash back into the heart.

Apex The tip of the left ventricle.

Arterioles Small blood vessels formed by the conduit arteries progressively branching; their function is to control blood flow to the capillaries.

Atherosclerosis The loss of the natural elasticity of the arteries caused by a progressive build up of fatty deposits (i.e., cholesterol, cellular waste, calcium, etc.) called *plaque* along the inner lining of the vessel. Age can cause stiffening of the vessel, which with plaque can cause the blood flow to slow down or even block the vessel, causing the vessel to rupture.

ATP-PC (also, phosphagen system) The system by which adequate ATP availability for the contracting muscle cells is maintained until glycolysis is fully activated (see Adenosine triphosphate).

Atrioventricular node (AV node) A specialized area of cardiac tissue located in the right atrium near the base of the interatrial septum. The AV node is involved in the reception, modulation, and propagation of the impulse from the SA node and upper chambers of the heart.

a-V̇O$_2$ difference (also, Arteriovenous oxygen difference) The difference in the oxygen content of arterial and venous blood. It represents the amount of oxygen extracted from the blood by the muscle or any other organ.

Base or posterior wall of the heart The area of the heart formed by the atria (mainly the left).

Beta (ß) oxidation The metabolic process of degradation and oxidation of fatty acids that is strictly confined to the mitochondria.

Beta cells Pancreatic cells that release insulin.

Bile A complex fluid (water, electrolytes, organic compounds) secreted from the liver that is integral to the emulsification of lipids.

Bradycardia A heart rate of less than 60 bpm.

Bundle of His A collection of heart muscle cells that are specialized to conduct electrical signals; located distally to the AV node and are part of the impulse-conducting system of the heart.

Calcium channels A type of excitable cells that allow small ions to permeate the cell membrane, in this case, calcium.

Capillaries Small, very fine, thin-walled branches of arterioles. Their main role is to exchange nutrients, fluid, oxygen, and carbon dioxide between the blood and surrounding tissues. (see Arterioles)

Carbohydrates Chemical compounds comprised of carbon, oxygen, and hydrogen. Carbohydrates can be simple (monosaccharides) or complex (polysaccharides).

Cardiac output The volume of blood pumped out by the left ventricle of the heart in one minute.

Cardiovascular disease (CVD) A general term that includes heart attack, heart failure, stroke, and peripheral artery disease.

Cardiovascular or cardiorespiratory fitness The capacity of the circulatory and the respiratory systems to supply the necessary oxygen for the working muscles during prolonged work.

Carnitine A nutrient derived from an amino acid that helps the body turn fat into energy.

Cases The participants in an epidemiologic study who have the disease being studied (see Controls).

Catecholamines The hormones epinephrine and norepinephrine. These have the following effects on the heart: increased heart rate (chronotropic effect), increased force of contraction (inotropic effect), increased rate of relaxation (lusitropic effect)

Chylomicrons Re-formed fats that are coated with a thin layer of protein and secreted into the blood stream.

Circumflex The branch from the left main coronary artery that wraps around the lateral portion of the left ventricle and branches off to the posterior wall of the heart.

Cohort A clearly defined group of individuals to be studied.

Complete protein A type of protein that contains all of the essential amino acids.

Compound lipids (also phospholipids) Triglycerides combined with other chemicals to form other compounds.

Concentric contractions Muscle squeezes (contractions) that occur when the length of the muscle involved in the contractions shortens.

Control In scientific studies, the group of people or animals without a condition or disease who are used to statistically compare with another group or groups with a condition or disease to test or define a hypothesis. (see Cases)

Coronary artery disease (CAD) (also coronary heart disease [CHD]) Disease of the heart resulting from atherosclerosis that afflicts the arteries of the heart (coronary arteries). (see Atherosclerosis)

Cross bridges Where the myosin heads project towards actin filaments in the smooth muscle contraction and relaxation process.

Cytoplasm (also, Cytosol) The watery environment of the cell.

Derived fats Type of fats formed from simple and compound fats.

Determinants The identification of factors that influence the occurrence of the disease.

Diastole The relaxation phase of the cardiac cycle. It begins at the end of systole.

Diastolic blood pressure (DBP) The pressure that the blood exerts on the blood vessels during the relaxing phase of the heart (diastole).

Direct assessment of blood pressure Use of a pressure transducer connected into a catheter that is inserted into an artery to measure the continuous beat-by-beat arterial blood pressure.

Distribution Identification of who is getting a specific disease as well as when and where the disease is occurring.

Duration The length of each exercise session.

Eccentric contractions A type of muscle contraction that occurs when the muscle involved lengthens.

Ejection fraction (EF) The percentage of the end diastolic volume that is pumped out by the left ventricle with every contraction; a tool to diagnose heart failure.

Elastin A protein found in the largest arteries in the body such as the aorta and the arteries of the legs that have thick, muscular walls. It allows the arteries to expand as blood is pushed through in systole and recoil during diastole.

Electron transport chain The second phase in the metabolic process where the hydrogen atoms released during the Krebs cycle enter the electron transport chain and significant quantities of ATP are generated.

Embolic stroke Results when a thrombus (blood clot) formed outside the brain is carried by the blood stream to the brain, where it lodges in a small artery. The thrombus blocks blood flow to critical areas of the brain and deprives brain cells of oxygen and nutrients.

Emulsification The first step of lipid digestion and involves the breakdown of fats into smaller fat droplets.

End-diastolic volume (EDV) (also, Left ventricular volume [LV-EDV]) The volume of blood present in the left ventricle at the end of diastole.

Endocardium The single layer of endothelial cells that line the interior surface of the heart (the one in contract with the blood) and valves.

End-systolic volume (ESV) (also, Left ventricular volume [LV-ESV]) The remaining volume of blood in the left ventricle at the end of systole.

Energy currency Refers to ATP because it can be gained and spent again and again. (see Adenosine triphosphate).

Epidemiology The scientific discipline involved in the systematic study of the distribution and determinants of disease or events in specified populations.

Epinephrine A hormone released into the blood stream by the medulla of the adrenal gland, a hat-shaped organ located on the top of each kidney, and has longer lasting effects on heart rate.

Essential fatty acids (EFA) Nine fatty acids that cannot be synthesized in the body and must be obtained through diet.

Excitation-contraction coupling The mechanical and physiological events fundamental to the sliding filament of the muscle cells.

Exercise A structured program designed to achieve a state of physical exertion of certain intensity, duration, and frequency.

Facilitated diffusion (also, carrier-mediated diffusion) The transport of molecules bound to a protein carrier across the cell membrane.

Fast response A type of action potential that occurs in the cardiac muscle cells and the conducting fibers (Purkinje fibers).

Fast-twitch fibers (also, Type II fibers) Mainly anaerobically-oriented muscle fibers. Their contractions are explosive, and generate greater force than Type I fibers, but do not last as long.

Fat soluble vitamins The A, D, E, and K vitamins are stored in fat within the body.

Fatty acid Long-chain compounds with straight hydrocarbon chains.

Frank-Starling mechanism of the heart The ability of the heart to adjust stroke volume to the changing volume of blood entering the ventricles.

Free radicals (also, reactive oxygen species [ROS]) Highly chemically reactive molecules, the action of which is potentially damaging to the DNA, proteins, and lipids, that leads to chronic diseases such as cancer and cardiovascular disease.

Frequency The quantification of the existence or occurrence of disease and the rate or risk of the disease in the population. Number of exercise sessions per week.

Functional syncytium Describes the condition when the heart functions as an entire unit.

Gated channels The state of the ion channel at a given moment (either an open or closed state) that allows or prevents specific ions from passing through the cell membrane.

Glucagon A hormone secreted by the pancreas that increases blood glucose concentrations.

Gluconeogenesis The formation of glucose from proteins.

Glucose A monosaccharide that is the final product of almost all dietary carbohydrates that enter the circulation after they pass through the liver.

Glucose transporters Protein carriers that transport glucose across the cell membrane.

GLUT-4 transporter A type of transporter found in the muscle cells. They facilitate glucose transport into the cell and are activated by physical activity and insulin.

Glycemic index (GI) An indicator of the potential of an ingested carbohydrate to raise blood sugar levels.

Glycogen The stored form of glucose found in the muscle and liver.

Glycolysis The process by which ATP is generated anaerobically.

Heat exhaustion A common heat illness usually caused by a decrease in blood volume consequent to profuse sweating and or inadequate hydration.

Heat stroke A life-threatening illness that occurs when the body's temperature rises to dangerous levels due to the inability of the body to dissipate heat.

Hemorrhagic stroke A blood clot causes a rupture of a blood vessel in the brain, depriving the immediate areas of the brain of oxygen and nutrients.

Hepatic triglyceride lipase The enzyme involved in the removal of triglycerides from very low density lipoprotein (VLDL) molecules, transforming them to low density lipoprotein (LDL) particles.

High density lipoprotein (HDL) The class of lipoprotein (smallest and most dense) involved in the transportation of cholesterol from the peripheral tissues to the liver for excretion or re-utilization of energy.

Hydrolysis A process by which the pancreatic enzyme, pancreatic lipase, splits most of the triglycerides into free fatty acids (FFA) and monoglycerides.

Hyperinsulinemia A condition defined by higher than normal levels of insulin secreted to maintain a normal rate of blood glucose transport into the cell.

Hypertrophic cardiomyopathy A pathologic condition seen in patients with primary myocardial disease or significant valvular disease. The structural cardiac changes in these individuals are usually much greater than those induced by exercise only.

Hypertrophy Visible muscle growth in skeletal muscles as an adaptation to an increased demand.

Impaired fasting glucose A condition defined by a blood glucose level between 100 and 125 mg/dl after an overnight fast. This range is higher than the normal blood glucose levels of 70 to 99 mg/dl but not high enough to be classified as diabetes.

Impaired glucose tolerance (IGT) A condition defined by blood glucose level between 140 and 199 mg/dl after a 2-hour oral glucose tolerance test. This level is higher than normal but not high enough to be classified as diabetes.

Incidence   The ratio of new cases of a disease per unit of time, often presented in terms of one year.

Indirect assessment of blood pressure   The use of a sphygmomanometer and stethoscope to measure the rate of heart beats per minute.

Inferior surface of the heart   The area of the heart comprised of both ventricles (primarily the left) that lies along the diaphragm.

Inferior vena cava   A large vein that returns de-oxygenated blood from the lower body (legs, pelvis, abdomen) to the right atrium of the heart.

Insulin   The key hormone that facilitates the transportation of glucose into the cells.

Insulin resistance   A condition defined as a state in which insulin requirements for the efficient transport of a set amount of glucose across the cell membrane are increased.

Intensity   The percentage of the effort exerted during a given activity as it relates to maximum capacity of the individual.

Intercalated disks   A specialized region of cardiac muscle tissue comprised of a very low electrical resistance tissue that connects myocardial fibers designed so to propagate the impulse from one fiber to the next virtually unimpeded. This allows all cardiac muscle fibers to contract nearly simultaneously when stimulated.

Internodal tracts   Special fibers in the heart on which the generated impulse from the sino-atrial (SA) node spreads rapidly throughout both atria.

Interventricular septum   The thick wall shared by the two ventricles.

Intima   The innermost layer of the blood vessel composed of sheet of endothelial cells that rest on a thin layer of connective tissue.

Ischemia   A condition that occurs when blood flow to a tissue (i.e., myocardium) is not adequate.

Isometric (static) contraction   A muscle contraction in which resistance is applied to the muscle or muscle group, but the muscle maintains a constant length and no joint movement occurs.

Isotonic (dynamic) contraction   Muscle contraction that is characterized by movement of the joint.

Krebs cycle   The first of the two phases in the metabolic process where ATP is formed aerobically. (see Adenosine triphosphate).

Lactate threshold   The sudden rise in blood lactate levels to approximately 2.5 times the resting level during incremental exercise. It marks the point where the capacity of the muscle to deal with the lactate internally is surpassed and a shift to predominantly anaerobic metabolism begins.

Lactate   The end product of carbohydrate metabolism via the anaerobic pathways (glycolysis).

Low density lipoprotein (LDL)   A class of lipoproteins that is the major carrier of cholesterol (carrying about 60% to 80% of all cholesterol in the blood) to the peripheral tissues. It is formed by the liver, gut, and triglyceride-rich lipoproteins (VLDL and chylomicrons) after triglyceride hydrolysis.

Left anterior descending (LAD) coronary artery   The branch from the left main coronary artery that continues downwards towards the apex of the heart.

Left bundle branch   The left branch of the impulse-conducting nervous system of the heart. It innervates and conducts impulses to the left ventricle.

Left main coronary artery   The trunk of the arterial blood vessel that supplies blood to the left side of the heart.

Length   The duration of time (weeks, months, years) that a particular activity is sustained.

Lipase Enzyme involved in the hydrolysis of dietary fats.

Lipoprotein lipase The enzyme involved in the removal of free fatty acids from very low density lipoprotein (VLDL) molecules.

Lipoproteins Transporters of cholesterol to the cells. They are comprised of proteins and fats.

Low extremity arterial disease (LEAD) A more precise term for peripheral vascular disease.

Maximal oxygen capacity or maximal oxygen consumption ($\dot{V}O_2$ max) The maximum amount of oxygen that one can utilize to do work.

Media The layer in blood vessels that contains smooth muscle and provides the mechanical strength and contractile power of the blood vessel. It is the layer responsible for diameter change (vasodilatation and vasoconstriction) of the vessel.

Metabolic equivalents (MET) A measure of energy output equivalent to the amount of energy expended per kilogram of body weight, during one minute of rest (basal metabolic rate). One MET is equal to 3.5 ml of O_2 per kg of body weight per minute, or 1 kcal per kg of body weight per hour.

Metabolic syndrome refers to a cluster of specific cardiovascular disease risk factors that include high blood pressure, elevated triglycerides, low levels of high-density lipoprotein (HDL), impaired fasting glucose, and excess abdominal fat. Insulin resistance is thought to be the underlying pathophysiology.

Mitral (or bicuspid) valve The valve situated between the left atria and left ventricle of the heart that regulates blood to flow from the atria to the ventricle.

Modifiable risk factors Risk factors for heart disease can be modified either by a change in the individual's lifestyle (e.g., diet and exercise) or by medical interventions.

Monounsaturated fatty acids Fatty acids that contain only one double bond along the carbon chain. Olive oil, canola oil, peanut oil, almond oil, and pecan oil contain mainly monounsaturated fatty acids. Monounsaturated fats remain liquid at room temperature but begin to solidify in cold temperatures.

Muscular endurance The capacity of the muscle or muscle groups to perform repetitive contractions over a period of time against a resistance, such as lifting a set amount of weight several times.

Muscular fitness The capacity of the muscle or muscle groups to perform tasks that require muscular strength or muscular endurance.

Muscular strength The capacity of the muscle or muscle groups to exert force during a voluntary contraction.

Myocardium The thickest muscular layer of the heart wall.

Myofibrils Small units that make up each muscle fiber; it is these myofibrils that contain the actual mechanism of muscle contraction.

Myosin A protein contained in myofibrils, involved in muscle contraction by bonding tightly with another protein actin.

Non-modifiable risk factors Risk factors for heart disease that cannot be changed (e.g., aging, genetics).

Norepinephrine (also noradrenaline) Hormone released by the sympathetic nervous system on to the pacemaker of the heart that acts to cause immediate changes.

Odds ratio The statistical number of chances that an event will occur in one group compared with it occurring in another group.

Omega-3 fatty acids (also, n-3 fatty acids or ω-fatty acids) A specific type of polyunsaturated fatty acids that are found in seafood (salmon, halibut, tuna), some plants, and nut oils. Their double bond is in the third bond counting from the end (omega) of the fatty acid. These essential fatty acids are crucial to brain function as well as normal growth and development.

Osteoporosis   A condition defined as a decrease in bone mass by 30% or more or having below the average bone mass of healthy individuals in their thirties.

Overload principle   This principle states that for adaptations of any physiologic system (muscles, heart and even brain) to occur, the imposed demand must be beyond the present capacities of the system.

Oxidation-reduction reactions (also, Redox)   Chemical reactions that involve an electron gain by one reaction species (reduction) and an electron loss (oxidation) by the other species involved in the reaction; free radicals are the by-products of these biochemical reactions.

Oxidative stress   A condition formed when the balance between formation of ROS and antioxidants is disturbed either by an increased production of ROS or a reduction in antioxidant species.

Pacemaker cells   The cells of the sino-atrial (SA) node endowed with the property of automaticity that depolarizes spontaneously in a rhythmic fashion.

Parasympathetic nervous system   The part of the autonomic system responsible for the opposite actions of the sympathetic system. Parasympathetic stimulation of the heart decreases heart rate and the force of contractions.

Peptide links   The connection (—CO—NH—) between the carboxyl group of one amino acid to the amino group of another to string together amino acids to form peptide chains.

Pericardium   The outer layer of the heart.

Peripheral vascular disease (PVD)   A condition that involves atherosclerosis of peripheral vessels (i.e., arteries of the legs) resulting in pain of the lower legs when walking.

Phosphocreatine (PC)   The compound stored in the muscle cells to quickly replenish ATP as it is used.

Physical activity   Any movement that requires skeletal muscle contraction and results in energy expenditure beyond resting levels.

Polypeptides   Chains of amino acids.

Polyunsaturated fatty acid (PUFA)   A type of fatty acids that contain two or more double bonds along the carbon chain. Corn oil, safflower oil, sunflower oil, and soybean oil are examples of PUFAs; they are usually in liquid at room and in cold temperatures (see Omega-3 fatty acids).

Potassium channels   A membrane protein that only allows potassium ions to pass through the water-filled membrane and into the cell.

Pre-Diabetes   A condition when individuals exhibit subtle abnormalities in blood glucose and insulin concentrations that is not high enough to be classified as diabetes. Through lifestyle management of blood glucose levels, an individual can delay or avoid the disease progression to type 2 diabetes.

Pre-Hypertension   A category of blood pressure (force exerted on arterial walls as blood is pumped) that includes individuals with systolic blood pressure (SBP) between 120 and 139 mm Hg and/or diastolic blood pressure (DBP) between 80 and 89 mm Hg. Left untreated, this will turn into high blood pressure, which will increase the risk of heart attack, stroke, and heart failure.

Preload   The stress on the left ventricular wall at the end of the diastolic phase, approximated by the left ventricular-end diastolic volume (LV-EDV) or cardiac output.

Prevalence   A statistical ratio that measures the number of people who have a disease or a characteristic out of all of the participants in a study at a given point or period in time.

Principle of reversibility This principle states that the level of fitness acquired through training will be lost if training is discontinued.

Prodromal Symptoms or occurrences that are usually experienced in the months and weeks leading up to a condition such as a heart attack.

Progressive resistance principle This principle states that the association between the workload and physiologic adaptations behave in a dose-response fashion. That is, a progressive increase in the workload will yield progressive adaptations beyond the present level.

Prospective cohort studies Studies that involve the selection of information of a group free from the disease of interest and the follow-up of that group to track the incidence of that disease over time.

Prostaglandins Potent hormone-like compounds that are derived enzymatically from fatty acids and have important functions in the body. These control blood pressure, contraction of smooth muscle, blood clotting, immune function, proper growth in children, and modulation of inflammation.

Pulmonary circulation The cycle that delivers deoxygenated blood to the lungs via the pulmonary artery to be oxygenated and sent on to the heart.

Pulmonary valve The valve that allows the flow of blood from the right ventricle to the lungs.

Purkinje fibers Specialized heart muscle tissue that transmit the electrical impulse first to the muscles that control the heart valves and then throughout the entire ventricular tissue.

Rate-pressure product An index of myocardial oxygen consumption (the metabolic demand of the heart) calculated by multiplying the heart rate times the systolic blood pressure (SBP).

Relative refractory period The time during which the cardiac muscle cells can depolarize prematurely if they are provoked by a stimulus of adequate strength.

Relative risk reduction The measured difference in rates between two groups (e.g., how much a risk is lowered in an experimental group versus a control group).

Relative risk A statistical measurement comparing the absolute risks of an event or developing a disease in two different groups of people relative to exposure.

Response-to-injury theory The theory states that atherosclerosis develops as a result of repetitive injury and ongoing inflammatory process of the inner arterial wall (endothelial layer) of large and medium-sized arteries.

Resting potential The electrical change differential between the inside and outside of the cardiac cell prior to excitation (at rest).

Retrospective cohort studies Historical scientific studies that examine the relationships between disease and risk factors after the disease has occurred.

Reverse cholesterol transport The process by which excess cholesterol from the periphery is transported to the liver by the high density lipoprotein (HDL) particle for catabolism.

Right bundle branches The right branch of the electrical impulse-conducting system of the heart. It innervates and conducts impulses to the right ventricle.

Right coronary artery (RCA) The artery that extends from the aorta to right side of the heart and wraps around it, supplying blood to the right heart, the inferior and posterior wall of the ventricles, and part of the interventricular septum.

Risk factor A parameter that can predict a future event.

Saturated fatty acids Fatty acids with all carbon attached to each other by a single bond and hydrogen atoms attached to most of the remaining sites of the carbon. Found in animal products (beef, pork, chicken, lard, butter, eggs, tropical oils, etc.), these fats are high in cholesterol and high density lipoproteins and add excess calories.

Simple lipids (also, neutral fats) Primarily fatty acids, triglycerides, waxes, and sterols.

Sino-atrial node (SA node) A specialized area of cardiac cells that initiates the impulse for the heart to contract (the pacemaker of the heart).

Sliding filament model Refers to the sliding action occurring within myofibrils that results in muscle contraction and relaxation.

Slow response A type of action potential that occurs in the sino-atrial (SA) and atrioventricular (AV) nodes.

Slow twitch fibers (see Type 1 Fibers)

Sodium channels A type of protein membrane that allows only sodium ions to pass through the water-filled membrane and into or out of the cell.

Sodium-potassium pump A cell membrane transporter that captures the sodium ions that leak into the cell and the potassium ions that leak outside of the cell and returns them to their respective environments.

Specificity principle The body's response and adaptation to a specific type of exercise (stimulus).

Statins A class of medications designed to attenuate the formation of cholesterol by the cells (cholesterol-lowering agents).

Stroke volume The amount of blood the heart pumps out with each contraction.

Superior vena cava The vein that returns blood to the right atrium of the heart from the upper body.

Sympathetic nervous system The part of the autonomic system that controls the body's response to stressful conditions via the release of norepinephrine (also known as noradrenaline). In the sympathetic stimulation of the heart, the system is responsible for increasing heart rate and the force of the contractions.

Systemic circulation (also, greater circulation or peripheral circulation) The circulation system that provides blood to all tissues of the body except the lungs.

Systole The contraction phase of the cardiac cycle; during this phase, blood is pumped out of the heart chambers and into the lungs and all other tissues of the body.

Systolic blood pressure A measurement of the force exerted on the arterial walls when blood is pumped through the body. Top measurement of blood pressure occurs when the heart contracts.

Tachycardia A heart rate above 100 bpm.

Tendons Tough connective tissue that attaches muscles to bones.

The specificity principle This principle states that the body will make specific changes to accommodate the specific demand placed upon it.

Thrombotic stroke Results when a thrombus (blood clot) is formed within the vessels of the brain, blocking blood flow to critical areas of the brain and depriving the brain cells of oxygen and nutrients.

Trans-fatty acids Unsaturated fatty acids artificially formed by the partial hydrogenation of vegetable oils (referred to in products as partially hydrogenated oils) added to processed foods to stabilize them for longer shelf life. Trans-fatty acids add cholesterol and low density lipoproteins (LDLs) to the diet, and increase the risks for heart disease.

Tricuspid valve The valve situated between the right atria and ventricle that allows blood to flow from the right atria to the ventricle.

Triglycerides   Comprised of three fatty acids attached to a glycerol molecule. They are mainly used to provide energy for the different metabolic functions.

Tropomyosin   One of the four proteins found in the myofibrils, involved in muscle contraction.

Troponin   One of the four proteins involved in muscle contraction.

Type I (slow-twitch) fibers   Mainly aerobically-oriented muscle fibers. They are engaged by the muscle to contract predominately when oxygen is available.

Unsaturated fatty acids   Fatty acids that are not saturated with hydrogen atoms and are derived from plants; in room temperature they are usually in liquid form.

Vein   A type of blood vessel that transports the non-oxygenated blood back to the heart via the superior and inferior vena cava.

Venules   A type of blood vessel that collects blood from the capillaries; they gradually join together and progressively form veins.

Very low density lipoprotein (VLDL)   A triglyceride-rich particle produced by the liver and the gut. VLDL enters the circulation as premature particles and is transformed into mature VLDL as it acquires cholesterol.

$\dot{V}O_2$max   The maximum oxygen utilized by the body during maximal work.

$\dot{V}O_2$ Reserve   The difference between the maximum oxygen uptake ($\dot{V}O_2$max) and resting O_2 uptake (see Maximum oxygen uptake).

Voltage-sensitive   The opening and closing of the cardiac channels that depends upon the voltage across the membrane.

Water soluble vitamins   Type of vitamins that are not stored in the body and must be consumed in the daily diet to prevent vitamin deficiency. They are thiamin (B_1), riboflavin (B_2), niacin (B_3), pantothenic acid (B_5), pyridoxine (B_6), biotin (B_7), folic acid (folate, folacin, B_8), cobalamin (B_{12}), and C.

Index

Page numbers followed by *f*, *t*, or *b* refer respectively to figures, tables, and boxes.